Ready To Go:

The History And Contributions of U.S. Public Health Advisors

BETH E. MEYERSON
FRED A. MARTICH
GERALD P. NAEHR

AMERICAN SOCIAL HEALTH ASSOCIATION
RESEARCH TRIANGLE PARK, NORTH CAROLINA

PO Box 13827
Research Triangle Park, NC 27709

Cover Design by Sally Zimmerman and Frank Chapman

Manufactured in the United States of America

10 9 8 7 6 5 4 3 2 1

Library of Congress Cataloging-in-Publication Data

Meyerson, Beth E., Martich, Fred A., Naehr, Gerald P.
Ready to Go: The History and Contributions of U.S. Public Health Advisors / Beth E. Meyerson, Fred A. Martich, Gerald P. Naehr.
p. cm.
Includes bibliographical references and index.
1. Centers for Disease Control (U.S.). Public Health Advisors – Popular works.
2. Epidemiology – Popular works.
3. Sexually Transmitted Disease – United States – Popular works.
I. Title.

Library of Congress Control Number: 2008927781

ISBN 978-0-615-20383-6

For the U.S. Public Health Advisors
of yesterday, today and tomorrow.

Table of Contents

Acknowledgements .... *i*

Introduction *1*

Chapter 1: I Want One of Those 7

Chapter 2: The Madam and Her Doctor *35*

Chapter 3: The Original Experiment *55*

Chapter 4: The Early Years *69*

Chapter 5: The Expansion *93*

Chapter 6: Winnowing *127*

Chapter 7: Ready to Go *163*

Chapter 8: The Silverbacks *207*

Chapter 9: The New Experiment *229*

Notes *241*

Index *287*

About the Authors *311*

I still carry a passport. I still have a bag packed. Old habits are hard to break.

Joseph "Spider" Webb
Public Health Advisor (ret.)

Acknowledgements

"There has to be a history of Public Health Advisors somewhere. We're talking about CDC. Someone is always publishing something." That was my comment to Fred Martich in 2001 during my dissertation research. I was writing about the impact of CDC federal assignees in state Sexually Transmitted Disease (STD) programs in my study of public health federalism, because, since 1948, Public Health Advisors had been assigned to state and local STD programs by the federal government to function at an operational level. Surely there was something in print about them? No such luck.

Fred, a Public Health Advisor, or PHA, was the deputy chief of the Behavioral Interventions and Research Branch in the Division of STD Prevention at CDC. We had known one another since my days as the state AIDS and STD director with the Missouri Department of Health. When I asked Fred to help locate a published history of PHAs, he informed me that I found the right guy, because he was also the treasurer of the Watsonian Society, an organization of CDC Public Health Advisors. Fred confirmed that there was nothing published beyond some videos and a few newsletter and newspaper articles. He shipped to me several documents and a video from the Watsonian Society archives so that I could write the chapter. Fred was pleased with the outcome. He shared the chapter with Jerry Naehr, a former president of the Watsonian Society who was on detail in the Office of the Director at the National Center for HIV and STD Prevention at CDC. Jerry knew the extensive history of all assigned field staff, present and past. Within a year Jerry and Fred would convince me to write a book about PHAs. This is how it all began.

That nothing had been written about PHAs ultimately was not surprising, because Public Health Advisors are known as "do-ers" and not scribes. Although the Watsonian Archives were immensely helpful to the task of writing a chapter about PHAs, they lacked the spirit which infused many a PHA story about the nature of the job. After much discussion, in 2003, we established the PHA History Project to chronicle the history and contributions of U.S. Public Health Advisors through their personal stories and extant archives. We moved quickly in order to reach several of the earliest PHAs: William "Luke" Hamlin, Delwin "Del" Hammons, Walter Hughes, Donald Lederman, and William "Bill" Watson. The need to reach these original PHAs outweighed other project considerations (such as funding). This approach initially worked because by this time Jerry and Fred had retired from CDC, and my company (Policy Resource Group, LLC) funded project startup costs and underwrote much of my salary while working on the project. Julie Eckstein, the Missouri project director for the Center for Health Transformation and former director of the Missouri Department of Health and Senior Services, secured the help of Healthy Communities St. Charles County to act as the nonprofit fiduciary agent for the PHA History Project in the event that funding might be forthcoming. The value of this contribution cannot be overstated, because without Healthy Communities, we could not have received contributions to the project. Our first two (and very generous) donations came from PHAs Bill Watson and Jack Jackson. Within weeks, word about the project had gotten out through the PHA network. We began receiving checks from individuals and organizations ranging from twenty-five to five thousand dollars. These donations sustained project operations, as we were able to underwrite transcription costs, travel to interviews, and ensure safe delivery of archives and artifacts to the project and back to their owners.

Financial contributions from individuals confirmed the project's importance. We would like to thank the following individual donors to the PHA History Project: Jeanne and Charles Alexander, Jack and Betty Benson, Jo Ann Bittle, Windell and Gail Bradford, Marcia Brooks, Richard Carney, Bill and Frances Doyle, Donald and JoDean Eddins, Robert and Patricia Emerson, Edith Gary, Delwin and Juanita Hammons, Anne Renee Heningburg, James and Dorothy Hicks, Jack Jackson, Sue and Van Jenkins, Carolyn Johannes, Gloria and Robert Keegan, Robert and Karen Kingon, Robert and Carolyn Kohmescher, Georgia and Kenneth Latimer, Joel and Frances Lewis, Martha

Martich, Dean and Constance Mason, Dennis and Barbara McDowell, Barbara Meek, Edward Mihalek, William and Julia Mitchell, Frank Meyers, Larry and Linda Posey, Roberto and Lyndy Potter, Kathryn Rauch, Norman and Anita Scherzer, Judith and Graydon Sheperd, Lynn Stafford, John and Mary Vadnais, Charles and Judith Watkins, William Watson, Brian Wheeler, and Jack and Barbara Wroten.

Organizations working with PHAs also contributed to the effort. We would like to thank the following organizations for their financial assistance to the PHA History Project: Booz Allen Hamilton, Inc, COMFORCE Technical Services, Family Health International, Information Network Systems, McKing Consulting Corporation, National Coalition of STD Directors, and Science Applications International Corporation. We also would like to thank McKing Consulting Corporation for the use of their offices to conduct several interviews in 2004, and the Council of State and Territorial Epidemiologists for the use of a conference room for a daylong author meeting in 2007. We are grateful to the Centers for Disease Control and Prevention for a grant that allowed us to devote full-time attention to writing the book during the period from April 2007 to June 2008. In 2005 CDC Director Dr. Julie Gerberding and Chief Operating Officer William Gimson agreed to help this history effort. The grant became a reality through the persistent efforts of Robert Delaney, then CDC's chief of staff; Robert Curlee, deputy director of the Financial Management Office (FMO), and Sara Schmit, previously with FMO.

Over the course of the project, we conducted one hundred forty interviews with Public Health Advisors and their close associates who were not PHAs. We spoke with several current and past directors of the Centers for Disease Control and Prevention, directors of centers and divisions within CDC, and directors of State Health Departments both current and past. We received emails and letters from dozens of PHAs, and many shared personal archives, memorabilia, and photographs. At least twice a year, I could count on a package from Ken Latimer containing copious notes and detailed descriptions of PHA work and history.

In our effort to produce a comprehensive history of Public Health Advisors and their contributions, we elected to interview PHAs from across the decades of hiring, across program service experience, from a variety of temporary duty experiences, and from the rich diversity of the PHA workforce. We used national meetings as an opportunity to meet with several PHAs from across the country, and we reached others whenever and wherever possible, including places where I was working for Policy Resource Group, LLC, such as in India, the Caribbean, or elsewhere in the U.S. Charles Joseph "Joe" Webb (PHA) and Brenda Drum hosted me for a day or two in Hugo, Oklahoma. John "Jack" and Barbara Pendleton allowed me to access the personal papers of Jack's aunt Lida J. Usilton. Lida's papers provided a tremendous breakthrough in historical knowledge for our research team.

Although we did succeed in making our PHA history representative, we could not interview everyone who graciously stepped forward to participate. And although every interview deepened our understanding of the work and history of PHAs, not everyone interviewed will see themselves in these pages. Further, although some terrific "war stories" helped express the essence of PHA experience, many could not make these pages because of the project's nature. As we reviewed the interview data, we found that we actually had two books in process. One focused on the history and contributions of PHAs (this book), and another focused on the war stories, which were primarily in Sexually Transmitted Disease work. This second book will be our next collaborative publication. It will not be for the faint of heart!

Throughout our project research, many people tolerated our continued requests for clarification and guidance: the late Jack Benson, Joseph Carter, Billy Griggs, Stacey Harper, Walter Hughes, Dr. E. Earl Kennemer, Robert Kingon, Jack Jackson, Kenneth Latimer, Bernard "Bert" Malone, Harold Mauldin, Pat McConnon, William Parra, Dr. David Sencer, Ferdinand "Ferd" Tedesco, Dr. Steve Thacker, William Watson, and Jack Wroten. Special thanks go to Russell Havlak, who waded through various iterations of chapters and provided expert advice as I crafted sections of chapter 6. Russ was always willing to provide counsel and eloquent explanation.

We thank our interview participants and those who submitted stories and archives. Without their participation and archival contributions, this project never would have had a chance. Thanks to Glenn Acham, Steve Adams, Kenneth Archer,

Rodney Armstrong, Dr. John Bagby Robert Baldwin, Steven Barid, James Beall, the late Jack Benson, Roger Bernier, Frank Berry, Joseph Betros, Steven Bice, Orlando Blancato, Raymond Bly, Dr. Gail Bolan, Richard Bowman, Windell Bradford, Marcia Brooks, Dawn Broussard, Kristin Brusuelas, Paul Burlack, Peter Buxtun, Kathryn Cahill, Joseph Carter, Mike Cassell, Dr. Willard Cates, Pamela Chin, James Coan, Dayne Collins, Richard Conlon, Gary Conrad, Dr. James Curran, Scott Danos, Lumbe Davis, Robert Delaney, Lori de Ravello, Kim Do, Bill Doyle, Heather Duncan, Dr. Donald Eddins, James Felton, James Fowler, Phillip Finley, Dr. William Foege, Daphne Ford, Tracy Ford, Louise Galaska, Kathleen Gallagher, Karen Gavin, Dr. Julie Gerberding, William Gimson, Joseph Giordano, Martin Goldberg, Kent Gray, Kevin Griffy, Billy Griggs, William "Luke" Hamlin, Delwin Hammons, Virginia (Bales) Harris, Russell Havlak, Mary Hayes, John Heath, Anne-Renee Heningburg, Carl Hickam, Dwan Hightower, Elvin Hilyer, Dr. Alan Hinman, Walter Hughes, Dr. Kathleen Irwin, Arthur "Jack" Jackson, Dr. Harold Jaffe, Bassam Jarrar, Van Jenkins, Robert Johnson, Robert Keegan, John "Jack" Kelly, Robert Kennedy, Stuart Kingma, Robert Kingon, Valerie Kokor, Glen Koops, Robert Kohmescher, Kathryn Koski, Jerry Lama, Dr. Michael Lane, Kenneth Latimer, Donald Lederman, James Lee, Robert Longenecker, Craig Leutzinger, Bernard Malone, Dean Mason, Harold Mauldin, Patrick McConnon, Dennis McDowell, Monte Meador, Barbara Meek, Frank Meyers, John Miles, Franklin Miller, Peter Moore, Linda Morse, Dennis Murphy, John Narkunas, David Newberry, Candice Nowicki-Lehnherr, Dr. Lori Leonard, Kevin O'Connor, Patrick O'Mara, Thomas Ortiz, Otilio Oyervides, John Paffel, William Parra, John Pendleton, Ted Pestorius, Francis "Frank" Piecuch, Alice Pope, Larry Posey, Edward Powers, Lee Ann Ramsey, Kathryn Rauch, Robert Ray, Dr. William Roper, Michael Sage, Louis Salinas, Melinda Salmon, Anthony Scardaci, Joseph Scavotto, Norman Scherzer, Steven Schindler, Mark Schrader, John Seggerson, Dr. David Sencer, Laura Shelby, John Shimmens, George Sides, Gregory Smothers, Lisa Speissegger, Dr. Patricia Simone, Jack Spencer, Kathryn Stark, Charles Stokes, Phillip Strine, Phillip Talboy, Dr. Steven Thacker, Victor Tomlinson, Dr. Edward Thompson, Timothy Thornton, Rita Varga, Dr. Thomas Vernon, Dr. Judith Wasserheit, Charles Watkins, William Watson, Alfreda Weaver, Charles Joseph (Joe) Webb, Stefan Weir, Gary West, Dr. Paul Wiesner, Wendy Wolf, and Jack Wroten.

Our research would not be complete without access to government archives. The Watsonian Society and the CDC Global Odyssey Museum provided unlimited access to their archives. Mary Hilpertshauser, the collections manager for CDC's Global Health Odyssey Museum, assisted us in our search for photographs and their background. Becky Sattlewaite of the CDC Archive Library helped us find publications. We are grateful to the Watsonian Society and to CDC for guidance and support during the research process, and for hosting events during the course of the project to help publicize the opportunity to collect stories and to announce the upcoming book release.

We also would like to thank those who reviewed portions or editions of the manuscript as we prepared for publication. Their careful review and candid feedback helped to bring this story to its present form: the late Jack Benson, who agreed to read a draft of the book though he was entering hospice, Windell Bradford, Dr. Richard Crosby, Jill German, Russell Havlak, Robert Kingon, and William Watson.

Our book project would not be possible without the expert help of those who are more technically inclined in all matters publishing. Editor Jonathan K. Cohen provided expert manuscript review; without which the reader would have to trudge through a book filled with errors or difficult wording. Janyne St. Marie made the tremendously detailed index possible. Anyone looking for a particular story or person in this book can thank Janyne. We would also like to thank our transcriptionists Barbara Alihosseini, Marcia Anderson, Lori Heilwagner and Barbara Ross for typing every single word from hours of interviews. Sally Zimmerman and Frank Chapman of Alice June Graphics, Inc. developed a superb book cover and related graphics. Huge thanks go to our publisher, The American Social Health Association (ASHA). ASHA's President and CEO, Lynn Barclay, has been a tremendous partner on this project and has been willing to work with us to make this book available quickly. We claim responsibility for any errors or omissions, despite all the expert technical help.

Finally, this project would not be possible without the support of our families. My spouse, Jill German, helped me strike a balance between my penchant for academic writing and the need to tell an interesting story. Fred was sustained during this effort by his patient and supportive wife, Joan; and Jerry was supported by his wife, Debbie. All three of us were supported by our many PHA colleagues and friends in public health.

We are grateful to all who made this effort possible and hope that we have helped continue a long discussion about the history and contributions of Public Health Advisors.

Beth Meyerson, M.Div., PhD
Lead Author

Introduction

This story begins with an experiment. The Madam and a quirky Ph.D. economist, The Doctor, circumvented federal hiring and personnel rules, stretched the limits of wartime government resources, and, in July of 1948, gave a small group of freshly-minted college graduates a chance to have a temporary job with the federal government in syphilis control on the Eastern Shore of Maryland. The Madam was not convinced that college men would do the dirty work. The Doctor knew otherwise.

These college men, who often dressed like door-to-door salesmen, started in venereal disease (VD) control, and quickly were recognized as an asset to immunization and tuberculosis control efforts once they arrived at the nascent Communicable Disease Center in 1957. By the 1970s, Public Health Advisors (PHAs) reflected the gender, racial, and ethnic diversity of the populations they served, and spanned the expanse of public health programs with a career trajectory that began at the patient level "in the field" and ended as part of the CDC management backbone.

Since the beginnings of their profession, PHAs have contributed immeasurably to the public health infrastructures of local and state health departments, and have served the CDC hierarchy with distinction. Public Health Advisors have been detailed throughout the world to eradicate smallpox, measles, and polio, and to address a host of other diseases and conditions. They are among the first responders in times of public health crisis or humanitarian disaster. Although PHAs have taken various career paths, traditionally each Public Health Advisor has been equipped with an accrued wealth of field and operational experiences, making him or her invaluable to CDC. Yet despite the importance of such unusual workers, CDC stopped hiring entry-level Public Health Advisors in 1994—just four years before the fiftieth anniversary of the series. By 1999, CDC was feeling the effects of this decision, as it relied on retired PHAs to serve in mission-critical roles in the U.S. and abroad.

This story begins and ends with an experiment. It is told for the benefit of history on behalf of the women and men who call themselves Public Health Advisors. PHAs are not the type to write their own histories or "toot their own horns," though some are master storytellers. Some such stories grace these pages, while others are best told in private company, but all eventually should be told because they shed light on this inimitable breed of public health worker.

Ready to Go: The History and Contributions of U.S. Public Health Advisors begins to tell the story of the Public Health Advisor. It is written for several audiences: PHAs and their close colleagues, past and current CDC employees, public health employees in state and local governments and ministries of health, students of public health, citizens concerned about community health, and those who hope to make a contribution through public service and might consider such an unusual and rewarding career in public health.

Chapter 1, titled "I Want One of Those," opens on the morning of September 11, 2001, as the CDC emergency operations team gathered to watch the second plane hit the World Trade Center. The chapter takes the reader on a tour of work experiences that define the Public Health Advisor—or "one of those"—and to the PHAs' uniqueness.

Chapter 2, "The Madam and Her Doctor," describes the historical basis for PHAs and begins with their "cradle": the Public Health Service Venereal Disease Division. Lida J. Usilton, known as the poker-playing madam to her "boys in the field," was a strong influence in the development of the future PHAs. "Doctor" Johannes Stuart, a Ph.D. economist known for his ingenuity as well as his quirkiness, was the program's "father." Together, the Madam and her Doctor began the experiment that later would contribute to the establishment of public health programs worldwide and would become a source of expert CDC managers. The chapter discusses the history of federal presence in venereal disease control, as well as precursors to PHAs such as the Public Health Commissioned Corps and the "New Dealers" who were hired and placed in local areas to mentor local and state efforts in venereal disease control. The chapter answers the question, "Why were PHAs needed?"

Chapter 3, "The Original Experiment," tells the story of an upstart group who served as the first "co-ops" in VD investigation on the Eastern Shore of Maryland in 1948. The VD Division recruited these men from colleges as an experiment because no one believed that the government could get baccalaureates to do "this kind of dirty work": VD patient interviewing and contact epidemiology. Stories from the remaining original PHAs and some of their early colleagues give a sense of the developing professional culture that endures even today.

Chapter 4, "The Early Years," introduces the reader to the original portal for PHA entry into service, venereal disease control work, which remains an important part of PHAs' work culture. This chapter describes the nature of early VD control work and how early co-ops and PHAs experienced the job. The reader also will learn how PHAs were soon deployed for various national efforts and research endeavors. The chapter describes how the Public Health Advisors made a place for themselves in the state and local public health arena, a working culture that previously had not known such unique public health professionals.

Chapter 5, "The Expansion," opens in 1957 when the "proud old VD program" moved from Washington, D.C., to the "little and upstart Communicable Disease Center" in Atlanta. The CDC recognized Public Health Advisors as important contributors to public health soon after they arrived there, and quickly recruited them to develop and enhance immunization and tuberculosis programs throughout the U.S. This chapter also highlights the expansion of the PHA cadre itself, and its transition from an all-white, all-male group to a mixed-gender, racially and ethnically diverse professional series.

Chapter 6, "Winnowing," describes the central aspects of the unique entry-level training for PHAs. The vast majority of Public Health Advisors are the products of years of fieldwork across many programs and in many different geographic locations. Moving frequently within the first several years of employment is a hallmark of the job, and creates a valuable worker with varied experiences. The training regimen, however, is difficult, and is the way to "weed out" those unsuited for the work. Less than half remain after the initial two years, due to the job's nature: harsh realities of public need, rapid deployment, and frequent moves. The resulting remnant is a group of public health workers and managers who are highly valued by CDC and international organizations, as well as state and local health departments.

Chapter 7, "Ready to Go," focuses on a sampling of PHAs' varied and rapid deployments. Over the years PHAs have been called to respond to outbreaks of disease such as hantavirus, Lassa fever, monkeypox, encephalitis, tuberculosis, measles, AIDS, smallpox, polio, Legionnaires', Guillain-Barré syndrome, SARS, syphilis, PPNG, babesiosis, and cholera. PHAs have been detailed for health campaigns such as Guinea worm, malaria, syphilis, diarrheal diseases, yellow fever, yaws, swine flu, and polio. They have been detailed in the wake of major events such as floods, hurricanes, volcanic eruptions, earthquakes, and the anthrax scare in the U.S. They even have been detailed as poll watchers in select Southern states during the 1972 and 1976 presidential elections. PHAs have been sent wherever such events occurred in the United States and in every conceivable foreign location: throughout the continents of Africa and Asia, and throughout South and Central America. The stories in this chapter sample the types of deployments PHAs have experienced since the 1950s, highlighting the contributions of highly-skilled, street-savvy professionals willing to intervene rapidly in any crisis.

Chapter 8, "The Silverbacks," discusses the contributions of PHAs after they have retired from CDC. Consistent with PHA culture, these retired PHAs are not found on the golf course. Instead they are serving international health organizations and state and local health departments, or are part of the experienced executive management cohort that straddles a widening human resource gap at CDC. This chapter examines the confluence and impact of events leading to the 1994 decision to discontinue hiring entry-level Public Health Advisors. The chapter's central theme is that PHAs are constitutionally committed to public health service, and that the silverbacks are standing in the management gap at CDC.

Chapter 9, "The New Experiment," suggests that the newly-created Public Health Apprentices may in fact be reinvigorating the proud old series. In telling this experiment's story and offering lessons from PHA history, this chapter argues that the CDC is making an intentional effort to integrate, structurally, culturally, and historically, the old and new experiments for the long-term benefit of health programs globally and of itself as an agency. This new experiment may prove to be a modern version of the system that provided a wealth of experienced, flexible, capable public health workers and leaders for efforts throughout the world. If so, this new cadre of men and women soon will be *Ready to Go* to contribute to the public's health today and tomorrow.

Whether it is through dirty work, problem solving, master management, or public health work, being a Public Health Advisor is not an ordinary work experience. We hope that this story will honor the men and women who have served CDC as PHAs over the years. We also hope to begin a wider conversation about the contributions of Public Health Advisors to public health, yesterday, today, and in the future.

Chapter 1

I Want One of Those

The team gathered in the CDC Emergency Operations Center five minutes after the first plane hit.[1] Members from toxicology, medical, and epidemiology silently watched the tragedy unfold.[2] Until the second plane crashed into the World Trade Center, they still thought this was a terrible accident. But after talking with officials in New York City, it was clear that this was a terrorist attack of some kind. Massive casualties and numbers of injured were expected. Emergency Operations Center director and Public Health Advisor (PHA) Kent Gray knew then that several decisions made six months prior were going to help CDC respond quickly now. One decision was to bring the Strategic National Stockpile (SNS) to CDC.[3] The other was to get FAA clearance for CDC planes in the event of aircraft grounding. FAA clearance was the idea of PHAs Steve Bice and Steve Adams.[4] After the Twin Towers fell, all non-military planes were grounded in U.S. airspace, with the exception of four: Air Force One and three CDC planes.[5] By 4:00 p.m. on September 11, 2001 the CDC planes were on their way to Ground Zero carrying emergency personnel, ventilators, and pharmaceutical supplies.[6]

Ken Archer's plane carried a team of six from the Stockpile program and four PHAs: Ken, Ron Burger, Dave Adcock, and Steve Adams.[7] Many on the plane had never been on a response of this magnitude.[8] The Public Health Advisors, however, were prepared. "Having been through training for this, I was prepared for just about everything," said Ken, who exactly four months prior had attended a tabletop emergency exercise in New York City called Operation "RED Ex," an abbreviation for Recognition, Evaluation, and Decision Making Exercise.[9] Ken's colleague Ron Burger was one of the few Senior Emergency Response Coordinators at CDC. He had more than fifteen years of experience in emergency operations. In his words he "had been to just about everything pretty big since 1972."[10] Ron's trouble, though, was that he had just returned from another response exercise and had taken his response gear out of his truck before driving to work. Unlike the others on the plane, Ron could not get back home before leaving for New York. So he left for this assignment of unknown duration with one shirt and one tube of toothpaste.[11]

There was plenty of nervous chatter on Ron and Ken's plane, but everyone grew quiet when they saw three F-16 fighter aircraft just outside their windows: two on the left and one on the right side of the plane. This was no escort. The jet fighters were checking things out to be sure the CDC planes were not part of an encore performance from the morning.[12] Ron looked at Ken "with eyes

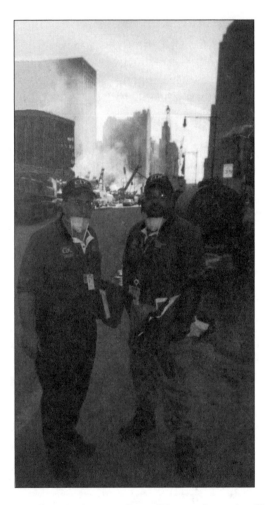

Steve Adams (Left) and Ken Archer near Ground Zero on September 12, 2001. Courtesy of Ken Archer.

the size of golf balls" and asked "Do they know we're friendly?"[13] Initially, they didn't, because FAA clearance for the CDC planes was unique and unexpected. After conferring with the North American Aerospace Defense Command, the fighter jets escorted the CDC planes on a straight line course to their destination, leaving them when the CDC planes reached Washington, D.C. airspace. The CDC pilots then commented that this was the first straight line path they had ever flown.[14]

The group breathed a collective sigh of relief as they took the new course to New York. Steve Adams, who at the time was deputy director of the SNS program, rose to address his colleagues. He knew that there would be next to nothing to supply their needs once they arrived because the emergency operations center in New York City had been taken out by the terrorists. FEMA was ready to rent new space for operations, but would not set anything in motion until CDC got there to approve it.[15] The best thing Steve could do was advise his colleagues on survival tactics. Ron Burger had already found snack food and drinks on board and asked the pilots if the group could take what they could fit in their pockets and knapsacks. Steve then told the group to open every compartment on the plane and grab all of the food.[16] Ron chimed in with additional advice: "Graze when you see food. Especially safe food." Ron knew that these snacks would likely be all they would have until the next day.[17]

The quiet of the deserted New York airfield was soon replaced with chaos once the CDC team landed and was escorted by police into the thick of things.[18] The epidemiologists went to the health department. Ken Archer went to help set up the emergency operations center. Ron Burger, who had served as the deputy director of the New York City Health Department in the late '70s and early '80s, also went to the health department which was just a few blocks from Ground Zero.[19] The work ahead for Ron and his other PHA colleagues would require the stuff for which PHAs are known: problem solving, ingenuity, dedication, and expert logistics. This emergency response would be like other colossal situations caused by flood, hurricane or disease outbreak. According to Ron, "[P]ublic health responds the same way no matter how the cat gets out of the bag…with all of the traditional, basic public health activities that we do so well."[20]

I Want One of Those

> *Dr. Fakhry Asad was the Egyptian physician [who] headed the Communicable Disease Division at the World Health Organization (WHO). He frequently visited the CDC and noticed the managerial role that Public Health Advisors played in the day-to-day operations of the agency. He suggested that the concept might be a logical one for WHO and would like to use his Division as a model for it. "I want one of those," he said. And so I came there... in November of 1984.*[21]
>
> William Parra, chief operating officer,
> Bloomberg Global Initiative to Reduce Tobacco Use,
> CDC Foundation
> Public Health Advisor (ret.)

"One of those" is a Public Health Advisor: a unique public health professional formed by a clustering of varied work experiences paired with personality traits that are selected for and honed by these experiences. PHAs are known for their "can-do" attitude, problem solving skills, ingenuity, and effectiveness. Like the Commissioned Corps preceding them, PHAs are assigned to local, state, national, and international posts in response to need. Unlike these predecessors and even their siblings in the Epidemic Intelligence Service (EIS), PHAs gain their broad skill set from the ground up. They begin their careers at the public health entry level with fieldwork and patient contact, building on this experience through service at virtually all levels of the public health system and in a variety of health programs.

Historically, most PHAs were initiated through venereal disease (VD) or Sexually Transmitted Disease (STD) fieldwork.[22] Even today, by the time they reach senior management levels in the public health system, PHAs have amassed experience in case finding and contact epidemiology, clinic management, personnel and fiscal management, program development, public health policy, and leadership. They gain these work experiences through several different placements in the U.S. and often abroad to ensure that they understand public health realities in rural and urban settings, high and low morbidity areas, resource-poor and cross-cultural environments. "One of those" means a public health worker who is well-rounded and intimately acquainted with program operations (how things run) because he or she has done the work personally. "One of those" also means a capable manager who possesses unique professional traits that are grounded in public health reality.[23]

Bill Gimson is the CDC's chief operating officer. He was prepared for his executive post through years of experience and several assignments in public health. His career is testament to the broad array of public health roles held by PHAs—roles which prepared him for the number-two job at CDC, just as they had done for other high-ranking PHAs before him. Bill remembers his modest start working as a VD investigator in 1974 in several diverse Chicago communities and then his transfer to New York City to work in Morrisania:

> In Chicago, I really got to know the African-American community pretty well. Then I worked on the West Side, which was in those days predominantly Puerto Rican, and then eventually moved to the North Side, which was gay white male... In 1978 I transferred to New York. They gave me Morrisania, which was the heart of the South Bronx in New York City. It really looked like a war zone.[24]

In 1981 Bill transferred with the Immunization Program to Puerto Rico. He was so successful that he became the Commonwealth's acting assistant secretary of health, in which capacity he functioned until 1985. Bill later served as the associate director for management and operations in the Division of Chronic Disease Prevention and Control at CDC, and in 1988 he joined the Financial Management Office to become the understudy of CDC's chief financial officer. In 2003, CDC Director Dr. Julie Gerberding appointed Bill as the agency's chief operating officer.

Bill Gimson's work experience is an example of the kind of job variety encouraged for Public Health Advisors. Not every PHA takes this path, and some are transferred more often than Bill. However, most share the exposure to the diversity of public health programs, governmental levels, geographic areas, and public health functions. Bill's start on the front lines of public health provided him with the tools to work effectively with people throughout his career, and gave him a lasting appreciation of public health operations from the ground up.

Not Your Typical Government Employee

> *I was in the Bronx. I was on the north side of Pittsburgh. I was out at midnight testing people in bars.... I was in jail. I did the interviews in there. I was in neighborhood health centers. I was in family planning clinics. I was in Chester in a Winnebago van in the middle of the night treating drug dealers with a doctor*

that we had to convince to stay with us. It is not the fact that I did that. It is the fact that when I came to the table with someone else, regardless of what they did, I could reach back into my experience and just say, "I have a sense of what you are talking about." And the bond then cranks up a bit. Somebody looks at you and they think, "Well, he is not a typical employee from the government to help you with your problem." [25]

Ed Powers
Public Health Advisor (ret.)

The broad public health experience PHAs gain in communities suffuses their professional approach and personality, even at the most senior management levels. Over several years, the PHA is exposed to the spectrum of public health through a series of planned transfers to a variety of work experiences across public health programs in different geographic areas. Bert Malone, director of the Division of Environmental Health Services with the Kansas City Health Department, explains that his experience as a PHA compounded with every assignment. His first assignment, in Saginaw, Michigan, set the tone for his varied work experience:

> We had responsibility for everything. It wasn't just case finding and case investigation; I was able to do all the education work in the community, and I was able to do all the administrative stuff in the office... I was able to do the clinical work, to do the exams on the males, and I did the laboratory specimen collection... Throughout my career I was blessed with opportunities that allowed me to do a variety of functions in each assignment. And it wasn't just one aspect of public health... I had broad experience early on in my career, and I looked for those opportunities when they presented themselves... We had opportunities—whether it was the Haitian refugees or whether it was the cruise boats that would pull into Miami or Lauderdale with concerns about a foodborne outbreak. It was having opportunities to do a broad variety of functions. I could build on each with successive moves and successive positions.[26]

Bert did not plan to leave his Catholic school teaching job in 1974 to become a VD investigator in Saginaw, Michigan, and four surrounding counties. It just worked out that way. His career brought him diverse geographic experiences—from Saginaw to Miami to Baltimore to Missouri—and these experiences occurred in the first ten years of his tenure as a PHA. After his stint in Saginaw, Bert moved to Miami to work in VD and Tuberculosis (TB). From Miami, he went to work in Baltimore in TB, and then to Missouri to work in TB, environmental health, and chronic disease prevention. Today Bert Malone is in Kansas City, Missouri directing environmental health efforts and lecturing in St. Louis as an adjunct professor at the Saint Louis University School of Public Health.

Like some of his federal colleagues, Bert opted to leave the federal service to become a permanent employee of the local public health system. The system of frequent relocation, rapid deployment, and varied program exposure is among the CDC's most important human resource contributions to local and global public health. While building its own federal management assets, CDC also builds local public health capacity by placing PHAs in city and state health departments and ensuring that they have broad public health exposure throughout their careers. When a PHA leaves federal service for local government employment, he or she becomes a more permanent member of the local health infrastructure. In this way the federal government contributes compounded public health experience that could not possibly be developed at the local level.

Every experience of every assignment contributed to Bert Malone's ability to be the public health leader he is today. Like other PHAs, he remains shaped by his initial field experiences. The field is where PHAs learn about community realities and begin to see potential for their own contributions to community health. These experiences linger indelibly and inform their perspectives and decisions in later years. Bert's field experience from thirty years ago with Haitian refugees was not far from his mind even as he sat in his executive office in 2004:

> Early in the Miami assignment, I think it was about '75 or '76, Haitians were literally arriving on rafts on the shore on Miami Beach. I was asked to help out the Feds even before the federal government really got directly involved in the resettlement of those refugees, just in the initial receipt of those individuals to bring them in for health screening. We worked with the Dade County Health Department to pick them up off the shores and bring them in for health screenings... And it really struck me at that point in my growth and my life, that here I was seeing people fleeing their homeland to get to a better life with literally nothing—I mean, literally dying as they hit the shores. And one guy did die of TB next to the Fontainebleau Hotel. It really made an impression on me, that they have this huge wealthy aristocratic facility and then here

> not less than a hundred yards away you've got people arriving on the shores destitute and dying. And I thought something's not right. Not that I can fix it, not that we can fix it, but it sure can impress upon you the global need for adequate public health.[27]

The PHA's exposure to public health begins in the field, which is to say, in direct contact with local communities. PHAs are initiated into their roles through fieldwork, which involves activities such as contact epidemiology or case finding, and blood testing or screening on a large scale. Fieldwork involves interviewing people with or potentially exposed to an infectious disease. It involves working with local public health departments, assisting with clinical services and prevention outreach. It involves trying to bridge the healthcare system's yawning gaps, into which many people fall. Fieldwork customarily happens on street corners, out of mobile vans, in drug-shooting galleries, under bridges—just about anywhere. For Ed Powers, a retired PHA who spent his career in sexually transmitted disease prevention, the PHA's work occurs even "in a Winnebago van in the middle of the night treating drug dealers with a doctor that we had to convince to stay with us."[28]

Fieldwork is a regular part of the PHA assignment to a local or state health department STD or TB program, and it can be part of a special detail assignment in response to disease outbreaks. Not everyone is cut out for fieldwork, because it is grueling and requires long hours. This type of work also confronts individuals with intractable human realities that continually evolve in the confluence of society's economic and social challenges. The PHAs who make it out of the field become tremendous public health managers, in part because they remain grounded in the realities that they have seen in the field. Such managers are unusual in health and public health policy, because often the senior-level people who are in positions to make change have not had these kinds of experiences. PHAs, however, carry the street into the executive suite.

Kevin O'Connor is the chief of the Program and Training Branch of the CDC's Division of STD Prevention. He has worked with the HIV and Hepatitis programs at CDC and has spent several years in the field working in STD control. As crack cocaine fueled syphilis epidemics in several parts of the U.S. in the 1980s, Kevin often encountered local private physicians who were ignorant of the obvious signs of syphilis because they had never seen cases prior to this time. He regularly worked in unusual places in order to bridge the gap between STD patients and the healthcare system. While assigned to Connecticut, his work frequently led him to crack houses. One particular Stamford, Connecticut crack house was home to at least thirty-eight cases of syphilis. Kevin set up shop there and "did bloods" (took blood samples), counseled sexual contacts and potential patients. The closer Kevin got to the community, the more he saw the lack of connection between STD patients and the healthcare system:

> When you smoke crack you have a lot of sex partners, so if you've been smoking crack you probably get three, four, or five partners a day… We had thirty-eight cases of syphilis related to this one crack house. One day I went in there and did nine bloods, and three of those ended up being brand new syphilis cases. One woman was eight months pregnant, and she had had gonorrhea in her first trimester. She had a doctor, and her doctor said to me, "Well, how'd you get involved?" He couldn't figure out where I came from. I said "Well, I was in the crack house and I was drawing blood, and your patient was there and she tested positive." He should have recognized her as a high-risk pregnancy because she had gonorrhea, but he didn't.[29]

Kevin's experience was not isolated. Although we are more than fifty years away from the World War II effort to be "fit to fight" (free from syphilis), we are nowhere closer to providing better public health service in STD because the healthcare system continues to respond differently to different people. In the 1980s Kevin prevented syphilis from reaching a baby born to his pregnant client who should have been under more diligent medical care. Dick Conlon had a similar experience a decade earlier while working with migrant populations at a Hunt's food plant in Toledo, Ohio. In Dick's case, a physician flatly refused to treat his patient, a pregnant woman with syphilis. Like Kevin, Dick reached across a gap in the healthcare system to provide for the health of this woman and her unborn child:

> A woman who'd had a prenatal blood test was seven months pregnant. Turned out she had secondary syphilis, and her gynecologist/obstetrician refused to treat her. He said he did not treat syphilis in his practice. To get her treated I had to drive from Toledo to Fremont, Ohio, to pick her up; take her back into Toledo, where they would treat her; and then take her back to Fremont. And then I did that again to get her re-tested a few months later. All this just because the doctor was stubborn and wouldn't treat her.[30]

Through these and other field experiences, the PHA bears witness to the challenges of public health—even in this country, with our so-called "world-class" healthcare system. This kind of service is an essential part of fieldwork. It goes beyond what the healthcare system is willing or able to do—even beyond what the public health system is willing to do. In 1992, Phil Talboy was assigned to Miami as an Emergency Response Coordinator during the Hurricane Andrew recovery process. Property damage was so significant that many people abandoned their homes. Swimming pools became rank mosquito breeding grounds, and housing material and debris became homes for breeding rodents. In the midst of the human devastation emerged hantavirus, a zoonotic pathogen communicated through aerosolized rodent excrement and causing hemorrhagic fever and renal syndrome.[31] A case of hantavirus was identified in a drug rehabilitation center, which meant that other patients and staff needed to be tested. Because the hantavirus vector is field rodents, rats had to be caught and tested as well. According to Phil, the Florida State Health Department staff refused to do any of the rat testing for fear of communicability and because, frankly, the job was dirty. Phil stepped forward. "I've always felt the role of the PHA is to do whatever's necessary to get the job done," he said.[32] His work resulted in the identification of a new strain of hantavirus—the Black Creek Canal Virus—with a huge positivity rate among rodents. "We caught more rats and mice than I ever want to see in my life." He continued:

> The state staff were reluctant to draw the blood because it was hantavirus. So as the PHA, I said, "I'll do it." I did most of the testing in a blown-out building on Homestead Air Force Base. I drew bloods in a self-contained suit in the middle of July in Florida.[33]

This and many other gritty field experiences inform Phil's current role as the deputy director of CDC's Division of TB Elimination. At first glance, he and other PHAs in senior management positions might strike you as scrappy, because behind the executive exterior one can see a public health professional forged in the field. This essentially means that PHAs are very practical managers and leaders, grounded in the aggregation of their observations over years of service. They know how the public health system works and how to get it to work better, and they are well-acquainted with the populations it serves. The availability of such an experienced manager means the difference between public health programs that work effectively and those that are unrealistic because the program architects or managers never actually worked in the field.

Dennis McDowell is a retired PHA who recently served as the acting deputy director of CDC's Caribbean Regional Office.[34] According to Dennis, he often had to draw upon his community expertise in this role because his public health colleagues had never served in the community, and therefore did not know much about the populations or their risk behaviors:

> While down in the Caribbean, many disease control experts were quoting outdated studies when talking about HIV transmission risk behaviors and risk groups: men who have sex with men and commercial sex workers and that sort of thing. And these people, my boss included, had never actually been to a house of prostitution and had never gone out to the gay bars. I've done all that in the past. So I personally have done the field work to understand first hand how HIV is really moving through the community, where people get condoms and how much they really know about their own risk behavior and how to reduce it. I'm comfortable doing that. It's not a big deal, but it's an important part of understanding the work we need to do.[35]

PHAs are effective in part because they learn to work in a variety of situations and can establish rapport with just about anybody. They use rapport-building skills in the course of daily work and in unusual tasks, such as working with outbreaks, where people must be honest about very private or less-than-stellar behaviors affecting the health of others. The ability to establish rapport is not innate—at least, that is the thinking when PHAs are hired and trained. As with Kathryn Koski, whose first day in the field involved a visit with Mexican transvestites, all PHAs become acclimated to working in situations and cultures that are new to them through repeated and entry-level job experiences working in communities. Today, Kathryn is the deputy chief of the Health Services Research and Evaluation Branch, in CDC's Division of STD Prevention. She credits her field experience as the place where she developed her rapport-building skills as well as her appreciation for the richness of community diversity:

> My first day in the field included a visit with transvestites from Mexico who were living together in this tiny apartment. There were six of them and they didn't speak word one of English. My Spanish-speaking colleague had to give them their STD test results and she took each one out individually and confidentially [counseled

> them]. Well, that left five of them with me. I didn't speak any Spanish and they didn't speak any English. So they must have sensed the need to put me at ease and just finally decided they were going to put on a show for me. And it was the most surreal thing. They got out all their clothes and gave me a little fashion show and showed me pictures of themselves in full makeup. It was great.[36]

Jim Beall had a similar cross-cultural learning experience in his work as a PHA. In the early 1980s he was "used as bait" on the airport prostitution circuit in Los Angeles, on Hollywood and Vine, in order to increase access to STD clinical services by sex trade workers. This was a new experience for "a Midwestern guy, but the work was invigorating and challenging." Jim would pose as a potential "John" and engage the prostitutes (male and female) in conversation about their sexual health, and would then refer them to the STD clinic for services. During his six-week assignment, Jim was able to refer countless numbers of men and women to receive needed treatment for STDs. This "fish out of water" was able to establish trust, build rapport, and serve as a health resource.[37] The field experience was also valuable because it exposed Jim to communities with which he had never before worked.

Through years of field experience in diverse communities, PHAs become able to establish rapport quickly in order to get to the heart of the health matter. The fact that they are part of the "government" and seek personal information does complicate the job, but PHAs become adept at building rapport through the repeated practice of developing relationships built on trust and confidences. A PHA's "currency," or effectiveness on the job, is a reflection of his or her credibility on the street. Having to build connections with people who might be very different culturally or behaviorally involves "getting used to it." Sometimes the work challenges core values, and yet, because PHAs are committed to the public health mission, they look beyond these issues to form relationships that will yield accurate information to ensure good health in the long run. Most people would not be cut out for this type of job because it would make them callous or negative. In the case of PHAs, the work makes them recall the competing issues that drive values in the lives of others. In doing so, it slows the rush to judgment that would otherwise take over. Wendy Wolf is the deputy director of STD Prevention and Control Services for the City of San Francisco. She recalls the competing priorities that challenge the client's health, and the importance of appreciating these challenges in the course of working with communities. "Unless you walk in their shoes, you can't know what they're going through," she says. The developing appreciation for client circumstance tempers the frustration that might emerge when, for example, a client refuses to seek needed health care. Wendy recalls a client early in her PHA career in 1970s New York:

> I remember this one woman as clearly as if I talked to her yesterday. She was a woman with secondary syphilis, a young single mom. She had symptoms of syphilis, she had a classic palmer-planter rash, and I never could get her in for treatment. I literally was out there at her house every day, and every day she would tell me, "Maybe I could make it in but I got all these other things that are more important to me to do."[38]

Wendy learned that many things compete with access to care, and that PHAs and other public health professionals must remain mindful of this fact: "There may be a million other things that are that much more important to them. For some of them it may be that they don't have money for dinner, or they may not know if they're going to be living on the street."[39]

Rapport-building is necessary because infectious disease fieldwork requires epidemiologic investigation to determine the source and spread of infection in order to stop an outbreak or to slow an epidemic's progress. Unlike other diseases, STDs historically have been intertwined with morality and cloaked in shame. Although disease investigation generally introduces one to myriad complex and competing value systems, STD fieldwork uniquely brings PHAs to appreciate the nexus of values and health. They learn that the public health mission is the focal point, and that although patient behavior may seem unbelievable, access to medical treatment trumps any need to shun or judge. This attitude, of course, contrasts markedly with the general public's perceptions. Historically, VD prevention and treatment were believed to reinforce bad behaviors.[40] Even today one can find physicians who refuse to recognize or to treat STDs in their patients. In theory, this practice seems inhumane; however, the challenging behavior that the PHA ordinarily sees may make this attitude more understandable, if still horrific. Joe Webb, a retired PHA who spent seventeen of his thirty two years with CDC in VD control, has seen it all. He says that PHAs learn early on that different world views and values should not prevent public health work. A focus on the greater mission keeps things in perspective: "You develop a rapport, so they tell you things they don't want to tell you, and they will tell you a whole lot more than you want to hear." Joe recalls a patient who infected his pregnant partner and ultimately their baby with syphilis:

> I once asked a guy with a syphilis lesion the size of a quarter on his penis, "When was the last time you had sex with this woman?" He said, "Oh, let's see, this morning before we left for the hospital." I said, "Why did you take her to the hospital?" He said, "Well, she was having a baby."[41]

Any PHA will tell you that the ability to establish rapport is a valuable skill that they call upon throughout their careers as they work with patient populations, public health leaders, private physicians, media representatives, the general public, and others. For Bill Parra, one of the first PHAs ever to be assigned to the World Health Organization (WHO) headquarters following Dr. Asad's request for "one of those," it was vital to establish relationships across cultures and within an organization that did not understand what a PHA was. Bill's ability to establish rapport served many purposes. First, it helped him get the job done. This ability set the standard for PHAs who followed, and helped establish a perception about PHAs and their value to the organization. "I had to work across cultures; I had to work across languages," he said. "I had come to understand culturally how you wrote letters and did things to get things done that didn't appear too brusque, too American-style." Bill could have had an easy assignment at WHO working for the American researcher Dr. Jonathan Mann, who was there to help establish the Global Programme on AIDS. However, this PHA was loyal to the assignment. He was there to assist the director of the Communicable Disease Division, even if this director did not understand that his role as a PHA was to serve temporarily until WHO decided to send him back to CDC. A temporary assignment was counter to the culture of the WHO, where professionals sought permanent appointments due to the organization's tremendous benefits. Bill became part of the WHO culture eventually and through the development of relationships. A sign of his effectiveness was his appointment as mediator between two "warring" programs: the Food Safety Programme in the Division of Environmental Health and the Veterinary Public Health Programme in the Communicable Disease Division. Disagreements occurred quite frequently during food outbreaks since the public health responsibilities between these two organizations were not clearly delineated. Bill was asked to arbitrate what he said was "like a relationship between the Palestinians and the Israelis":

> I had to work back and forth between these two leaders and win their respect. They couldn't even be in the same room. We had to

> decide what was the proper role of one and what was the proper role of the other, how they perceived it, how they might ultimately agree to share responsibilities in ways that would be productive when there was an outbreak of any kind. And we worked at it for about six months. It was really difficult. But we got it done.[42]

Bill Parra used his extensive complement of professional skills at WHO to bridge major communication gaps in order to "get the job done," a focus that is a central part of PHA culture and reputation. Another more recent example was the case with the anthrax scare in 2001. During that autumn, letters that possibly were contaminated with anthrax were sent to Senator Tom Daschle in Washington, D.C., and to journalist Tom Brokaw in New York. PHAs were on the scene at both sites to help bridge a communication gap between law enforcement and scientists that threatened the success of the response. Phil Talboy, Bill Gallo, Harald Pietz, and Joe Posid were detailed to New York as part of CDC's response. Although it was not a glamorous task, these PHAs spent their first night computerizing thousands of anthrax sample analyses so that results could be obtained more efficiently. Phil remembers that the "big story" was that they got an important job done in a very short time, reinforcing the PHAs' reputation:

> When we arrived, there was a big room set up at the city health department down on Worth Street. We walked in, all the EIS Officers were there doing their surveillance work, and somebody looked up and said, "Who are you guys?" We responded, "We're the PHAs." And a big roar in the room went up, "The PHAs are here. Finally we can get some work done!" On that particular day, a member of the New York laboratory staff told me they needed sample results entered into the computer system so that the lab staff could start giving out results. They had five thousand samples to get through, and it was really hard to go by hand through the records. I promised them we would get it all computerized by 6:45 the next morning. There were three of us and we worked all night and got all that data in as promised. We upheld the tradition that "the PHAs are here and the job will get done."[43]

During their twenty-three-day assignment in New York, these four PHAs also stopped a contamination cycle created by the clash of police operations and epidemiology. When Phil, Joe, Bill, and Harald arrived in New York, they found that most of the laboratories had been "spammed," or contaminated, because of the way police had handled the samples. "The police were coming in and taking the samples, labeled with yellow sticky notes Number 1, Number 2, Number 3, etc., and throwing them in a broom closet in a red biohazard bag," Phil said. The PHAs quickly fixed the problem by setting up a laboratory system that both police and epidemiologists could live with. Phil continued:

> Since the anthrax event was a crime, we had to set up the chain of custody for all the samples. We set up a holding area so that they could decontaminate the items to be tested. We figured if all those samples were positive, they would spam the whole laboratory. One of the laboratories was already spammed from the Brokaw letter.[44]

The reputation of PHAs among current and past CDC directors, local and state health directors, and colleagues is that PHAs get the job done. They are extremely effective, dependable, and mission-oriented. You can count on them. They are willing to roll up their sleeves and get their hands dirty, irrespective of their current public health role or position. When faced with a task, PHAs demonstrate ingenuity, adaptability, and commitment. It is as if the task allows them to focus their cumulative public health experience and know-how.

Since their beginning in 1948, PHAs have been so effective that they have been recruited to work in several programs across CDC and other health-related organizations inside and outside the U.S. federal government, and they have been given positions of significant authority when CDC needed effective managers to develop a program ex nihilo or during national or international health crises. Three PHAs, Bill Watson, Jack Jackson, and Bill Gimson, served as CDC deputy directors. Several PHAs serve and have served as deputies and directors of branches, divisions and also centers at CDC. Others chose to remain in state and local health departments running divisions or programs, and a few, like Steve Bice, have had the helm of major national CDC initiatives, such as the Strategic National Stockpile and the Emergency Operations Center.

Steve Bice began his CDC career in 1971 as a VD investigator in Los Angeles. He is one of the few PHAs who completed training to be an Epidemic Intelligence Service officer. For several years Steve worked out of CDC's San Francisco regional office responding to outbreaks and other health situations throughout the U.S. He also focused on the Pacific territories. There he worked with a variety of diseases, including cholera and leprosy: "I cut my teeth doing some epi work out there, plus there was always the ubiquitous typhoon and post-typhoon response."[45] He left CDC to work for what were then the Health Services Administration and the Health Resources Administration, setting up the National Community Migrant Health Centers Program. Steve also worked in the Office of the Secretary of Health and Human Services, expanding health services in the Pacific following the Compact of Free Association in 1986.[46] He returned to CDC as deputy director of the hepatitis branch and shortly thereafter was recruited to coordinate the Emergency Response Group, which eventually became the Strategic National Stockpile Program. In 2003, CDC Director Julie Gerberding asked Steve to direct all emergency operations for CDC. At the time, Steve did not think that CDC was ready for the kind of emergency operations he was used to dealing with.[47] He accepted the job because he got the green light to move in unconventional ways—at least for public health culture—to ensure that emergency operations were as effective as they could be. As Steve reflected on his career, he said that two things helped prepare him to be the quintessential PHA, "the go-to guy":

> There are two things that may sound contradictory, but they're not: they're complementary. First is organizational skill, knowing how to organize to accomplish tasks. You know you can get the job done. You have a certain amount of confidence, and that comes with the years of experience out in the field working with state and local people who really are the front edge of the sword in all ways. But the second is that you also know your place. They are complementary. You know who you work for, you know how to work within a system, and never get bigger than your britches.[48]

PHAs "know who they work for." Although their activities are often unconventional, PHAs understand hierarchy and can work within it. Steve refers to "incidence command," a phrase that describes the system of managing multiple agencies in a rapid-response environment. Although this management style is well understood in an era of bioterrorism, it is important to note that such a hierarchical way of working is anathema to public health culture, which values a decentralized authority and management structure characterized by collegial scientific and medical discourse. In situations of rapid response or where efficiency is critical, the PHA culture of "knowing who you work for" is paramount to success. Perhaps it is less about knowing who they work for than being so deeply committed to the mission that the PHA sheds his or her current title, rolls up his or her sleeves, and falls in line to get the job done. The work, says Steve Bice, is nothing to be snooty about:

> You come to understand that if you have to roll up your sleeves and get dirty to help people be healthy, then that's what you have to do. That's what you should do. If a health officer wants somebody to do bloods in an HIV clinic and you're willing to do it, then roll up your sleeves and do it. If a health officer says, "My nursing staff is falling-down tired, could we just have about ten of you guys giving shots so we could get over this meningitis?" well, gee, can't you? I would think we can and we will.[49]

PHAs have been trained over years of placements to do whatever was requested, even if it meant risking life and limb. In careers such as the military, police, or fire safety, such behavior is not unusual. But such a willingness to expose oneself to risk is not expected of public health workers. It is not surprising, then, that from the perspective of some in public health, PHA colleagues might be a bit too hierarchically inclined. This is a central misunderstanding of the PHA, because the difference is that PHAs do well in hierarchy while using their own ingenuity to get the job accomplished. The focus is on the mission. These are men and women who do not cling to their job descriptions and say, "I'm not supposed to do that." Instead, PHAs "roll up their sleeves" to help get the job done.

Such commitment to the mission helps Anne-Renee Heningburg in her work with the CDC's Global Immunization Program. She began her career in New Orleans in 1979 doing VD work. From there, Anne-Renee transferred to Michigan, New Jersey, and Los Angeles. In 1995, she joined the polio eradication effort, and has worked in Geneva, Uganda, the Philippines, Nigeria, Zimbabwe, and the southern Sudan. At the time of her interview in 2004, she was working in India in logistics and management to help ramp up polio efforts. When asked what she did specifically, Anne-Renee said she did "whatever came up – the usual PHA stuff."[50] As the Technical Officer in Lucknow, Uttar Pradesh, Anne-Renee had to bring order to the chaos of polio efforts. In 2004, Uttar Pradesh had yet to interrupt polio transmission, so the World Health Organization launched a massive buildup of surveillance medical officers. These professionals were technically strong; however, they were not good managers or organizers. Enter Anne-Renee: "I was handling management issues in their regional office, trying to get their staffing up to speed, building an office that fit all the people who were working there, doing a number of things along those lines. Helping out with training, communication, whatever came up—the usual PHA stuff." Holding a master's degree in public administration from Harvard did not prevent Anne-Renee from rolling up her sleeves and helping out. She saw how what Steve Bice called "snootiness" prevented important work in polio. Anne-Renee has seen this time and again—in India, the Philippines, and Africa. In her opinion, the PHA's contribution is to make things happen in these kinds of contexts: "Okay, this is what we need to do; this is what it takes to do it. Now how can we get these two together to make it happen?"[51]

In these types of roles PHAs develop management and operations acumen, making some of their best contributions to public health at the management level. Dr. Alan Hinman, senior public health scientist with the Task Force for Child Survival and Development, knows the importance of PHA management skill. Paring such skill with science has been a powerful public health contribution. He saw this at the beginning of his career as an Epidemic Intelligence Service officer on his first of many outbreak assignments, and he saw this in his service as the New York State Epidemiologist and head of Communicable Disease Control. This observation was reconfirmed when he re-joined CDC as the director of the Immunization Division in 1977 and subsequently director of the National Center for Prevention Services (1988-1995). In these roles he was paired with PHAs Harold Mauldin, Jack Kirby, Bill Doyle, Windell Bradford, Tony Scardaci, and Steve Barid. For Alan, these PHAs have set the bar of excellence:

> One of the best things CDC did in the smallpox program was to team an epidemiologist and a Public Health Advisor in the long-term assignments they made overseas. The epidemiologist was the bright guy who has these weird ideas, and the Public Health Advisor was the guy that sees how you can actually get it done... What I mainly think of is a series of very successful partnerships that bring results; bringing together the scientific/medical and the programmatic to achieve things like eradicating smallpox, eradicating polio, interrupting measles transmission in the United States, and a whole series of other really important public health advances. Public Health Advisors have been an integral part of that.[52]

Those who sing the praises of PHA management skill are their scientific colleagues who would have stumbled in their positions at CDC without the help of their "number two" or deputy. Although scientists are often placed in leadership roles at CDC, there is recognition that the agency cannot run effectively without operations expertise. CDC unlocked a secret to success when it paired PHAs and scientists in the 1960s. Bill Watson, a PHA who was Executive Officer of CDC at the time,[53] saw the need for operations expertise in the Smallpox Program. The program was faltering in the hands of scientists who did not have management or logistics background. D.A. Henderson, the lead scientist on smallpox, was reluctant to accept the help, but would later be completely convinced of the practice.[54] Following this success, the scientist-PHA pairing became a central management philosophy of CDC.[55] Dave Sencer, director of CDC at the time, recalls the management innovation:

> A big change in perception of Public Health Advisors occurred probably in 1966 or 1967 with the smallpox program, where the program was built around what they call the operations officer and the epidemiologist. And this opened the eyes of many of the scientific types at CDC to the value of having a combination of talents that can be put to work on the same problem. And I think that was sort of a bellwether [of] the change.[56]

Dave knows the value of keeping one's hands dirty. Even as CDC director, Dave continued to keep his TB skills fresh by reading chest x-rays.[57] He found a kindred spirit in PHAs who served alongside him. Bill Watson was his deputy and second in command at CDC for several years. After Dave left CDC in 1977, Bill served in the same capacity under CDC Director Dr. Bill Foege, who entered his role as director from the Smallpox Program, where for years he worked alongside PHAs. Bill Foege recalled:

> I went from that to being CDC director with Bill Watson as the deputy. He made that a much easier job than it should have been. I used to say that I trusted his judgment more than mine. It was the case that when I would be gone, and he would be acting director, I never once had to revisit a decision that he made. It was such a good relationship that [I could] have absolute trust in what he was doing. And in fact the working relationship was so good that he and I then went on together to the Carter Center, the Task Force for Childhood Immunizations.[58]

CDC is a scientific organization. Scientists are generally at the forefront of activity. A PHA's contribution to this system lies in being the "number-two" to the scientist, bringing operational and managerial knowledge to move the science forward and translate it into community-level solutions and services. Scientists and physicians are the first to tell you that they themselves are not very good managers. When taking on a major role at CDC, the first thing many do is to pair up with a PHA. Dr. William Roper, CDC director from 1990-1993, recalls the management value of PHAs:

> It had been deeply embedded in the fabric of the organization that people who were trained in management were key to the operation of the Centers and the various other programmatic units at CDC. And it was then and is now an important part of the way CDC does business, to have, in many cases, a physician or other science leader for an organization and have that person have as their number two a Public Health Advisor who is trained in management and the administrative aspects of the job.[59]

The administrative contribution of PHAs beyond CDC was exemplified by Bill Parra at the World Health Organization (e.g. "one of those"). However unlike CDC, the WHO did not continue to use PHAs at headquarters. The outcome today is "painful to watch" because scientists are left to "organize endless administrative details," says Dr. Kathleen Irwin who recently retired from CDC and now coordinates global policy on use of Human Papillomavirus vaccines at the WHO. "WHO has relied heavily on CDC for the last four decades to perform complex activities well and efficiently. Perhaps this is largely due to the practical know how of CDC PHAs."[60] During her career at CDC, Katy worked with PHAs in several capacities, primarily research, and recently management. She believes that having a PHA on the management team ensures that research projects run smoothly and are completed on time. PHAs also help to translate "research-ese" for use by program managers and the public. Without PHAs, "it would be a mess."[61]

> PHAs make it happen. They make the logistics of doing research and program evaluation much easier; they make our projects better managed. They let scientifically trained people do the scientific tasks for which they're skilled, and handle administrative, fiscal, or other tasks so scientists don't fumble them. They manage our funds better. They can make projects happen that, without their entrée, without their connections, without their understanding of the practical applications of public health, would never yield useful results to communities. I shudder to think what would happen if PHAs with these skills were no longer a central part of this agency.[62]

Pat McConnon is the executive director of the Council of State and Territorial Epidemiologists. He began his career as a PHA in 1967 working in an STD clinic in Cincinnati, Ohio. His career took him throughout Ohio, then to

Virginia, Minnesota, and to CDC headquarters in VD control. In 1981 Pat began a two year assignment in Thailand as part of the refugee resettlement effort (see Chapter 7). In 1984 he was appointed the deputy director for the newly-formed National Center for Chronic Disease Prevention and Health Promotion and Reproductive Health. In 1989 Pat was detailed to the Carter Center to work for two years in Nigeria on Guinea worm. He returned to Atlanta for what "seemed like two months of staring at my computer," and was, to his gratitude, detailed as the operations officer for hantavirus in 1993. At the time, an unknown pathogen was killing Navajo Indians in the Southwest United States. It was his role to "keep things moving down there." When Pat speaks about his role in partnership with scientists, he recognizes that the PHA's value is to keep things on track, given many scientific colleagues' lack of operational experience. When CDC places a PHA on a scientific team, they essentially are saying to the scientists that "these guys are going to help you so you can do your job. Otherwise, trust me, you won't be able to do it."[63] Pat is used to being the PHA among scientists, and the hantavirus assignment was no exception. His role was to help get the science under way:

> I was the only non-scientist among about thirty people. They were all chomping at the bit to get going, but there at the Holiday Inn they didn't know what to do or where to go. "Well, what do we do now?" It's like the dog that caught the bus or something. I said, "Well, you know, we need some offices, we need photocopy machines, we need a secretary, you need technical support, you need some local people who can get you into and around on the Reservation," because when you went in there the Navajos were shooting at news media helicopters. So everybody was a little worried about what kind of reception you were going to get when you went and knocked on a door and that sort of thing.[64]

PHAs are able to work well in the scientific pairing because they translate information for decision making. Steve Bice calls this "a wheat and chaff thing."[65] Their value also appears in multidisciplinary contexts, because they speak the language that is shared by decision makers, and they simplify complex concepts that are intrinsically a bit jumbled for use in decisions. Often PHAs are there to manage the scientists, because the scientists are focused singularly on their goal at the expense of other things. The FBI, for example, has come to the CDC for help because CDC scientists have compromised crime scenes. The scientists are concerned with disease and intervention. The FBI is concerned with crime. The PHA is the type of worker who can "crosswalk" between disciplines,[66] just as Phil Talboy and colleagues did with anthrax decontamination in New York City and Steve Bice did in his role as the Health and Medical lead for the Hurricane Andrew response. Steve stood in the gap between the integrated emergency operations culture of decision making and the scientific culture of discourse. This was no more apparent than during Secretary Andrew Card's briefing by several response partners. Steve recalls:

> I stood up and gave the brief for Emergency Support Function #8, Health and Medical. As we finished, a physician got up and wanted to talk, and Card said, "I've had the briefing from Health and Medical." "Yes, but Steve isn't a physician." And Card said, "I just had a complete briefing from Health and Medical. I don't need another briefing." There were several concerns voiced already about post-hurricane public health issues. We had framed up around those issues and interdicted most of them. We could talk a lot more about problems, which this physician felt was important to do; but within the larger context of putting that community and state back on its feet, Card didn't need an in-depth discourse on epidemiology post-hurricane. It just wasn't contextually appropriate. Not that he wasn't interested. Not that he didn't care on one level. But he had larger, overarching decisions to make.[67]

The Problem Solvers

> *The series truly fits a definition of public service like no other job. I'm sure that almost every PHA cringes at the description of "bureaucrat" because we just never could see ourselves as bureaucrats. You picture a bureaucrat as someone very necessary but sitting still. PHAs, if they were doing their jobs, were never sitting still, were never satisfied, were always looking for a challenge, always questioning, looking for answers. The PHA is looking at the horizon and beyond, looking out into space so to speak, thinking, "Where's the next problem going to be?" We are problem solvers. We can find a solution around any barrier.*[68]
>
> Dick Conlon
> Public Health Advisor (ret.)

Problem solving is a skill, sometimes learned and sometimes innate. The PHA's ability to quickly size up a problem and creatively solve it is unmatched in public health. PHAs have contributed their problem-solving skills to a variety of public health problems, ranging from small issues, such as reaching hard-to-reach communities to provide health services, to setting up massive immunization and screening programs at a moment's notice. Anne-Renee Heningburg speaks modestly about her problem-solving acumen: "At the bottom, functionally, it's just figuring out how to move things forward. You just have to learn the obstacles and how to get over them."[69] For Anne-Renee, the problem was getting polio immunizations into Sudan after a last-minute loss of transportation for the vaccines. At the eleventh hour, the plane scheduled to deliver the vaccine broke down. This was a problem of epidemic proportion. Polio immunizations must be given in the community during precise time periods. National Immunization Days (NIDs) are planned with this in mind. Coordinating a national immunization effort is challenging enough, but Anne-Renee's challenge was heightened because Sudan was in the midst of civil war. Getting the polio vaccine into Sudan would require a large plane called a "Buffalo," the kind developed for use during the Vietnam War. In 1998, only seventeen such planes were in use. The Buffalo scheduled for Sudan broke down five days before the NID was to begin. Heningburg used her creativity and social network to secure a plane for the effort:

> One guy I came across who had kids in my friend's Boy Scout troop worked for the World Food Program's Somalia program. They also were using Buffalos. I asked if could I "borrow" a Buffalo, though I was sure he would say no because their mission was delivering food in Somalia, not polio eradication in southern Sudan. He said, "No way," but he knew about a Buffalo in Somalia with a contract that was ending, and it might be available for two weeks. I found the owners, who after lots of negotiation agreed that they would accept a contract. So I asked UNICEF to make another contract. Though their contracts group wasn't meeting for another three weeks, we found a way to do it in two days. Working through all the challenges, using the informal network, convincing people to abandon the "business-as-usual" methods, I got this Buffalo which delivered our supplies, and the NIDs happened as planned. So the team referred to this as my Buffalo, and somebody took a picture of it for me. To me it represents the PHA credo: "Just lay out the obstacles, and we will figure out how to get around them."[70]

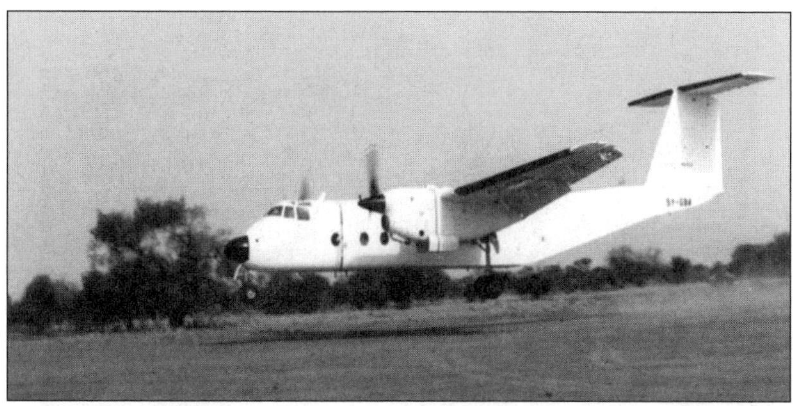

Anne-Renee Heningburg's "Buffalo" landing in Lokichoggio, Kenya, the base for Southern Sudan's polio operations.
Courtesy of Anne-Renee Heningburg.

Dr. William Foege, CDC director from 1977 to 1983, had his share of experiences with PHAs. Most of his work was with global programs, and it was here that he saw the importance of having public health workers who understood how to deliver and manage a program. Although PHAs had been around since 1948, the concept "didn't catch on for a long time, and it is part of why we're in such a hole right now of not being able to deliver things in global health."[71]

> I think of Andy Agle, who has just passed away… I've known him since 1966, when we started working together in Africa. Andy is a good prototype of the field Public Health Advisor, because what you really needed in West Africa in smallpox was a person who understood problem solving. The science was actually secondary. Andy worked in some of the toughest places in the world. I first knew him when he was working in Togo... He worked in Nigeria, Afghanistan, Bangladesh, the absolute most difficult places in the world, and he continued to thrive because he was a problem solver. Instead of getting frustrated by the things that went wrong, he would very calmly try to figure out a way around.[72]

PHA problem-solving skills are honed over several years of field assignments in challenging or nearly intractable situations. As Jerry Lama learned, the job is not nine-to-five, and requires a creative approach in order to find people who need treatment.

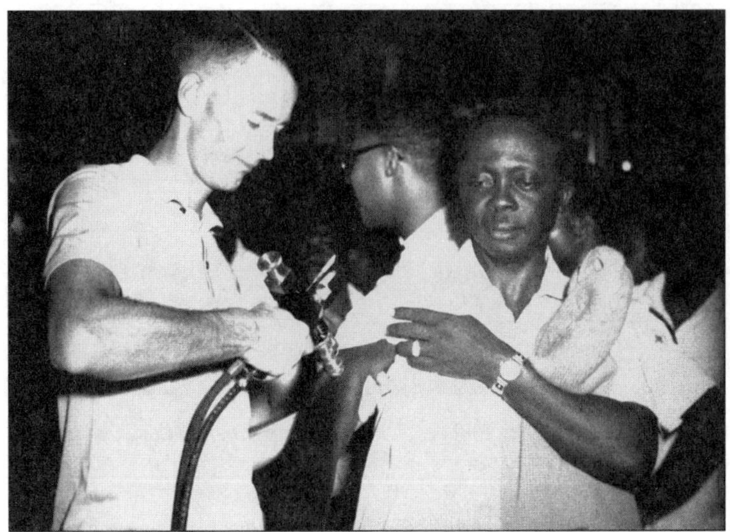

The late Andy Agle (PHA) vaccinating Dr. Beaunie Challenor against measles in Togo in 1967, prior to the kickoff of the Global Smallpox Eradication Program.
Courtesy Joel G. Breman, Centers for Disease Control and Prevention, Public Health Image Library.

> You spent a lot of time finding out when it would be best to find your contact if they were only named in a public place, like a bar or a street corner. And you worked those hours necessary to find the person. Sometimes Sunday morning was the best day to go into a particularly dangerous housing project because the bad guys were still sleeping. So you got in early, did your work, and got out. You learned to set your own hours, set your own priorities, and you learned very, very quickly that problem solving is a fun skill that did really make you feel competent and confident, and it's something I enjoyed.[73]

The sense of empowerment is part of the highly developed "can-do" attitude for which PHAs are known. This spirit pervades the series. When most people think of a "can-do" attitude, they recall post-World War II American self- and cultural efficacy: we can do anything we put our minds to. People talking about PHAs refer to their willingness to do anything based on broad experience in problem solving and public health service. It is about "getting the job done," and it involves confidence in the ability to do so. "Can-do" is also a willingness to "give it a try," and across CDC people celebrate this spirit as a central characteristic of PHAs. Current CDC Director Dr. Julie Gerberding credits PHAs as being one of the core groups of contributors to such a spirit at CDC:

> I think the Public Health Advisors have really been one of the pillars of the can-do spirit at CDC. They are the people we go to when there's a new problem to solve and we need experienced and trusted people who can provide the structure and support for getting the job done right. Examples in recent years have been with the smallpox vaccination program, the anthrax attacks, situations where there's a sudden public health threat or public health emergency and we can't send the junior squad into the field without the kind of maturity senior leadership can provide.[74]

When Dr. Asad requested "one of those," he had only a glimpse of what a PHA might bring to the headquarters of the World Health Organization. A glimpse is all that he would have until Bill Parra's arrival, because PHAs are not the type to broadcast what they contribute. In fact, PHAs are often transparent in the organization—whether at WHO or any other public health organization. This transparency is historic and dates back to the beginning of the PHA series, when in 1948 a statistician named Lida J. Usilton and an economist named Johannes Stuart thought a federal infusion of VD personnel into local health agencies would help control syphilis in the U.S. As it turns out, the "Madam and her Doctor" were correct. Their decision to initiate an experiment of co-ops on the Eastern Shore of Maryland would reverberate throughout public health for decades to come.

Chapter 2

The Madam and her Doctor

By the mid-1940s, U.S. efforts to control syphilis were not going well. There was a need for a new kind of "soldier" in the war against syphilis. In 1948, Lida J. Usilton and Dr. Johannes Stuart launched an experimental program using federal assignees as local VD interviewers and investigators. These assignees later came to be known as Public Health Advisors. For the experiment to get off the ground, personnel rules had to be stretched, government regulations and practices had to be worked around, and somebody had to do the dirty work. It all began with a poker-playing Madam and her Doctor who tried to solve a problem.

Syphilis was the problem. It had been seeded in the population with the return of American troops after World War I. By the close of World War II, local state and federal VD efforts were afoot. Although the private sector was engaged in the fight against VD, it would end up abdicating its role, and the federal government would become the primary driver and funder of efforts to eliminate syphilis and other sexually transmitted diseases in the U.S. This federal role, however, was not fully possible until the time of Roosevelt's New Deal.[1]

The Venereal Disease Division of the U.S. Public Health Service (PHS) served as the federal headquarters for VD control. The Army Appropriation Act of 1918 established the Division with two million dollars and a mandate to "work through state health departments to control the spread of social disease."[2] A portion of the funding included one million dollars for grants to states to establish VD prevention and treatment efforts.[3] The state grant portion of this federal appropriation was eliminated in 1926, a time when the "win the war against VD" mentality had faded and was replaced by government fiscal austerity and social temperance.[4] The forty-four states that had developed VD programs were on their own to finance them, as it would not be until 1935 that the VD Division could once again contribute grant resources to state and local VD control efforts, particularly syphilis. Many states did not replace the lost federal revenue for VD control because they lacked fiscal capacity and political will to fully underwrite VD efforts. The VD Division closely observed local attempts to address VD, and later would conclude that state and local governments were not appropriately and consistently responding to the threat of VD, particularly syphilis.[5]

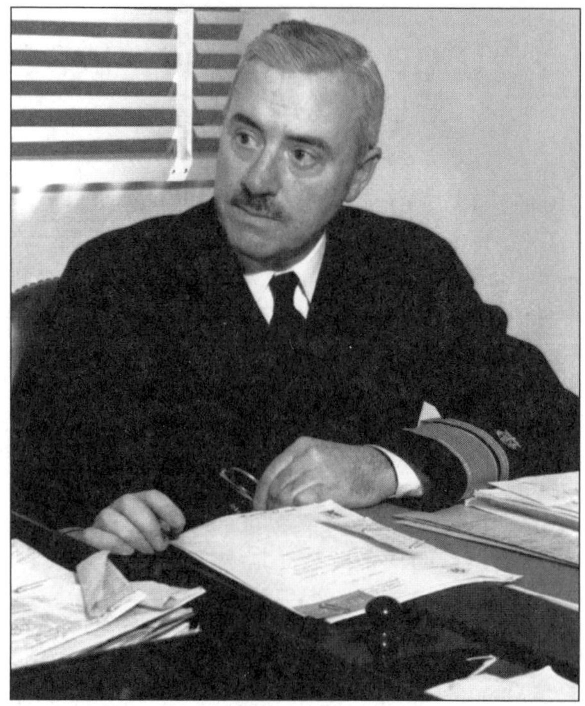

U.S. Surgeon General Thomas Parran during his tenure as Surgeon General, 1936-1948.
Courtesy of the Centers for Disease Control and Prevention, Public Health Image Library.

When Thomas Parran became Surgeon General in 1936, he brought with him experience as a director of the VD Division and a commissioner of the New York State Health Department. Infused by the zeal of the New Deal era, Parran renewed the federal government's work with and through states despite the lack of sufficient federal funding for VD control. VD was on the rise due to lack of attention, and Parran made sure that his vision of eradicating syphilis was communicated through the mass media. By the time *Reader's Digest* had published his July 1936 article entitled "Why Don't We Stamp Out Syphilis?" several syphilis epidemics had spread throughout the U.S.

In *Reader's Digest* and in his 1938 book *Shadow on the Land* Parran exhorted the public to shed moralistic views preventing syphilis control. He argued that syphilis should be a major public health concern for several reasons: it was contagious and spread by a series of person-to-person epidemics, it affected more Americans than car accidents, and it was cheaper to treat than tuberculosis.[7] U.S. health surveys in 1935 indicated that at any one time, 683,000 persons were under treatment and observation for syphilis. This same year saw 518,000 new infections, 100,000 of them among persons under twenty years of age.[8] It was estimated that one in ten persons would have syphilis in their lifetime. The disease was devastating if untreated, causing more than fifteen percent of all blindness, fifty percent of perinatal blindness, and eighteen percent of deaths from heart disease. In the late 1930s, 60,000 children were born each year with congenital syphilis.[9]

Thomas Parran is credited with leading the first national effort to eradicate syphilis. This effort resulted in increased national attention and increased federal appropriations, and it set the course for VD control efforts for the next two decades. Dick Bowman, a fiscal officer for the VD Division in the 1940s, recalls the increase in VD funds:

> The upward spiral in the appropriations for VD began really in '38, '39, with the Surgeon General's issuance of the book Shadow on the Land. Shadow on the Land had the very famous slogan, "syphilis strikes 1 in 10"... It means over the lifetime of ten people, one will acquire syphilis, at some moment in time... that was the beginning of the upward spiral of the VD funds.[10]

The Lafayette-Bulwinkle Act of 1938, otherwise known as the National Venereal Disease Control Act, essentially federalized VD control efforts, which since 1935 had been conducted by states, with the help of about ten percent of the Title VI appropriation of the Social Security Act.[11] This infusion of federal funding helped to renew the VD control efforts, which had been stopped in 1926. Parran's leadership changed the way VD was approached. Program and policy emphases no longer would be on sex education and the syphilis prophylaxis campaigns of the social hygiene era. Instead, the central efforts would become clinical and epidemiologic, including health surveys, treatment demonstrations, scientific research, and contact epidemiology.[12]

Another important shift occurred with the federal government's role in public health. The VD Division's work soon would involve not only grants to states, but also the assignment of personnel to the Public Health Service regional offices to advise states with their grant programs. These personnel were called "co-ops,"[13] as they were seen as the human resource associated with a financial "cooperative agreement" between the federal government and a state. The VD Division also began detailing health officials directly to local health departments to help them develop VD education and treatment programs. By 1939 PHS had deployed personnel to work in another venue: mobile rapid treatment programs for syphilis.[14] These PHA predecessors served as "mentor, partner, and counselor to the health departments of the nation,"[15] and the mentoring soon became the philosophical basis for the Public Health Advisor in 1948.

With the help of federal resources, states established diagnostic services, VD clinics, epidemiology programs, mass blood testing, research in VD diagnosis and treatment, and, eventually, rapid treatment centers.[16] Grants to states reinforced the shift to clinical and epidemiologic emphases, and the focus of VD control would remain primarily clinical and epidemiologic until the advent of public health social marketing and behavior change programming in the 1980s.[17] With grants to states came federal guidance and program support. Dick Bowman managed many of the state VD grants in the 1940s. He recalled that they would be flexible with some states because these states could not financially match the federal grant for VD programming:

> Before 1940 [grants to states were] done on a formula basis... that had elements of population, extent of the problem, the ratio of how much money the state appropriated to help that was allocated to the venereal disease. All those elements went into the formula... [T]he change came in the early 40's, going to a part formula and part program project grant... [VD Division staff] worked with the states to set up the projects. Most of the projects required matching funds, but as we said, "We'll let them pretty much match with the other side of the street" because they didn't have that much flexibility. They put in as much as they could:... the personnel, their facilities, all of that was used for matching if it became necessary... The first project grants were for [the purchase of] penicillin.[18]

With the help of the VD Control Act, the VD Division became a mammoth presence in the Public Health Service, and it was ensured that the Division would grow into one of the federal government's largest health arms. The VD Division was assigned to the Bureau of State Services within the Federal Security Agency during a reorganization of the Public Health Service in 1943.[19]

At that time it was comprised of research, laboratory, and statistics programs. Grants to states were handled out of the statistics branch. By 1948 the VD Division would have several staff assigned to the regional PHS offices to work with states.[20] According to Bill Watson, one of the original Public Health Advisors, the VD Program dwarfed all PHS programs:

> The VD program [was larger] than NIH, and very proud of the whole traditional program of the Public Health Service because what they had tried in World War II had worked... They had a budget bigger than NIH, and they had a budget far bigger than CDC. Of course, at that time CDC worked with malaria control.[21]

Grants to states were managed by a master's-trained biostatistician by the name of Lida Josephine Usilton. Lida was hired as a clerk with the War Department while working her way through college at Washington University. During her undergraduate studies, she was made chief of Analytical Medical Statistics in the Veterans' Bureau. In 1927, she joined the VD Division of the Public Health Service as principal statistician, and in that role she established a national VD reporting system that would guide the administration of the VD Division and articulate the need for continued federal support of VD control efforts.[22] By the time she directed the VD Division's granting effort to states, Lida Usilton had established herself with solid credentials in the PHS and had helped Thomas Parran write his seminal book *Shadow on the Land*.[23] She also became known as the "Madam." According to her nephew, former PHA Jack Pendleton, the reference to "Madam" was an analogy to the VD arena. A brothel's madam was in charge while taking care of her "girls." In Lida's case, the Madam was in charge and took care of her "boys."[24] Regional office VD staff and future Public Health Advisors were proud to count themselves among Lida's boys. Walter Hughes was one of them. He recalls Lida as a visionary and powerful leader:

> She was commanding and knew what she was talking about... She was really the sparkplug for the whole operation. If she called, that took precedence, I tell you. There was nothing more important to me than the assignments and what she wanted. She had such vision. You didn't hesitate.[25]

Lida Usilton was a leader, a highly skilled negotiator, and a pioneer in VD control. She set the course for VD surveillance, epidemiology, and case finding, and worked with others to initiate the national network of rapid treatment centers for syphilis.[26] That Lida directed the Operations Branch of the VD Division with such power is notable when one recognizes that she was a non-M.D. in the midst of a physician-dominated Public Health Service and VD Program,

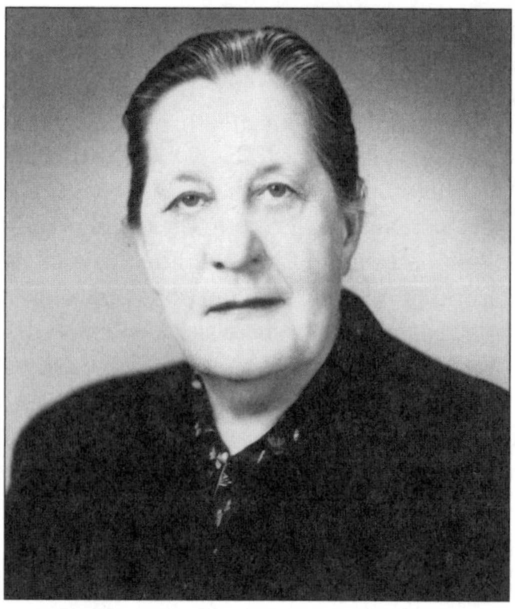

Lida J. Usilton, circa early 1950s.
Courtesy of John Pendleton.

and a woman in the midst of a male-dominated field and hierarchy. During this period, the VD Division served as a "boot camp" for future PHS leadership[27], and Lida Usilton was an important gatekeeper. It was known that "if you served in the VD Division with Lida Usilton, you could be Surgeon General some day."[28] Jack Pendleton recalls that Lida's role as a gatekeeper was not appreciated by everyone, particularly the male and medically-trained hierarchy:

> There was some resentment by the medical people, that here was this woman in there, and non-medical. I believe on paper there was an M.D. Chief of the Division, and Lida was the CEO.[29]

Many credited the national strides in VD to Lida, though she herself was not one to take credit. The New York Times called her a "pioneer, explorer, inventor, guide, teacher, and worker in the field of VD control."[30] In 1954, when she received the prestigious William Freeman Snow Medal from the American Social Hygiene Association, hundreds of letters from every conceivable location offered congratulations and accolades for her contributions to VD. In contrast, Lida's acceptance speech urged others to enter into government service, and claimed that the prestigious award was "more a tribute to my many co-workers in this field than to myself."[31]

Lida Usilton was a pioneer as a female leader in government in the 1940s. Often working as the only woman among men, she paved the way for others. Although colleagues and future field staff would express surprise at a female boss, they soon would be convinced of her able leadership. William "Luke" Hamlin, an original PHA, was a newly-minted co-op when he experienced his first female boss in Usilton:

> We were meeting with Dr. Johannes Stuart, and at some point of the day he said, "I want you to meet my boss, she's available now." Still being so naïve, I couldn't conceive of a female being boss back in 1948. We met her, and she was very imposing.[32]

Lida Usilton was liked by her colleagues and known for having many Washington connections, among them a friendship with Eleanor Roosevelt.[33] This ability to be connected in Washington was shared by her assistant, Dr. Johannes Stuart, and it resulted in increased VD appropriations and access to resources which were unheard of in the immediate postwar era. Dick Bowman recalled that Lida's way of working in Washington involved hiring political family members to keep VD on the agenda. In one case, she hired the son of Representative Frank Keefe, the Chairman of the Appropriations Committee for Public Health.[34]

Many early Public Health Advisors would speak of being "called before the Madam" for a job review when she visited a state for grant purposes.[35] PHAs were part of the human resources that the federal government gave to local and state health departments, and a review of the job was important. Disease trends might require a shift in resources, and the "audience with the Madam" was often the time when a Public Health Advisor would hear about a potential transfer. Ken Latimer and Joe Giordano were among the early PHAs. Ken recalls a meeting with Lida Usilton in 1951. He came "before her and her entourage, which was kind of like coming before the queen at that time."[36] Joe describes the "curious phenomenon":

> At the end of the year...you got a telephone call saying, "the Madam is coming." ... She interviewed all the boys, the co-ops, in the state who were graduating at the end of that first year. There might be ten or twelve of them, and that's about what there was. Here she would sit in her hotel room... and one by one you'd be paraded in front of her. The question she would ask is, "Well, how'd you like to go to Puerto Rico?" You'd been primed before her visit, and you were told that when she asked that question, [you should] say, "Ready to go!" Because if you say you're not, chances are you weren't going to graduate. So if you said you were, you didn't get to go [to Puerto Rico], but you were going to be transferred.[37]

The Washington staff and the regional office VD staff had a legendary esprit de corps. The Madam was a poker player, and while fun was had, business always

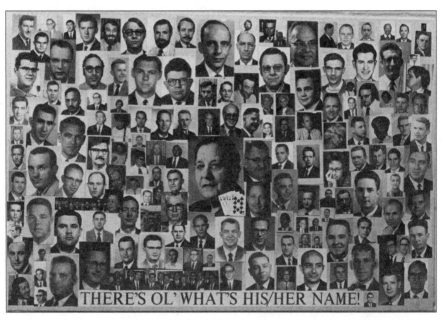

THERE'S OL' WHAT'S HIS/HER NAME!

Montage created circa 1960s of Public Health Advisors, some EIS Officers, Dr. David Sencer (top middle) and Lida J. Usilton (middle). The playing cards were part of Lida's notorious reputation among field staff as a poker player. Circa 1960s. Courtesy of David Sencer.

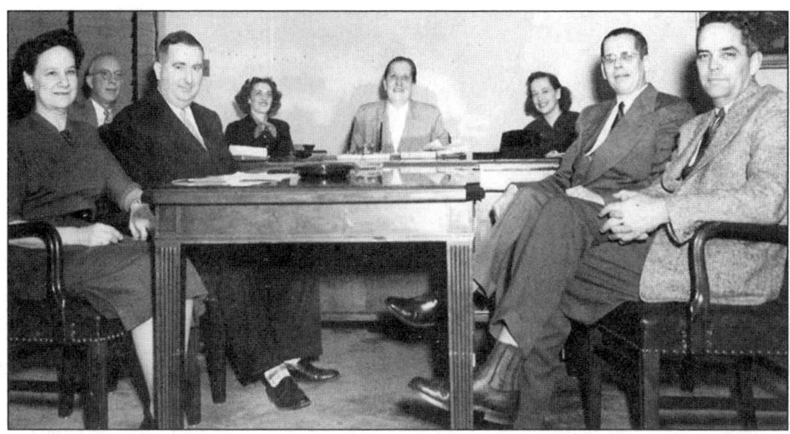

Lida Usilton and staff. Circa late 1940s. Left to Right: (unknown), Jim Donahue, Johannes Stuart (back left), Nita Rupkel, Lida Usilton, Margurite Gully, Dick Bowman, Don Reidesel.
Courtesy John Pendleton.

was done. Jack Pendleton recalls Lida holding her own in poker games with health officers, "people at the top level," and some VD Division staff. He recalled that the gender stereotypes would not quite fit for Lida. Although men were expected to mix business with pleasure, women were not, and certainly not with men:

> It did seem funny, the whole concept of a bunch of men sitting around with their collars open, and all the drinks on the table, sharing cards around, and this woman sitting over there, winning a few hands. You could see that she's talking to Dr. Jones here right now, and tomorrow morning she's going to be talking to Dr. Jones about his co-op budget.[38]

Lida's right-hand man in Washington was Dr. Johannes Stuart. He was Lida's assistant program officer and is credited as an architect of the Public Health Advisor program. This "tall Dutchman" from Grand Rapids, Michigan, sought out a job in government in the early 1940s following a Ph.D. in economics from the University of Chicago.[39] Dr. Stuart was commissioned as a captain in the army and worked for a period of time in Puerto Rico.[40] He met Lida Usilton after hearing about a job in the VD Division while working at the Department of Agriculture.[41] The two were quite a pair from the start. Bill Watson, who served as an assistant to Stuart ("Stu") in the early 1950s, recalls their meeting:

> Stu heard about a job in the VD program and came over and interviewed with Miss Lida J. Usilton... They got around to talking about compensation, and she made him an offer, and he said, "No, thank you," and started walking out. And she called somebody on her staff and said, "Go get him!" [They] brought him back, and she offered him what he asked for.[42]

Dr. Stuart functioned as an assistant to Lida, though, according to Bill Watson, titles were never Stuart's interest. He perceived himself to be an advisor to the VD program, and would become invaluable to it and later to the CDC as its first Washington Office staff member. Although Stuart did not leave behind much in terms of written archives or photos, he did leave a mark of personality and creativity on those with whom he worked. Johannes Stuart was known as a character, as one who liked to take risks, and as a man with a strong social conscience.[43] Bill Watson recalls Stuart's hiring of an internment camp survivor in order to "set things right":

> When I went to Washington Johannes had a young woman working for him... She and her family had been in one of the American/Japanese internment camps. It was right after the war, and hiring Japanese was not a thing that many people did. But he did. And in retrospect, I think he sized up the fact that we had done an injustice on the whole thing... And there he was, righting that wrong in his small way. That was so typical of him.[43]

Dr. Stuart believed that government service was an honorable calling. Bill Watson recalls that in the early 1950s, while working in Washington, Stuart was crushed to find that one of the VD field staff was convicted for taking bribes from a brothel:

> One of our guys assigned to Idaho had been caught and indicted for taking bribes from the bawdy houses. [Stuart] went out for that trial, and the man was found guilty and sentenced to prison. He came back to Washington and sat down behind his desk and looked at me and started to cry. He was anything but a softie, but he cared so much about government and about this program.[45]

Getting things done for the VD Division required imagination as well as perseverance, and the Madam and her Doctor exuded these qualities. When the VD Division was ramping up the Rapid Treatment Centers for syphilis, they needed cars to transport patients. This was a time during World War II when cars were not available, yet Lida believed that with a little persistence Stuart could get surplus cars. Such creativity and persistence would be passed on through history to become a central trait of PHAs. Dr. David Sencer recalls this story as told to him by Johannes Stuart:

> Miss Usilton said, "Stu, go to the Pentagon and get us cars because we've got to transport patients to the Rapid Treatment Centers." So Stu goes over to the Pentagon, and he starts here, and he gets moved here, and he gets moved there. Finally, late in the afternoon, he ends up with a Colonel who could do it. So he's sitting there talking to the Colonel, and the telephone rings. Colonel answers it. "It's for you." Stu picked it up. It was Lida, who said "Stu, it's likely to be muddy. Make sure you get chains." So Stu said to the Colonel, "And we need chains."[46]

Like Lida, Dr. Stuart was an advocate for the VD Division. He was known as a very imaginative person with a will to "push the envelope to get around regulations" so that the public health task was accomplished.[47] Some of this was commitment to the vision of VD control, and part of it was Stuart's cunning. According to Dave Sencer, Johannes "loved to connive."[48] Over the years, he became the "go-to" guy in Washington, able to get anything done by calling the right people. According to Dick Bowman, Stuart was a "master" at handling Congressional mail and complaints. "He could write ten pages of beautiful language that ended up saying absolutely nothing."[49] Stuart often parlayed his Ph.D. to his advantage, having his secretary page him in various meetings and places just so that people would wonder how it was known that a "Doctor Stuart" was there.[50]

Johannes Stuart would have a long career in the Public Health Service, and he would be remembered principally as an architect of the Public Health Advisors. While Lida had her boys, Stuart was the father of PHAs. Together, the Madam and her Doctor led a staff that was committed to making things in VD control happen at state and local levels. These men and women who initially worked out of the PHS regional offices were "New Dealers": professionals hired under President Roosevelt's New Deal.[51] As such, they had a zeal for public service. Many joined the Public Health Service as VD staff during World War II,[52] and some were part of the commissioned corps.[53] Unlike the Public Health Advisors who followed them, the regional office VD staff in the 1940s was made up of relatively high-ranking people, and they did not have field experience—that is, experience conducting contact epidemiology or working directly with VD patients.[54] The first of the VD staff in the regional offices were all men with the exception of one woman, Mary Rheubotham, who was called "Mother Mary."[55] They included Larry Brennan in the KC Regional Office,[56] Tom Davis in New Orleans,[57] Mary Rheubotham in the Dallas regional office,[58] Bob Shannon in Chicago,[59] Art Callan in San Francisco, and Henry Getz in New York. These VD regional staff served as liaisons for the state VD programs to help oversee the funding for the Rapid Treatment Centers, grants, and the assignment of personnel to states. They were hard-working professionals who believed in government service. Bill Watson remembers several of these men and women:

> I had enough experience working with them to get a good indoctrination about government. They really were believers, and their heroes were all the people who had started the NYA, the National Youth Administration. They believed in government, they really did… I remember lectures I got: "Now you will be managing Federal funds, and you are entitled to your paycheck and reimbursement for official travel that is approved and that's all. And never use your public office for private gain." They really believed that and they operated that way.[60]

The work of the VD Division in the 1940s involved funding a few education campaigns, identifying effective diagnostic and treatment tools for syphilis and gonorrhea, and funding the treatment of syphilis.[61] The primary focus was strengthening the public health and medical response to VD. This was a significant job due to the nature of syphilis treatment prior to the advent of penicillin, and because of the shift in public attitudes about VD after penicillin use became standard for syphilis treatment.

Prior to 1941 and before the time of penicillin, the treatment for syphilis consisted of arsenotherapy: an injected compound of bismuth and arsenic administered over a twelve-to-eighteen-month period.[62] Only ten percent of patients completed treatment because of the long, arduous regimen and the drug reactions, which included death from arsenic.[63] Public health and medical communities did not do much to improve treatment completion rates. As the 1940s progressed, syphilis treatment lacked wide support because the sway of moral arguments in the United States characterized it as reinforcement for immoral behavior.[64] This was a significant shift from the view of syphilis treatment for American service personnel, which held that chemoprophylaxis kept our troops "fit to fight."[65] Increasingly, state boards of health viewed treatment as "not practical" or as leading to promiscuity due to its availability, and this viewpoint prevented the development of strong VD control programs at the local level. Many private physicians shared this emerging public view of VD, refusing to

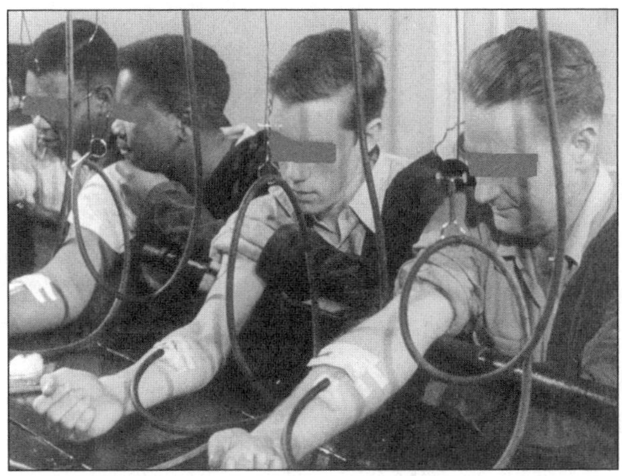

Intravenous rapid treatment for syphilis. Circa 1940s.
Courtesy of Ken Latimer.

treat their patients with syphilis or hiding the diagnosis as a paternalistic act to cover a husband's indiscretion.[66] Even after the advent of a five-day intravenous treatment for syphilis in 1941,[67] private physicians were loath to administer it.

In 1943 the federal government established Rapid Treatment Centers, or "RTCs," throughout the country to provide inpatient, hospital-based treatment for syphilis in a six-to-eight-week period to accommodate post-treatment observation, vocational rehabilitation, and a variety of adjunct health services. Most RTCs were state-operated with funding from the federal government,[68] and helped to reduce syphilis by assuring treatment completion under the supervision of highly specialized syphilologists. The centers also demonstrated the effectiveness of treatment to a skeptical medical community.[69] Lida Usilton and her VD Division colleagues joined forces with the Federal Works Agency and state health departments to establish a national network of RTCs, to help staff them with local and federal medical personnel, and to support them with "Lida's Boys." Eventually there would be more than sixty RTCs located in "Civilian Service Corps camps, remodeled small hotels, sanatoriums, hospital buildings, and special wards in hospitals."[70] Mass blood testing would identify people in need of treatment, and these people would be sent by bus to the nearest RTC. Initially local health department personnel or VD regional office staff assisted the effort. When Public Health Advisors came on the scene in 1948, one of their earliest activities was mass blood testing, follow-up, and RTC support. Harold Mauldin, an early PHA, recalls his experience leading a mass blood testing initiative in Baton Rouge, Louisiana in 1948:

> I headed up a team of mass blood testing. I organized testing, followed up on those found to be positive, and referred them to Rapid Treatment Centers. We had two Rapid Treatment Centers in Louisiana at that time, one at Charity Hospital in New Orleans as well as one for the middle part of the state... I set up and chartered the first Greyhound busload and sent them down to the Rapid Treatment Center in New Orleans... When we did the blood testing, and got the results back from the laboratory, I'd go to their homes and bring them in. I brought them over to the courthouse, where I loaded up the bus... You had Medical Directors assigned by the Public Health Service... Dr. Holman Wherit was the Medical Director at that time down there.... Of course, I had called Wherit before sending them down and asked him if he could take a busload, and he said yeah, but he thought I was talking about one of these little ten, twelve... It got down there with forty-seven [people] or whatever the crap it was. I filled the dang bus slap up out of east Louisiana Parish. They had no health department up there, so I filled that daggone bus up, and they got down there and he went crazy. He had to put them in the halls... He didn't have room.[71]

Ideally, Rapid Treatment Centers provided efficient and safe treatment for syphilis while being a "home away from home" to the visiting patients. Often treatment centers offered services related to other venereal diseases and conditions, mental health services, screening for conditions such as TB, and even child care.[72] Contact epidemiology, or identification of a patient's sexual partners, was conducted at the centers to help halt the spread of syphilis. Joe Giordano, a PHA in the early 1950s, recalls how PHAs worked in the Rapid Treatment Centers:

> [T]he patients were interviewed at the Rapid Treatment Center, contacts were elicited, and often within a matter of days, that contact might appear at the same Rapid Treatment Center for treatment. The population of the Rapid Treatment Centers came from

> a variety of places. It came through routine blood testing; it came through contact tracing… I think a big one was from the testing that was taking place relative to the military. If a person went for an induction examination and was found to have a positive blood test, now that was another source.[73]

Jacksonville, Florida's, RTC was a contrast to other Rapid Treatment Centers. It was a result of Johannes Stuart's ingenuity in response to a problem emerging in Ocala in 1946. That year, a fire closed a hospital-based RTC in Ocala, leaving hundreds of patients in need of care. Johannes Stuart solved what would have been a great problem, as no other locations existed for immediate use. He arranged for the former naval ship *Ernest Hinds* to provide the service. The *Hinds* opened on Jacksonville's Northbank on July 1, 1946, and quickly was crowded with patients from all over Florida. More than twelve thousand people were served in the seven months that it operated.[74] The *Hinds* never would have served in this capacity were it not for Johannes Stuart and his ability to find a workable solution and to handle potential obstacles. Bill Watson recalls the story:

> They needed a Rapid Treatment Center in Jacksonville, Florida, and there was no building available, so Stu came up with the idea, "Well, let's get a hospital ship from the Navy and bring it to Jacksonville"… There are all kinds of stories about that ship being loaded close to a bridge where people could ride over and see, and somehow it was scandalizing. Stu had it towed from the West Coast through the Panama Canal and out to Jacksonville… They couldn't charge another government agency for the ship itself, but they sent us a bill for towing. Of course, we didn't have any money then. So Stu somehow maneuvered around that. He was a genius at getting around that kind of thing. We never had to pay that towage fee, either. [75]

Among the early tools to fight syphilis, contact epidemiology was the weakest and would become the initial opportunity for the PHA contribution to public health in the late 1940s. As with any communicable disease, syphilis control depends on finding individuals who have been infected so that they can receive treatment. In public health this is called "case finding." There are three primary methods of case finding: contact investigation, education of populations to encourage voluntary testing, and (in the 1940s and 1950s) "mass" blood testing or "screening" for syphilis.[76] Contact epidemiology, also called contact investigation or contact tracing, involves identifying and locating all persons who are contacts of a patient to ensure that they are examined and, if infected, treated. Dr. Samuel Grubbs was one of the earliest to use contact tracing to control VD. In 1917, with the help of local businesses and a grant from the Red Cross, Dr. Grubbs established a system of testing, contact tracing, and isolation (of prostitutes primarily) in Newport, Virginia, military installations.[77] Despite contact tracing's successful application to control VD and other major communicable diseases, such as tuberculosis, diphtheria, polio, and typhoid, it was not used uniformly in VD control until the late 1940s.[78] This was due in part to the "moralizing" of syphilis since the social hygiene days, the lack of resources to conduct it, the lack of standardized approaches, and physician resistance.[79] Private physicians generally eschewed contact epidemiology because it was seen as adjunct to medical treatment, and because it was perceived to intrude on the physician-patient relationship.[80] This was a particular challenge in the fight against syphilis because physicians would choose not to report new cases of syphilis so as to avoid performing or cooperating with patient interviewing.[81] Although some attempts were made to educate medical professionals through postgraduate education in syphilis epidemiology at places such as Vanderbilt University, these programs were neither widespread nor well-attended by the majority of physicians.[82] Further, the hegemony of physicians in public health meant that views about field epidemiology would influence the way local public health resources were focused and used. These difficulties were noted as early as 1938 and persisted until the late 1940s, when the VD program shifted to ensure a more effective and standardized effort with contact epidemiology.[83]

Contact epidemiology's task was not simple. Social custom and individual embarrassment often prevented the identification of sexual partners. If sexual partners were not identified early, they could not be assessed for their own infection or be offered treatment, and they could infect others.[84] Special skill was and is required to work with people newly diagnosed with syphilis, to help them understand their diagnosis, and to identify others who may have infected them or who were infected by them. The job does not end once sexual contacts are identified, because the VD investigator needs to find these persons in order to offer them a test for syphilis and help them access treatment if infected. The task is further complicated by the quality of information received from the initial patient. Locating information for sexual contacts may be scant at best due to shame, forgetfulness, or just lack of information about a sex partner. Examples of such information might be "the girl who frequents the red door bar downtown," or "a guy who said he was a brush salesman from Topeka." An infected patient might have been sufficiently inebriated that all he could recall is that his partner "had a five-year-old boy with a broken leg in the local hospital."[85] Stopping the spread of syphilis requires the cycle of treatment, contact identification and location, interviewing of sexual contacts, and bringing them to treatment if infected. The process is repeated for every new case of syphilis.

In the 1940s, the basis for contact investigation was found in local laws enacted around the time of World War I. Where these laws were present, they required physicians to report VD cases to local health departments, and required local health authorities to identify the existence of VD cases in their jurisdictions.[86] In the late 1930s strategies for identifying sexual partners ranged from "involuntary" approaches using state law as a hammer to force the patient to identify partners, "tactful persuasion" involving trust-building with the patient, and a call to the "greater good" for epidemic control, to having no approach at all—that is, nothing was done to identify possible contacts for the purpose of stopping the chain of infection.[87] Without the help of private medicine, the job of contact epidemiology fell to public health departments, though not many were engaged in the effort in the early 1940s. The few that were—New Jersey,[88] Chicago,[89] New York City,[90] and Memphis/Shelby County, Tennessee—also evaluated ways to improve performance the task.[91] Much of the discussion at the time involved the type of workers necessary for the job of contact epidemiology, the scope of work, and the task's importance. It is clear from the literature of the time that public health and private medicine had yet to be convinced of contact epidemiology's importance. Historically, medical personnel associated with public health clinics or (infrequently) physicians' offices engaged VD patients to identify their sexual contacts. As early as 1922, the New Jersey Department of Health used nurses who were also called "medical case workers."[92] These workers primarily interviewed VD patients to persuade them to disclose their sexual contacts. This was essentially where the effort stopped, as the literature from the 1920s to early 1940s discussed ways of engaging patients to assist sexual partner disclosure and is silent about locating these contacts. By the mid 1940s, contact epidemiology was conducted by many health departments with nurses and non-medical follow-up workers who received the names of sexual contacts from physicians and clinics and located them for examination and for treatment if infected.[93] With the shortage of nurses in 1943, the State of Tennessee began to employ non-medical staff called "VD investigators." There were two classifications: a junior investigator required an equivalent of a high school education, and a senior investigator required an education equivalent to a college degree.[94] Other health departments used a social worker to conduct patient interviewing and contact epidemiology. In contrast to social workers today, these professionals did not possess a particular degree or training but would ideally possessed a medical understanding of syphilis, a broad education, and an appreciation for socio-cultural differences. These new investigators were assigned to Rapid Treatment Centers for one or two weeks for an orientation and then to a county with a strong VD investigator for intensive training. This training would be followed by assignment to a county health department with supervisor oversight.[95] These worker requirements and training regimen became part of the required preparation for future Public Health Advisors. In 1938, characteristics for social workers (primarily female) included:

> (A) broad and general education, a psychological understanding of people... a knowledge of varying standards of living and the characteristics of racial groups. A flexibility of thought and open-mindedness, with enthusiasm for her work and a constant desire to learn are essential. She should have been adequately grounded in a basic knowledge of the etiology and medical treatment of syphilis and gonorrhea as well as an understanding of their relationship to other diseases... The social worker should be able to work successfully with various professional groups—medical and social, public and private."[96]

Even as some local health departments were engaged variously in VD patient interviewing and contact epidemiology, the outcomes were not stellar, because new syphilis cases were not identified soon enough—if at all. In 1947 the Arkansas State Board of Health and the U.S. Public Health Service conducted an experiment in three Arkansas counties to evaluate simple improvements to the approach of contact investigation. The study, known as the "100-Day Experiment,"[97] demonstrated an eightfold increase in productivity (for example, in identification of new syphilis cases from contact tracing) following changes in procedure and patient prioritization. The study emphasized changes in procedure and in focus of investigation because at the time no local resources were available to increase personnel. The study found that increased emphasis on interviewing, cooperation, and coordination of case interviewing and investigation, good supervision, training, and prompt location of contacts would markedly improve outcomes related to case finding and treatment. Success here and with syphilis for decades hence was measured by the productivity in case finding and treatment from every new case of primary and secondary syphilis. The study's subtext, however, was that the elements of good training and supervision, proper prioritization of new syphilis cases, and high-quality patient interviewing were not happening throughout the United States. Although the authors of the 100-Day experiment suggested that the issue was one of procedural change and focus, it appeared that the real problem lay with the quality of the local workers and their training. Perhaps the issues were related, because at the time, public health focused on all stages of syphilis and not on early syphilis. Bill Watson recalls what so many early PHAs observed:

> Most of the contact epidemiology was being done by state people, and they weren't very good at it either. I found that out when I got to be state rep in South Carolina... They were not college graduates. They were political flunkees. When I went to South Carolina and I'd make my rounds to the county health departments, I'd find these political appointees with just a big stack of investigations just sitting there not done! But they knew the local senator or representative, and usually came from a family who had connected them. They considered the job—well, they don't really have to work. This was a political appointment.[98]

Local health handling of syphilis was so poor that there was no way of knowing whether people were notified if they were potentially infected with syphilis. Patient records with identified sexual contacts were forwarded to health departments by clinics and doctors; however, local public health VD investigators did not generally follow up on them. It was not uncommon for these referrals to be found filed in a desk drawer, never seeing the light of day.[99] The problem did not rest only with local investigators. Some clinics and physicians made no effort with newly-diagnosed patients to identify their contacts or report their diagnoses to local health authorities. VD control efforts were so inconsistent across the U.S. that it was not clear that anything except testing and treatment was being done efficiently. Without consistent disease reporting and timely contact epidemiology, the effort to control syphilis would be akin to using a spoon to empty an ocean. Lida Usilton told her staff that mass blood testing efforts and skilled contact epidemiology would be necessary to eradicate VD, and that the federal government needed to step in and show how contact epidemiology should be done.[100]

Quality and preparedness of local health department staff were not the only issues standing in the way of syphilis control. Many local health departments could not handle any additional concerted effort in syphilis. In 1943, five years prior to the publication of the 100-Day Experiment, Lida Usilton obtained the list of people rejected from the military on the basis of a syphilis infection. She reasoned that the VD Division and local health departments needed to follow up on these recruits' sexual contacts in order to stop syphilis in the civilian population. At the time, the military was doing nothing but treating their infections.[101] The size of the follow-up effort was massive due to the backlog of cases that were never followed up from selective services testing.[102] Dick Bowman recalled the impact of the agreement between the VD Division and the Selective Service:

> In the early days they would reject all the positives [from the service]. So the positives were pulled and referred to the states... So what was the problem? Well, the problem was [that] there was not the manpower to follow up on that quantity of positive blood tests... The question was: how do we get the manpower to do it? The immediate problem was that the states and the Division had personnel ceilings. They didn't have room to hire people, and neither did most of the states.[103]

The Selective Service records follow-up put intense pressure on local health departments. In New York City alone, it was estimated that during wartime the local health department received approximately twenty-five thousand positive test results annually from civilian and armed forces for follow-up. Local public health agencies just didn't have the human resource capacity to conduct public health follow-up for this effort or for the contact epidemiology effort in VD generally.[104] Local and state health departments increasingly looked to the federal government's VD Division for guidance and resources to fight syphilis.

By the mid-1940s several things were clear. The federal government was emerging as a leader in VD control. They were placing human resource capacity in the PHS regional offices and in the Rapid Treatment Centers, and they were funding local and state VD control efforts. Despite the added federal resources, local public health infrastructure was neither qualified for nor capable of the contact epidemiologic task. With such poor and inconsistent contact epidemiology efforts, syphilis would continue unabated throughout the U.S. To break the chain of syphilis, a more standardized approach with qualified field epidemiologists would be needed. The Madam and her Doctor would have an answer to this problem: the Public Health Advisor.

Chapter 3

The Original Experiment

The war was over, and the VD program had a need for people. It had been a very active program during World War II, and at that time was the largest program in the Public Health Service. But after the war, the manpower situation changed... They had a problem. The civil service registers from which they would recruit were all filled up with former corpsmen from the military, and [Johannes Stuart] didn't think that, based on his experience, this was the kind of person that he was looking for to do VD work. Over some opposition he sold the idea that he ought to start recruiting young college graduates.... There were people in the Public Health Service who didn't think that was feasible... In those days, they weren't convinced at all that you could recruit people to do this kind of dirty work from the college graduate pool.[1]

William "Bill" Watson
Public Health Advisor (ret.)

Johannes Stuart and Lida Usilton reasoned that in order to get the fight against syphilis back on track, there needed to be an infusion of federal personnel at the patient level, conducting syphilis screening and contact epidemiology; however, it was not clear who among the federal workforce would agree to do this type of work. The "New Dealers" working for the VD program in the PHS regional offices functioned at senior management levels, and therefore would not be good choices. The Madam and her Doctor would have to find someone else to do the job.

Assigning federal personnel to deliver services in state and local health departments had not previously been done, but by the 1940s, the federal government had positioned itself to do so. Twenty years previously, federal interest was limited to the interstate spread of disease to supplement state activities within their boundaries.[2] By the 1940s it was clear that restricting federal attention to interstate VD transmission would not be sufficient, as state and local VD control efforts were variable at best.[3] Communities needed and wanted the federal government's help. This help eventually would come from a new type of public health worker who embodied the sentiments of Dr. Joseph Mountin, PHS Director of the Bureau of State Services under Surgeon General Thomas Parran. According to Mountin, the Public Health Service could offer a worker who would "perform many of the routine operations" in addition to the customary activities of consultation and mentoring.[4] The new initiative gave the states human resources focused exclusively on syphilis screening and contact epidemiology, since these were the weakest elements in the fight against syphilis. Jack Pendleton recalls the rationale to provide states with federal personnel ("co-ops") to perform routine VD control activities:

> Not all states had the money to control syphilis. Co-ops would give them a step in the right direction. We also helped the VD Division prove that contact epidemiology was an acceptable, successful effort. We were demonstrating a concept that we wanted to spread nationally.[5]

In 1948 a unique public health professional, personifying an amplified federal VD control effort, was born. A handful of Public Health Advisors were hired as an experiment in July of that year. Others were added to their ranks within weeks, and by the late 1950s an effort would be afoot to provide every state with a PHA. The term "PHA" would emerge in the early 1950s, once the workers were established as part of a federal series. In 1948, co-ops were known primarily as epidemiologists or VD investigators because they began their work at the entry level of public health: interviewing VD patients, following up on their sexual contacts, and conducting blood testing.[6] Entry into public health through the portal of VD fieldwork would become a central aspect of PHA culture.

Hiring a federal worker to do VD field work was not a simple task. New Dealers and veterans were on the federal register awaiting jobs. According to Bill Watson, "after the war, registers for government jobs were jammed up with veterans who had special privileges, and it wasn't working out very well for the VD program."[7] Finding the "right" federal workers to do this kind of job in VD was a challenge. Johannes Stuart believed the VD Division should hire college graduates to conduct VD interviews and contact epidemiology. In those days, however, college graduates were uncommon, and Stuart would have to convince Lida Usilton that a cohort of college-trained professionals could and would successfully do the job that locals and the people crowding the federal registries could not do well.[8] Although the federal civil service rolls were loaded with people wanting federal jobs, not many of them would be interested in this type of work, if they truly understood the job. Getting around the civil service registry by hiring college graduates would control the quality of contact epidemiology and avoid a high dropout rate and subsequent program cost. This point was not lost on Stuart the economist.

The Madam gave the nod to the plan, and Johannes Stuart spearheaded an effort to bring on new federal VD investigators. Stuart's plan to hire college graduates would help circumvent the federal register.[9] According to Bill Watson, Stuart "never objected to any of the [personnel] rules of the bureaucracy, but saw [them] as a challenge, and found a way to get around them and stay legal."[10] Actually, Stuart did not really circumvent rules, but used the system of excepted service appointments which was just becoming an established practice of the federal government. With the excepted service, a federal agency could appoint personnel without using the customary recruiting and competitive procedures.[11] There was perhaps a second purpose for the college degree requirement: it reflected emerging thinking among experts about the qualifications for VD investigating.[12] Such opinion was relatively recent and not widespread, so it appeared novel when Stuart sought to require a baccalaureate. Would anyone with a college degree do this kind of work? Don Lederman was interested. He was the first to receive an offer by Stuart for this unusual job:

> I was the first co-op hired by Johannes Stuart. Stuart contacted Syracuse University in New York, and I heard about the position from my political science professor. I was still in college when I was brought to Washington to interview for the position.[13]

Although Stuart wanted to hire young college graduates for the task of contact epidemiology, he was careful not to hire "would-be doctors" because they would not remain in the program.[14] Successful candidates possessed a liberal arts degree and had a certain personality that contributed to their success with patients, health departments, and physicians. A liberal arts background served the PHAs well, as they became public health generalists, able to adapt to changing public health situations and needs.

Co-ops were recruited for the experiment from universities in South Carolina, Maryland, and New York.[15] According to Bill Watson, Stuart ran the recruitment program "right out of his hip pocket. He did a lot of the interviewing himself. You didn't get in and you didn't get promoted without Stu's stamp of approval."[16] This project was Stuart's baby. Lida Usilton often would say, "You brought a cradle in here, Stu,"[17] because the new recruits were seen as young pups among the VD program's old dogs.

The first people hired for the experiment were Stathan "S.A." Boudreaux, Marvin "Paul" Connor, Cy Erlich, Lamont Gill, Luke Hamlin, Don Lederman, and Bill Watson.[18] These men answered interview notices that were posted with alumni and job placement offices at their colleges and universities. Bill Watson was a recent graduate of the University of South Carolina when he almost missed his chance to be interviewed by Johannes Stuart. He got a notice from the alumni office that someone from the Public Health Service would be in Columbia interviewing interested candidates for jobs. Bill was not in the market for a job because he was expecting to attend law school in the fall. He went for the interview, though, because it was "an excuse for me to go to Columbia to see my girlfriend." Bill recalls:

> Stuart almost missed me. He had interviewed several people and was in the process of leaving and in fact he was walking out the door; and I said... "You haven't talked to me yet." He said "Oh, you're here to talk to me." And I said yes, and so we had this long conversation.... He didn't tell me much about the job at all. If he had I would have probably said no, but he was such a fascinating guy that I was taken with him. He asked me all kinds of questions but nothing that had to do with VD or public health or anything. We talked about cabbages and kings and everything else.[19]

Bill returned home and was working on his family farm when he received the job offer. "I was called off the tractor to take a long-distance call from Washington, which was unheard of in those days. It was Stu, and he wanted to know if I was interested in a job."[20] Johannes Stuart would so impress Bill that he would abandon his plan of law school for a job as a VD investigator in Maryland. Bill would take the night train to Washington to report just after the July 4th holiday. On that train he would meet Luke Hamlin, another recruit from South Carolina. Luke recalls being fairly naïve when he was hired out of college. As a very young student majoring in Spanish language, he thought that after graduation he "would be appointed Ambassador to Spain." When this opportunity was not forthcoming, Luke set his sights elsewhere, though he certainly did not anticipate a job in VD:

> I saw on the college bulletin board that Dr. Johannes Stuart was going to be in Columbia... I had to go home and see what VD was by looking in the dictionary. I went to interview on a Thursday, and he called me on the following Monday asking if I wanted to work in Maryland as a VD investigator. I was flabbergasted to be offered a job, but I didn't know where Maryland was... It didn't take me too long to think about that.[21]

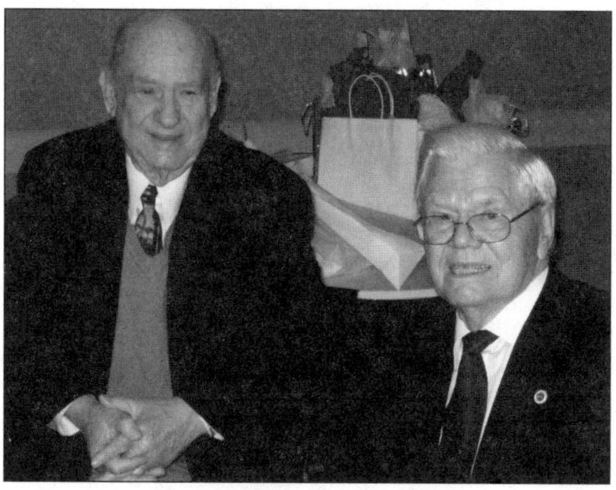

William "Luke" Hamlin and William "Bill" Watson. Two of the original PHAs at a dinner of the Watsonian Society in September 2007.
Courtesy of Fred Martich.

That Luke and Bill would ride the same train to Washington was not the only coincidence among the initial co-ops. Stathan "S.A." Boudreaux and Bill Watson knew one another previously. Both were World War II veterans who had served in the same personnel unit at Fort Benning, Georgia, and both had been prisoners of war in Germany at the same time.[22]

The new hires started the job after the July 4th holiday in 1948. They first were sent to Gallinger Hospital in Washington for orientation, and then met the boss, Lida Usilton. Many were housed in a local Washington boarding house in DuPont Circle. S.A. Boudreaux was joined by his wife and their small child.[23]

Hamlin noted that the co-ops could not go through DuPont Circle to get to work because the city was building a subway at the time. Boudreaux was the only co-op with his own car, so he would take the group to work.[24]

None of the original co-ops had any background in VD control. They had to learn all about VD so that they could be conversant with patients, the public, and physicians. They had to learn how to interview patients so that they could identify others at risk for syphilis, and they eventually had to learn how to conduct mass blood testing campaigns. Their initial training consisted of ten days of thorough introduction to contact epidemiology.

Interview training was conducted by Bob Swank, one of the authors of the 100-Day Experiment and an "ace interviewer" who would go on to make many lasting contributions to interview training efforts for the VD Division.[25] Swank joined the VD Division in 1941 after working for the VD Epidemiology Unit of the District of Columbia Health Department, and after several years in the mental health field in Massachusetts, New York, and Connecticut.[26] He directed the VD training school located at the Alto Rapid Treatment Center in Alto, Georgia, from 1950 to 1951, and then served on the VD staff for the Georgia Department of Public Health as a federal assignee. Bob Swank became synonymous with VD

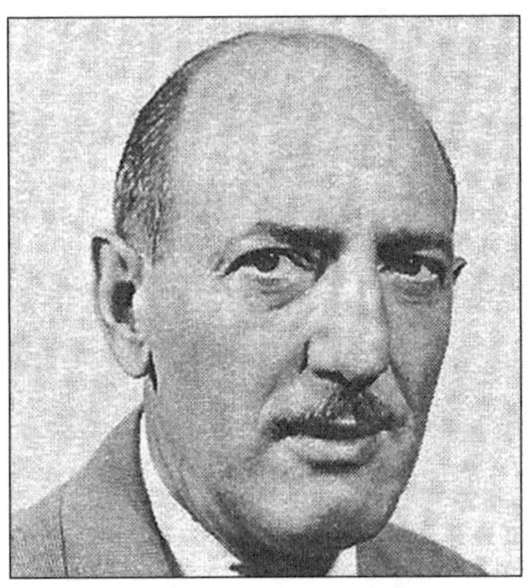

Robert Swank. Photo from CDC Contact newsletter, June 1, 1962.

interview training. During his tenure with the VD Division, he continually enhanced the interview process and methods through collaboration with Masters and Johnson of the Institute for Sex Research (see Chapter 6).[27]

The new co-ops visited VD clinics in Bethesda and Washington, DC, in preparation for their assignments in a VD clinic. They received lectures from renowned syphilologists about the clinical aspects of syphilis so that they would be able to educate patients and work with physicians who were less than knowledgeable about the disease. Unlike those who followed them, these original co-ops were not initially trained in phlebotomy, the drawing of blood through venipuncture. This soon would change, because the co-ops were called upon to draw blood in the field and conduct mass blood testing in the community.[28]

Following the training period, the co-ops were sent out to the field to be VD investigators. Determining where they would start their work was an important decision. Although state and local health departments might welcome improved VD control efforts, the "trial" placement of co-ops could not happen just anywhere. Varied opinions about federal presence and involvement in local public health efforts meant that there was not a consensus about the placement of federal workers to take on operational activities in states or local areas at the time. In addition, Usilton and Stuart did not know whether locals would accept this type of worker.[29] The location for acclimating the co-ops would need to be carefully selected and have full local support. The Eastern Shore of Maryland was chosen because the VD Division had ties there. Bill Watson recalled that a retired physician and former Assistant Surgeon General of the Public Health Service was located in the Eastern Shore region.[30] Bill was assigned to Pocomoke City. Luke Hamlin was assigned to Salisbury. Don Lederman was assigned to Centerville. Bill's assignment was close to the family of co-op Paul Connor, and the two often returned to Connor's family home in Baltimore to spend the weekend. Bill spent his first assignment enjoying Ocean City as a "young unmarried guy."[31] Meanwhile, Luke Hamlin focused on making ends meet on the meager income of a co-op in Salisbury, Maryland. He found a room for four dollars a week and would scour the local tomato groves for leftover green tomatoes. "The groves had contracts with canning factories. After they picked the tomatoes, we'd go get the rest."[32]

As they went off to their assignments, the co-ops were given automobiles to help them get around in the field. In 1948 cars were hard to come by, but the Madam and her Doctor made sure the co-ops had just what they needed.[33] Getting a car was a big deal, especially for Cy Erlich and the young Luke Hamlin. Cy never had driven a car and would need to be taught to drive before the group could start their work on the Eastern Shore. Luke was nineteen, and having a 1947 Ford complete with the Federal Security Administration seal made him feel like the "King of Russia."[34]

The co-ops were assigned to VD clinics in their respective locations, where they conducted interviews with newly-diagnosed clinic patients and then tried to locate their sexual contacts and bring them in for testing and syphilis treatment. Bill Watson recalled working with a local health department physician who was quite knowledgeable in diseases, but did not trust that penicillin was effective against syphilis. Such an attitude was shared among a remnant of the VD field at the time.[35] This particular physician insisted on keeping three patients on the outdated treatment of arsenic and bismuth. When the physician asked Bill to conduct the spinal taps for his patients, he politely refused.[36]

The co-op experiment was well-designed from the start. Stuart assigned a supervisor to work with the newly-minted co-ops, and a local statistician to measure their success.[37] Success in contact epidemiology was measured by several indices, among them a contact index (how many sexual contacts are identified per new syphilis patient), epidemiologic index (the ratio of the number of infected persons identified through contact investigation to the number of patients diagnosed), and brought-to-treatment index (how many of the newly-diagnosed were brought to treatment from the field).[38] Measuring contact epidemiology's effectiveness was standard practice for the VD Division, and it was an important element of the experiment because the new VD investigators would focus on finding new cases of syphilis. This experiment was serious business. One of the co-ops was found cheating on his indices by writing up cases on people who were in the local cemetery. He was summarily fired, and the remaining co-ops got the message "real quick."[39] Bill Watson recalls that at the time the co-ops did not realize they were "that much of a guinea pig" in such an important experiment.[40]

The Doctor's hunch was correct, and the co-op experiment was a success. College graduates would in fact be attracted to this work; they would excel at it and therefore contribute to the fight against syphilis. In 1951 Stuart wrote that reductions in syphilis resulted from contact investigation because, like sonar, it "finds the submerged, hidden cases that lie ready to extend infection or to develop late disability and death." He extended the metaphor to argue for contact epidemiology's cost benefit and stated that although contact investigation was an expensive tool requiring competent personnel, it was one of the most effective tools to control syphilis.[41]

Within four months of their hire, the new co-ops found themselves transferred to other Maryland communities and eventually to other locations throughout the U.S.[42] The repeated transfers from one place to another would become the hallmark of the PHA experience. Accepting an appointment as a co-op meant that you understood you would be moved quickly and often, because like any public health resource, co-ops were to go where the need was greatest. Bill Watson was moved to Annapolis to lead statewide efforts in VD. Luke Hamlin remembers being transferred to La Plata, Maryland, after serving four months in Salisbury. After six months in La Plata, Luke and his new wife were transferred to Louisiana, and then to Wichita, Kansas:

> In June of the first year we got transferred to the Dallas region. Bill [Watson] got transferred to Arkansas and we got transferred to Louisiana... So we went to New Orleans and then got transferred to Monroe, and we were there just four months, [then] transferred to Shreveport... and then to Baton Rouge for about a year. I was only there four months until the next place. I remember coming into the office one night from a field trip in Louisiana and saw on my desk the orders to move to Wichita. This was January of '52.[43]

Within a year of the July 1948 hiring, two of the original co-ops would leave for other work opportunities outside public health, and one would be fired for cheating on his contact numbers.[44] Those remaining include names that by now have made the public health history books. Bill Watson, primary among them, went on to a remarkable public health career, retiring as the deputy director of the Centers for Disease Control and Prevention in 1984. Bill felt that his contribution to public health was in part a personal one, grounded in his family experience. At the age of twelve, he lost his ten-month-old sister to pneumonia following an infection of pertussis or whooping cough. His contributions to immunization efforts later in his career would in some small way answer the need his family had so painfully identified:[45]

> I had a ten–month-old sister who got whooping cough and developed pneumonia and died. I will tell you that brings home the im-

> portance of immunization. The impact that had on my mother, and my father too, but my mother, in particular, never got over that child's death. She had lost a beautiful ten-month-old, as healthy as she could be, who died of whooping cough.[46]

Luke Hamlin would remain with the VD program until 1962. He then took his skills to the Health Mobilization and Disaster Preparedness Program, which focused on preparing for a nuclear attack. Luke later transferred to the Emergency Medical Services Program and retired from the federal service in 1981.[47] S.A. Boudreaux remained with VD Control until 1964, and then worked in the Kansas City Regional Office with the Accident Prevention and Poison Control Programs. He later transferred to the Environmental Health Program and remained there until his retirement in 1979. Don Lederman worked with the VD program until 1960, when he transferred to the Emergency Medical Services Program in the Bureau of Medical Services. He retired in 1979.

Others soon followed in the footsteps of the initial co-ops. In the fall of 1948 Walter Hughes was assigned to the Mississippi Health Department as the supervisor of VD control, or what PHAs would call the "state rep."[48] Delwin "Del" Hammons was hired in August 1948 after learning about the job from his cousin, who was a postmaster in Monroe, Louisiana. Johannes Stuart called Del and arranged for him to interview with Tom Davis out of the PHS Regional Office in New Orleans. After his interview with Tom, Del spoke with The Doctor by phone:

> He asked me two or three questions, and I answered them, and then he said, "When could you start with us? We got some jobs in several places, and we really need somebody in West Virginia."… We talked over the little details about everything and when I could start and where I was to report. That was August 9th, 1948.[49]

Del trained for two weeks and then was assigned in Parkersburg, West Virginia, to the Wood County Health Department. The health department was very small and was located in a small house. It had a part-time health officer and a periodic clinic. Del served several surrounding counties that did not have health departments. He was the VD public health infrastructure in this area, and he focused on syphilis interviewing and contact epidemiology. The assignment was an important introduction to public health infrastructure and community need:

> They had me investigating. The patients were usually factory workers. Some lived up the mountainside or behind the mountain with no road to the place. You had to walk to locate them and get them in. That was a difficult thing because a lot of them didn't have cars or transportation.[50]

The VD Division would hire eighteen more co-ops by 1950.[51] All early PHAs began in the field, working in conjunction with a Rapid Treatment Center or a VD clinic in a health department. A central part of the experiment was the temporary nature of the job offers. The early co-ops were given "excepted appointments," meaning that they were not civil servants, did not get benefits, and did not have federal classification.[52] According to Dick Bowman, co-ops received a federal check, but nothing else. They were to abide by state vacation rules. The job was "pegged at the level of a GS-5 which, I think it was like $2,000 back then... It was felt that getting college graduates would justify the '5' level."[53] Co-ops paid for their first move with the federal government, and unlike the original co-ops, those who followed had to furnish their own automobile. The late Jack Benson, hired in 1950 as the twentieth co-op, had to purchase a car quickly in order to take the job. Like Bill Watson, Jack almost missed an opportunity to interview with Johannes Stuart. It was a surprise to learn that he had to be sworn in by an officer of the PHS commissioned corps before he could start the job. Jack drove thirteen hours from North Carolina to Atlanta in order to interview with Stuart. He was directed to drive back to North Carolina within two days to be sworn in, and to return immediately back to Atlanta to attend training with Bob Swank:

> Dr. Stuart was coming down from Washington on Thursday evening for interviews. Being without a permanent job at the time and just having graduated from school, I drove to Atlanta. His plane was late. It was about seven o'clock that evening when the interview finally took place... Back then it was a thirteen-hour drive to Raleigh, North Carolina... I found this character by the name of Horace Holmes and wasn't sure that he was the individual to report to because he was listed as a Captain Horace Holmes. We didn't know that Public Health Service had a Commission Corps. So he took us under tow, and we went out and he found an agricultural person employed by that culture who promised to swear us in. We had to raise our hand and take a little oath. And

> then that evening we turned around and were sent back to Alto, Georgia, to Bob Swank's interviewing class.[54]

The ability to have co-ops in the field in the late 1940s for VD control was surprising in view of what was going on in Washington with the VD Division at the time. In 1948 Dr. Theodore Bauer became chief of the VD Division and soon after had to effect large budget reductions. The use of penicillin to treat syphilis had rendered the Rapid Treatment Centers unnecessary. Twenty-six government-operated VD hospitals had to close.[55] The VD Division would be reduced in its financial, infrastructure, and human resource power that year, but the co-op experiment survived. The program's temporary nature probably helped it survive the budget cuts because it functioned largely under the radar in those years. With excepted appointments, the co-ops would not really be "on the books" as federal government employees. Such a temporary existence might trouble many new employees, but not the early co-ops. Despite the lack of job security, they had faith that their job would prove valuable to the VD Division, and that they would become a permanent part of the organization. This confidence was remarkable given the time and the Division circumstances. Joe Giordano, hired in 1951, recalls how strange this confidence must have looked to the modern person:

> We had no civil service status whatsoever. We had no civil service protection. We paid Social Security, and the fact of the matter is that we could be terminated at any given time for no reason whatsoever... [I]f you look at it in retrospect, and were not part of that era, you might be very, very critical; but the fact of the matter is that we're talking about a program that was in its infancy. It had a lot going for it, and you needed that kind of flexibility to get this program off the ground and rolling. You needed that kind of flexibility in terms of selection of people. You didn't know if they were going to work out, you didn't know whether the states were going to find them acceptable or what have you.[56]

Once it became clear that the initial and subsequent co-ops were successful, the VD Division moved to legitimize the effort. Lida Usilton felt that they could not continue to attract qualified people without a civil service classification. According to Dick Bowman, the VD Division created the federal job classification GS-685, termed "Public Health Advisor," to legitimize this new public health role:[57]

> We worked with Betty Grantling, who was the personnel officer assigned to HEW, as it was then... She said, "Well, we'll have to set up a new series." At first they were going to call it Public Health Representative, and then they decided, "Well, Public Health Advisor is a simpler title." So she set up this series. She consulted with the VD staff as to what the job required.[58]

The series' precise creation date is not known, though it is thought to be sometime between 1953 and 1956.[59] Dick recalls that there was no adjunct classification that could be used for the co-ops. Once the series was established, co-ops would need to be examined for their qualifications. The final step toward legitimacy was taken in 1964, when the Civil Service Commission and the General Counsel of the Department of Health, Education, and Welfare (HEW) approved the crediting of co-op service to an employee's retirement.[60] Dick remembers that he, Lida, and Johannes Stuart were examiners:

> [O]nce it was set up and approved by the Civil Service Commission, Miss Usilton, myself, and Johannes Stuart were made Civil Service Examiners so that we could go through the applications and set up those that qualified for the job... As soon as this was established the co-ops were converted, and it wasn't until a few years later that we were able to give the employees credit for the co-op years by paying the retirement of the years that they were under co-op. [W]e had a little trouble doing that.[61]

Finally the use of the GS-685 series made the co-op part of the federal government. From that point on, new entry-level hires would accept a temporary appointment with the understanding that eventually they would need to take and pass the Federal Service Entrance Examination (FSEE).[62] Early hires to the program remained co-ops for one year, sometimes longer, as a mechanism for training and weeding out. The term "co-op" later was replaced by "associate." Whatever the title, the meaning was clear: it was a training and introductory period for the new hires. The co-op appointment would allow program flexibility to ensure that the right people were hired for the job.

Chapter 4

The Early Years

The battle against syphilis was the reason Lida Usilton and Johannes Stuart initiated the 1948 experiment to place co-ops in local areas as VD investigators and patient interviewers. It was immediately clear that the experiment was a success because the co-ops were adept at syphilis case finding and patient interviewing. By the mid-1950s, syphilis rates were the lowest they ever had been.[1] The infusion of this type of human resource helped to cause a major reduction in syphilis rates in the early 1950s, and it helped change the local public health approach to controlling syphilis. Despite the epidemiologic success with syphilis, all was not smooth for the early PHAs. As the new co-ops were being introduced to public health, the public health community was being introduced to the PHA. Accommodating this new type of public health worker into VD programs staffed primarily by nurses and physicians was not easy, and the new co-ops had to make a place for themselves in state and local public health departments. During these early years, some areas appreciated all the help they could get, while others were a bit skeptical and did not trust the "male interviewers."[2] Health departments and private physicians needed to be convinced that skilled patient interviewing and case finding were effective tools to reduce syphilis, particularly once syphilis treatment was widely available. They also needed to be persuaded that PHAs could be trusted with their patients.[3]

The new co-ops were college-educated, and many had been World War II veterans. They were also all white men until approximately 1954, when the first African American male PHAs, Al Billingslea and George Love, were hired.[4] Another seventeen years would pass before the first women PHAs—Penny Friedberg, Susan Bass, and Janella Apodaca—were hired in 1971 (see Chapter 5).[5] The all-white and all-male cadre contrasted with local health department VD investigators, even in the 1940s. Local VD program staff included female nurses who conducted some patient interviewing and field epidemiology, and local health personnel in the South often included African American male VD investigators and assistant investigators.[6]

By the end of the 1950s, PHAs also were distinguished by their uniform: a black suit, a hat, and business shoes. According to Bob Emerson, "we modeled our garbs" –black, dark blue or grey suits – "after the FBI in those days."[7] Ray Bly quickly got the message about the required dress when he was hired in 1956 to work in St. Louis, Missouri: "We want you to wear a suit and a tie. We don't care if you wear the same one every day; we want it clean, neat, well-pressed, with your shoes shined, and your hair cut."[8] The uniform was designated to communicate professionalism and respect for the role and for the patient, though some thought it made them look like door-to-door salesmen or FBI agents. Even so, all early PHAs strictly adhered to the uniform despite the contrast with the fieldwork. Jim Fowler recalls how difficult it was to maintain professional attire when drawing blood in the tobacco fields of North Carolina:

> I would be looking for people out in the tobacco fields, going out across those rows with highly-shined cordovan shoes, and sweating like mad in ninety-nine-degree temperature and one hundred percent humidity. Sometimes we were allowed to leave our jackets. When we'd find someone we were looking for, we would draw blood right there. Well, in order to draw the blood you'd have to lock the person's arm with your elbow near the side. Always at the end of the day, you had a large gummy black residue on your white shirt because when you pick tobacco, there's a resin that occurs, and that resin combined with the sweat and the dirt.[9]

The uniform was standard until the 1970s, when it became more effective to dress comfortably while working in the community. John Shimmens was glad to see the change, because the uniform was a dead giveaway: "Everyone knew we were the VD guys." The necktie was also a danger, especially to John. He was a new PHA in 1959 when he was almost "hung like a chicken" with his tie by an angry bartender after returning to a bar three or four times looking for someone named "Janey," who was the source of more than a few cases of syphilis. From that time on, even until his retirement, John always wore clip-on ties:

> I went into this one bar—a pretty scuzzy place—and asked for "Janey." It was important to find her, and this was about the third or fourth time I had been in there. I got a little bit pushy with the

> bartender, and said, "You know, you've got to have this girl come into the bar here." And he was very tired of seeing me. He reached across the bar, grabbed me by the tie and pulled me up like a chicken and yelled, "I told you she ain't here, and I ain't going to do anything more about it!" I came back and I thought "I'm never going to wear a rope around my neck again." From that day to this day, I don't even own a necktie.[10]

The PHA culture that began to emerge in these early years was different in two other respects from the local public health environment. The PHAs themselves were energized and driven to succeed—often creating opportunities for friendly competition in case finding or blood drawing. This delight in competition was carried from assignment to assignment and became embedded in the PHA experience. Second, the PHA was assigned to a local area for a limited amount of time. They were transferred multiple times, particularly in the early part of their careers. These differences would become part of the unique contribution PHAs made to local public health, as the local systems could not possibly replicate employee exposure to geographic and program diversity, nor could local health (by definition) stimulate and sustain a national culture of competition for excellence.

An additional and enduring part of the PHA culture was and is experience with sexually transmitted diseases. PHAs were shaped by their initial experiences in public health at the VD patient level. The challenges and harsh human situations associated with this work would leave an indelible sense of reality that would inform PHAs' service throughout their careers. New co-ops spent their time interviewing VD patients to identify their sexual contacts and worked with communities to conduct blood testing. They took scant amounts of descriptive information and nonetheless found sexual contacts in the field to offer them a test for syphilis, and, if needed, VD treatment. Their training (see Chapter 6) allowed these PHAs to collect blood samples in the field, diagnose syphilis, and masterfully conduct patient interviews so that syphilis chain would be broken. Because of their day-to-day involvement with syphilis, early PHAs were often more adept than private physicians at diagnosing it.[11] Both of these elements—the experience and the training—became a central part of PHA culture.

The early co-ops worked in state and local health departments and Rapid Treatment Centers to conduct contact epidemiology and engage in mass blood testing on a county-by-county basis.[12] They were placed in "core project areas," initially located in North Carolina, South Carolina, Maryland, and Georgia, to receive initial training and coaching.[13] Not every recruit could handle the raw and personal nature of VD: the issues were sexual, the discussions with patients were candid, the life situations were challenging, and the signs and symptoms of disease often were disgusting. Successful PHAs accepted VD's realities, developed the skills to interview and locate patients and contacts, and did not wince or faint when observing VD's signs or symptoms. In 1953 Pete Campassi was a new co-op receiving training at the Rapid Treatment Center in Florence, South Carolina. He recalls seeing other co-ops faint at the sight of genital ulcers common to the bacterial disease granuloma inguinale (GI). Pete and other neophytes were shown a patient with GI under the watchful eye of Bill Watson, who was by then South Carolina's state rep. Pete remembers having to hide from Bill his reaction to the open sores and expansive lesions on the patient. Others were not so discreet:

> They figured out how to weed you out in a hurry… It was in the middle of the summer in hot hospital barracks, military barracks. The first day they take you into a room where a person is being examined… and those who didn't pass out stayed in the program. Those who passed out or turned green, that was the end of it. They were through.[14]

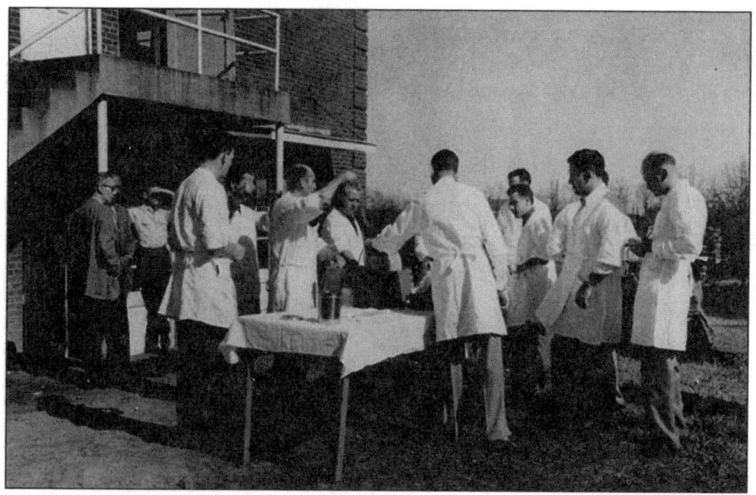

New hires learning how to draw blood at the Beale Street Clinic in Memphis, Tennessee. January 1957.
Courtesy of Bill Doyle.

Early PHAs and co-ops did a lot of mass blood testing, because in the late 1940s and early 1950s, it was believed that syphilis was sufficiently widespread.[15] Syphilis screening often was conducted along with other health screening efforts, and the public generally participated. Georgia was among the first states to conduct health screening on a massive scale for conditions including syphilis, beginning as early as 1945 in Savannah, where persons would be screened for syphilis and receive an x-ray examination for tuberculosis.[16] These types of community-wide efforts would involve the health sector and businesses as well as churches. PHAs would be sent to an area to organize screening efforts on a county-by-county basis. According to Bill Watson, testing was well-received by the communities:

> We had teams that we would form to go county by county, and these were managed out of the state... They would go into X county and organize that county. [They would] go out into the street corners and the bars and everyplace else; out in the country, churches and so forth, to general stores... to try to get everybody to come in and get a blood test for syphilis. We got a very good [reception].[17]

Early blood testing efforts occurred at places of work, schools, and even churches.[18] Luke Hamlin recalls that in 1949 he had to screen Shreveport, Louisiana, school children for syphilis because rates of congenital syphilis were quite high. He drew the blood of children as young as kindergarten age and witnessed the telltale syphilis symptom of "Hutchinson teeth"—notched and almost screwdriver-shaped teeth—among several children:

> We blood-tested both in parochial and public schools, starting off at the beginning of the day with the kindergarten children and working ourselves up to the end of the day because it was easier: the larger the children, the bigger the veins. The parochial school children would stand up there with their arms up and not move. Very disciplined. Other schoolchildren were unruly and scared and crying and everything.[19]

As a new co-op in 1951, Ken Latimer initially was assigned to help local blood testing efforts in Arkansas. He recalls having to drive around the state to each of the districts in a "kidney-buster," a Chevrolet Carryall wagon loaded with blood testing supplies and equipment, complete with a public address system and a phonograph to stimulate interest. Ken would broadcast songs developed specifically to announce the availability of syphilis treatment, such as That Ignorant Cowboy or Good News. "It was like the Pied Piper. People would flock out of their houses and dance down the street behind us,"[20] he said. Those who tested positive for syphilis would be treated and interviewed so that sex contacts could be offered testing and treatment. Ken recalls:

> Our co-op year in Arkansas consisted of mass and selective blood testing programs to detect untreated syphilis… We passed out VD comic books like Little Willie and That Ignorant Cowboy, as well as other disease information booklets. We distributed "I've had my blood test" buttons and free samples of Dentyne chewing gum to everyone receiving a blood test.[21]

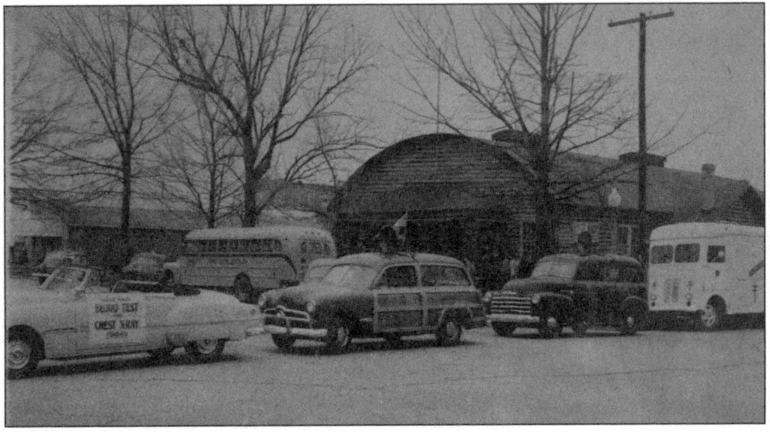

An Arkansas Tuberculosis and syphilis screening event, circa 1950s. A "Kidney Buster" is shown as the middle car in the photo.
Courtesy of the Centers for Disease Control and Prevention Global Health Odyssey. Originally donated by Deane Johnson. Photograph by W. W. Mundy of Dermott, Arkansas.

While in Arkansas, Ken was chosen to be involved with what he called the "last of the great mass blood testing surveys." In 1952, he and fellow PHA Harold Mauldin were screening employees at an Arkansas sawmill for syphilis when a local health department worker drove out to the site and told Harold that he had a "call from Washington." It was the Madam. When she called, it was important business. Harold returned to report that he was going to Puerto Rico to initiate a blood testing project there. Ken said he would be interested in joining him, and would have his chance to express his interest to the Madam directly while at a VD meeting in Chattanooga, Tennessee, two months later. He got his wish and spent the next three Christmases in Puerto Rico:

> I came in and I sat down in the center of this group, and they asked me questions and became acquainted, and asked me how I would like to go to an island, and I said, "I would love it." Lida said, "When you get back to Arkansas, you can anticipate being transferred to Puerto Rico."[22]

From 1951 to 1955, more than fifty PHAs were assigned to screen for and treat syphilis in Puerto Rico.[23] Harold Mauldin formed several public health teams and organized a central registry with the help of seven local assistants.[24] The teams were comprised of VD Division laboratorians, physicians, PHAs, and statisticians paired with local nurses and clerks.[25] They focused on screening, treatment, and interviewing. Reflecting on his sixteen-month assignment, Harold thinks that more than one million persons were tested for syphilis:

> Every day we had hundreds coming in from all over the dang island. We had a runner with a vehicle from the field... PHAs headed up the field teams, and we had nurses and clerical individuals... We blood-tested everything that moved, I guarantee you we did. Good Lord, I'd taken blood on infants in the scalp.[23]

The testing teams traveled around in a well-stocked kidney buster complete with educational materials, a sound system for music, and testing equipment. Testing occurred at places of employment, churches, community gatherings, and house-to-house. Teams offered testing to anyone; however, their efforts were targeted at those in the sexually-active age groups. Following shortly behind them was the medical rapid treatment team.[27] The testing and treatment teams traveled all over the island, staying as guests in local homes when there were no motels. Ken Latimer and his screening team cycled twice through the community:

> There was Woody Hayes and Bob Hagler and myself. We were "team captains." We had two nurses and three clerks. We went out to prearranged locations and did blood testing in every nook and cranny on the island and every barrio and playa, and the islands off the coast of Puerto Rico. During that time I'm certain we saw more

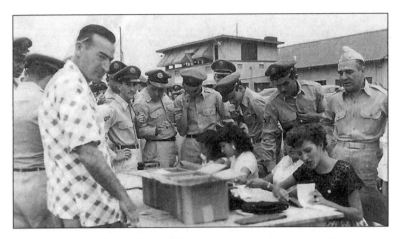

PHA Sam Glenner, Puerto Rico, 1953 while screening the National Guard. (Left, with pencil in ear).
Courtesy of Ken Latimer.

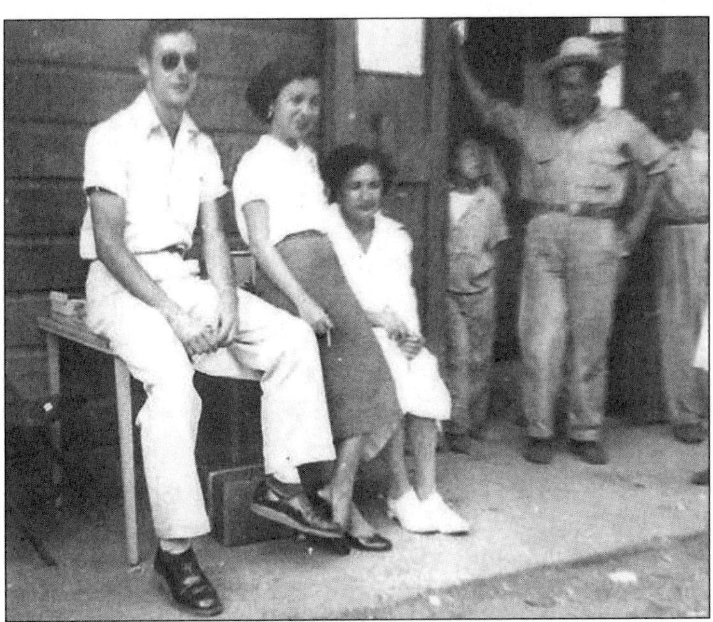

Ken Latimer (left) with team members Clerk Lydia Rosa Martinez, Nurse Mercedes Vierra De Terron. Ciales, Puerto Rico, February 1953.
Courtesy Ken Latimer.

> of Puerto Rico than people who were born and raised there. We went completely around the island blood-testing, and then about two weeks behind us was the medical rapid treatment team.[28]

As with the Puerto Rico screening project, early PHAs served as a ready and deployable public health workforce to help the VD Division address a variety of priorities. Prior to the introduction of penicillin and Rapid Treatment Centers, VD programs across the country were engaged in "case holding" to assure that patients completed treatment so as to render them no longer infectious. After penicillin's advent for syphilis treatment, patients no longer needed to be observed. This opinion was slow to develop, given the lack of knowledge about penicillin's efficacy at the time. How long, for example, would it take for people to be cured of syphilis? The modern reader might find it unnecessary to doubt antibiotics' curative ability. In the late 1940s and early 1950s, however, the practice of medical care and treatment for syphilis had become solidified as long-term treatment.[29] Treatment "relapse," or re-emergence of infectious syphilis due to incomplete or insufficient treatment, was an issue at the time, since it had occurred with the various prior treatments for syphilis. The prevailing belief was that patients would relapse within two years of treatment in the case of primary or secondary syphilis. To help the medical community move into the new syphilis treatment era, the VD Division initiated the Blue Star Research Study to evaluate penicillin. The study followed 560 patients with secondary syphilis on a monthly basis for the first year (1951), quarterly for the second year following their treatment, and for several years afterwards.[30] Blood tests confirmed whether patients were cured. Patient follow-up would not have occurred without a ready group of PHAs who were able to follow study participants even as they moved to different communities during the study's course. As would be expected, penicillin was found to be curative for syphilis, and patient holding and post-treatment follow-up were found to be unnecessary. This was a tremendous public service, particularly in view of syphilis treatment's historic burden for patients. Researchers credited the success of the Blue Star study to the "diligence of the investigators."[31] Jack Benson was a Blue Star investigator who followed his patients for twenty years, "going out every three months to get them in for an examination."[32]

The Blue Star program was not the only special assignment for early PHAs. In 1949, the VD Division began an effort to evaluate penicillin treatment among U.S. service personnel who had been treated a few years before. Half a million members of the Armed Forces had been treated for syphilis between 1940 and 1946. Unlike subjects in the Blue Star Research Study, these people were not recruited for the study at the time of treatment.[331] With the Syphilis Follow-up Program, veterans' names were distributed among the PHAs in the field for follow-up contact. Contacting these persons would prove to be a challenge for the PHAs' tact and diplomacy, because these veterans were not expecting to hear from them, and because several years had passed since their syphilis treatment. The follow-up task was massive. Within a two-year period, from 1949 to 1951, PHAs located 81,715 service personnel who had been treated for syphilis during the war.[34] Ken Latimer remembers that he and other Arkansas co-ops were given hundreds of names and addresses. They had to contact these people and obtain their consent to be re-examined and tested for syphilis in a local clinic or by their private physicians. He remembers the challenge of contacting these people after so many years had passed. For him, though, maneuvering through the confidentiality issues was "just another day in the life of a VD investigator":

> As you can just imagine, there were all sorts of challenging situations for us. The original dates of treatment were five or more years before. And now you were dealing with complex and challenging medical confidentiality situations. For example, in my district we had a bank president, a sheriff, a school principal, a well-known community leader, and many others. In addition, many of these individuals were now married with families.[35]

Jack Benson was also among those asked to locate the former service personnel. He was working out of Fort Bragg in North Carolina at the time and recalled that it was not easy to contact someone "out of the blue," remind them of their syphilis infection and treatment, and ask them to see a clinic or a physician for re-examination and testing. The follow-up situation was "quite touchy," but co-ops were trained in the techniques of patient interviewing and were prepared to help a person move beyond surprise and potentially shame to focus on their health and that of their families. If treatment was not curative and there were complications, this would impact a person's family or the community from an infection standpoint. In theory, the concern was laudable. In practice, however, things could be tough. Ken, Jack, and other PHAs who served in this effort demonstrated the value of their training. Jack recalled the importance of getting the chance to talk with the person and explain the purpose of the contact:

> A lot of these people had become businesspeople, managers, and it was quite touchy... We would come out, notify them confidentially that this was a follow-up and the records showed they had syphilis in the service. We wanted to be sure that they knew and would go to a physician... It was a little surprising to some of them and a little tough to deal with, but for the most part, they understood once you had a chance to talk.[36]

The Blue Star and Syphilis Follow-up programs would not have been possible without the steady buildup of the PHAs. By 1951, there were at least twenty-six co-ops in Arkansas[37] and seventeen in North Carolina.[37] By this time, PHAs were contributing to the local public health effort by providing needed help with VD investigation, patient interviewing, and mass blood testing. They supplemented the local investigation effort (if there was one) and helped to refocus syphilis control efforts toward finding the early cases. Through their assignments, the successful PHAs became adept at making a place for themselves in the local or state health departments, and they learned to wear "two hats." PHAs were by definition federal employees, yet they were detailed to function in a state or local government structure representing the local interests. They also were to represent the interests of the federal government, because, as co-ops, they were part of the federal government's cooperative financial agreement with states or local areas. They answered to both the local or state governments and the VD Division of the Public Health Service—which at the time meant the Madam herself. By 1951, Del Hammons was managing new co-ops. He stressed the significance of understanding the assignment's dual nature and the importance of representing the government to which one was assigned:

> We wanted a co-op to get acquainted and be a part of that local staff even though they were Fed[s]. Everybody understood the assignment, like nurses and all. "He's one of these VD people and he's federal."... The locals looked upon us as Feds, but we were representing the state when we'd go out there, and we made that very clear.[39]

The buildup of PHAs in the early 1950s occurred as much of the World War II-era infrastructure for VD control was being dismantled. Advances in syphilis treatment hastened the close of Rapid Treatment Centers. Medical schools that once had departments specializing in syphilology closed, and by the late 1950s, so did many of the extant VD clinics. Private physicians who were less than supportive of contact epidemiology efforts had more reason to resist relationships with public health now that penicillin could easily cure syphilis.[40] It appeared as if the only remaining local syphilis control effort was provided by PHAs assigned throughout the U.S.—that is, until federal funding was threatened in 1953. That year, it looked as if all the PHAs would need to go home. In the minds of some, federal funding for VD control no longer was necessary.[41] There was curative treatment for syphilis, and disease rates had plummeted by 1953. The saying went: "As the disease comes down, it's the program rather than the disease that gets eradicated."[42] This is precisely what occurred, and the blame lay squarely at the feet of the Eisenhower Administration. The decision to cut the VD Program was made by the newly-appointed (and first) Secretary of the Department of Health, Education, and Welfare, Oveta Culp Hobby. Bill Watson recalled that the Department made the decision based on the numbers of current syphilis cases. The thinking was that "syphilis was down to 5,000 cases a year, and so we don't need a national program anymore. States can handle this."[43]

Without an appropriation, everything would stop. There would be no money to pay the federal VD field staff. The news had to be shared with PHAs, who by 1953 were stationed throughout the U.S. and in Puerto Rico. Several resigned in response to the news, but others, like Jack Benson, "hung on" to see whether things would reverse themselves. He was hired briefly by the State of North Carolina to weather the storm:

> The VD Division would move us back at their expense to someplace near to where we might want to get out of the service because the grant money was not appropriated for that coming year. There was a slot in Burlington, North Carolina, and I was transferred back there... I was there about eight months and just felt, "Well, I will just hang on."[44]

Ken Latimer was working in Puerto Rico when he received the news about the VD program's elimination. The group of VD Division staff working in Puerto Rico was shocked by the news.[45] Like Jack Benson, Ken held out hope that the program would survive because the service was needed, and it would not be the last anyone saw of syphilis.

Bill Watson was working as the state rep in South Carolina when the threat to funding occurred. "Morale just plummeted," he said. Bill asked Tom Davis from the PHS Regional Office to come and boost the staff's spirits. Instead of a pep talk, Tom came over and said, "Anybody with a brain in his head will go find another job."[46] Those who stuck it out were rewarded within eight months when an effort in Washington returned the VD appropriation to the budget. Bill Watson recalls that Dr. Ted Bauer, then the director of the VD Division, recruited help from the State of Georgia to try to reverse the situation:

> Ted Bauer called the state health officer in Georgia, knowing that the Senior Congressman on the Appropriations Committee that dealt with public health was from Georgia, and asked if the head of the VD Control program in Georgia could come up and meet with him. Well, he came to Washington, D.C., and we talked, and then he went over to Capitol Hill and met with the Congressman and came back and said, "You know? They put their trousers on the same way we do!" He had persuaded that Congressman to put the money back.[47]

Not every penny of the VD program budget was returned, though a sufficient number of PHAs had resigned during the threat of program cuts that there was no need for an additional personnel reduction.[48] By 1955, VD control activity resumed. The program was hiring co-ops, was again transferring PHAs, and was initiating new programs.[49] This time, though, the focus was not syphilis. It was gonorrhea.[50]

When syphilis was a priority, the local VD staff would focus on gonorrhea and the PHAs would focus on syphilis. Once syphilis incidence was reduced, the federal focus switched to gonorrhea. When Ray Bly began his career in 1956, his assignment was to focus primarily on gonorrhea:

> We really devoted most of our time to gonorrhea. We were interviewing gonorrhea patients, mostly males so they would get us to the female, who was probably asymptomatic. We also did some physician visitation and worked with laboratories, and we had a public clinic that was open five days a week and then on Saturday mornings.[51]

The PHAs' emerging "can-do" attitude held that the VD control system which helped to reduce syphilis—screening, contact epidemiology, other methods of case finding, and access to treatment—would also control gonorrhea.

Controlling gonorrhea, however, was much more difficult than syphilis because the incubation period was shorter and the organism, Neisseria gonorrhoeae, mutated, complicating curative treatment.[52] Further, the gonorrhea infection cycle was difficult to break because symptoms among women were not easily identified. To address the challenges, in 1956 the VD Division initiated a pilot initiative in large cities called "Peppy Epi." The initiative would apply the intensity of syphilis focus to gonorrhea.[53] "Peppy" referred to a rapid public health response to gonorrhea in order to get the sexual contacts in for treatment. PHAs employed the tools of the time, which included telephone calls and a "Western Union machine," the precursor to the facsimile machine. By this time Jack Benson was working in San Francisco as one of the few PHAs out on the West Coast.[54] He made an unusual arrangement with the telephone company to facilitate patient contact:

> I had a confidential relationship with the telephone company's special agents to give me the addresses of clients where we might only have a phone number. They could also tell me the room where the phone was connected. Each evening, nondescript telegrams would be sent to potential clients/patients urging that they report immediately to the clinic... It was surprising the response we received from those appearing at the clinic the next day or telephone calls we received where we could then discuss the need for exam. This added effort to get a quicker response was successful in helping to reduce cases of gonorrhea infections. Once in the clinic, new cases of syphilis would also be found during the complete screening exams.[55]

Jack Wroten was a Peppy Epi when he began as a co-op in Fulton County, Georgia, in 1957. The workload was heavy. He and others would interview up to one hundred fifty people and close up to two hundred gonorrhea case investigations in one month's time. Jack recalls the work as "pretty much around the clock" for the one year that he worked on the project.[56] His focus soon shifted back to syphilis, because by 1959, gonorrhea was reduced nationally as a result of the Peppy Epi efforts,[57] and syphilis was increasing, marked by outbreaks in Houston in 1957, in Arkansas in 1958, and Shreveport, Louisiana, in 1960.[58] By the mid 1960s, national efforts were again under way to eradicate syphilis.

The PHA experience in the 1950s would forever mark their work in sexually transmitted diseases: syphilis and gonorrhea would continue despite their major efforts. As syphilis was reduced in the early 1950s, gonorrhea was on the rise. Once gonorrhea was reduced in the late 1950s, syphilis would reemerge. The battle against gonorrhea would continue to the present time and become complicated by drug resistance. Syphilis would be fueled by crack cocaine's introduction in the 1980s, and epidemics would continue to spark across the U.S. in the 1990s and early 2000s. The battle against VD was without end.

Just prior to the Houston syphilis outbreak of 1957, Johannes Stuart was considering how PHAs might help control VD at the U.S.-Mexico border. He decided to join health screening efforts that were occurring in conjunction with the Bracero Program, which was initiated in 1942 between the United States and Mexico to allow Mexican agricultural laborers—"Braceros"—to cross the border and work temporarily in U.S. agricultural fields and, for a brief time, on railroads. The Bracero Program was in response to increasing U.S. demand for seasonal agricultural workers during World War II and Mexicans' need for agricultural employment.[59] More than four million Mexican agricultural laborers were hired temporarily by U.S. farms and growers. The majority of Bracero workers were located in California, Arizona, and Texas, though workers were sent to many states.[60] The program lasted until 1964 and was the largest guest worker program of the twentieth century. U.S. border entry points for the workers were few, and thousands of laborers entered the U.S. through a hurried process of security and health screening before being chosen for jobs.[61] The medical exam's purpose was to control for communicable diseases, such as tuberculosis, and to assure that the workers were physically fit to do the agricultural and railroad work.

When Johannes Stuart asked Bill Watson to go to El Paso, Texas, to start screening for syphilis, Bill had to admit that he had never before drawn blood. Unlike the co-ops who followed him, the first co-ops were not trained in phlebotomy. After a bit of training, Bill and four other newly-hired co-ops arrived at the Bracero Center in August 1956.[62] The PHA team drew surprise from quarantine officials who were handling the x-ray process for tuberculosis. The officials were concerned that the small crew from VD would hold up the medical examination process. The team was up for the challenge, and drew blood from more than three thousand workers on one occasion. Bill recalls the initial reaction to the arriving PHAs:

> The doctor who was head of the quarantine office said, "Now the one thing that you can't do is back up on the x-rays." And the very

> opposite happened. We got them through the blood testing line quicker than they did with the x-ray line.[63]

Bill Griggs was among the five PHAs sent to El Paso for the feasibility study of syphilis testing for Braceros. Two months after he was hired in 1956, Griggs was asked to go with Bill Watson. Like Watson, Bill Griggs remembers the response from their Quarantine colleagues to the potential delay that syphilis testing might create during the medical examination process:

> Dr. Lyman, who was head of the Quarantine office at that point in time, said, "When are the other twenty guys coming in?" We said, "We're it." And he said, "We can't make it work. You cannot slow down the line." These people come into the border area, they get deloused, and they go out to the reception center. They strip to the waist, and they start through processing. The first thing they got was a short-arm exam; then they got a 70 mm chest x-ray. We inserted the blood testing line right after the short-arm. They got there at six o'clock, and literally they were through with chest x-ray by eleven-thirty or twelve. I mean, these people went through that fast, six hours, 3,000-4,000 people.[61]

By the summer of 1958, PHAs were working with the Bracero program in El Paso, Hidalgo and Eagle Pass in Texas; El Centro, California; and Nogales, Arizona. PHAs would test on average three thousand eight hundred workers a day.[65] Bracero Centers were also established in Mexico, and Bill Griggs was sent with a PHS commissioned officer to testing stations in Monterrey, Chihuaua City, and Guaymas to review the quality of activity. Bill said this was probably the first international assignment for PHAs. At these centers Braceros were given a physical screening, they were vaccinated for smallpox and reviewed for any deformity that might prevent them from working in the field. While in Mexico, Bill found that smallpox vaccinations were risking the Braceros' health by repeated use of non-sterile vaccination equipment:

> The first time I was there, they were smallpox vaccinating people with straight pins. They were using two steel cups. Alcohol was in one of the cups. The other cup was filled with straight pins. They picked the pins out of this one cup, used them and then placed them in this other cup. When the one cup got empty they just

> swapped cups. So some of these sorts of practices we obviously changed. We made available to them vaccination needles and suggested more stringent sterilization be used.[66]

Whether they worked in gonorrhea or syphilis, the PHAs in the 1950s found the job to be rewarding and challenging. Frequent transfers exposed them to a broad spectrum of community situations. The work was difficult. It required tremendous interpersonal and interview skills, the ability to learn and apply both medical and epidemiologic information to control VD, and personal sacrifice. Many PHAs were on the road for much of their early years, traveling from community to community in pursuit of VD. Early in his career, Jack Benson found himself in the role of a traveling syphilis tester. The experience would take him away from his family for almost six days out of every week. It was in 1954 when Jack was transferred to Lansing, Michigan, to work for the state health department.[67] There, he conducted syphilis screening and patient interviewing out of a refurbished trailer that he pulled around to large employers, such as cement factories or machine plants, to offer employees a test for syphilis. Shortly thereafter he was assigned to work in Detroit:

> I went out every day and up and down the streets and would park at some of these bars at night and early evening and beg for electricity to plug in the trailer so we would have lights... A nurse and a clerk and myself were pulling that thing.[68]

Detroit was far from Lansing, where his family first was relocated for the Michigan assignment. The job required Jack to take the train from Lansing on Sunday afternoon, work in Detroit all week, and return home Friday around midnight. "It was a week in, week out proposition," he said. His experience was not unusual for PHAs. The job required them to move from place to place, and to work long hours. When it came to case finding and screening, it was necessary for public health workers to be available and in the community at all hours of the day and evening in order to reach people. Long hours became a standard experience among PHAs, as did working in all types of conditions. Ray Bly recalls the "primitive conditions" in which he would conduct blood testing. As a trained phlebotomist, a PHA could draw a sample of blood to test for syphilis. This was a very helpful skill when people were located far from medical care, or if they did not have the chance to go to a clinic or doctor for a blood test. PHAs drew blood in every conceivable location: in a bar, in an alley, or in Ray's case, "at night in front of the headlights or under the dome light of a car."[69] He recalls a scare he had around 1958 when screening for syphilis at a labor camp on Long Island. He was working late at night, going from cottage to cottage offering workers the chance to test for syphilis. "The lighting was questionable," he said:

> One evening we were out there just going from cabin to cabin blood-testing. We were testing with Sheppard tubes. When the needle is in the vein you break a glass tip in a rubber sleeve attached to the needle and the blood tube. This releases the vacuum and draws the blood into the tube. The tube and needle are replaced in a glass top for transporting. Lighting was poor in the cabin. I was putting the top back on the needle and missed the opening -I stuck the needle right under the cuticle of my thumbnail. Blood was dripping off of the end of the needle. I was worried about the possibility of some form of infection, including hepatitis. We went out behind the cottage and bathed the thumb with green soap and alcohol, and really milked the blood out of my thumb. That took care of the problem.[70]

From 1948 until the late 1950s, PHAs waged the battle against syphilis through organized efforts in contact epidemiology and through targeted and mass screening programs. A remaining and important component of a public health response to syphilis involved the engagement of private physicians. Just as Surgeon General Thomas Parran had noted in the 1940s, private physicians' role in syphilis control had yet to be fulfilled.[71] They needed to report their syphilis cases to health authorities so that contact epidemiology could occur, and they needed a certain level of knowledge to be able to recognize syphilis and know how to treat it. In the early 1950s, when Ken Latimer visited Arkansas physicians as a co-op, the purpose was to ask permission to interview their patients who had tested positive for syphilis.[72] Ken recalls that although he was well received, public health authorities generally were reluctant to engage private physicians. This hesitation was an artifact of the development of medicine and public health, where private physicians did not recognize public health epidemiologic activity as important in the practice of medicine, and felt that public health activity would interfere with the physician-patient relationship (see Chapter 2). Despite concerns about interacting with private physicians, VD control required public health to establish an organized mechanism or program that would engage physi-

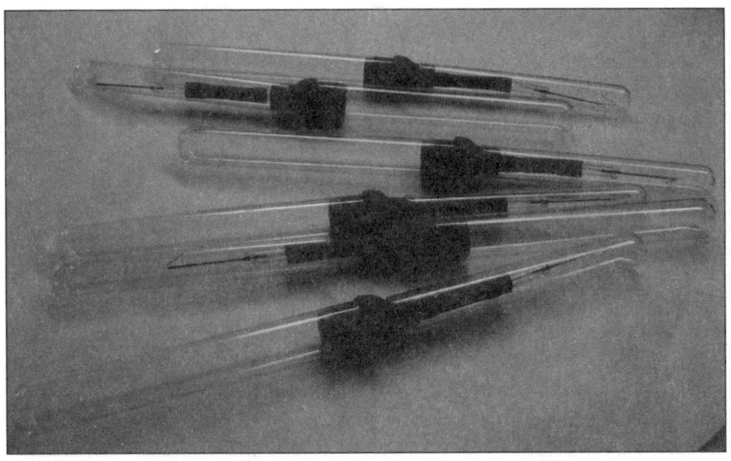

Sheppard tubes used in the 1950s to 1960s to draw blood samples in fieldwork. Courtesy of the Centers for Disease Control and Prevention Global Odyssey.

cians in VD control. Joe Giordano recalls how the Physician Visitation Program was initiated in the mid 1950s:

> At least in the very early years… no one would dare call a private physician to discuss with that private physician his or her patient, much less ask permission to interview. In about the mid-'50s that program got off the ground in a rather organized way... What we found out was that there were obviously enormous numbers of people who were being seen by private physicians, in all walks of life, and that… you could work with private physicians in terms of gaining permission to interview that patient.[73]

Early PHAs found that many physicians were not sufficiently educated to recognize and treat syphilis, so PHAs were trained to provide a Darkfield Microscopy Service to them. Darkfield microscopy was used to identify *treponema pallidum*, the bacterium that causes syphilis. A sample from a chancre or syphilis lesion was examined through an indirectly-lit microscope. If coiled shapes called spirochetes were seen, they would indicate the bacterium's presence. Jack Benson often provided this service to local physicians in his jurisdiction. He took a sample from a patient's chancre, read the darkfield, and then returned to the physician with the slide to teach him or her how to identify the spirochete and therefore diagnose syphilis. According to Jack, "A lot of physicians just did not have the experience [and] couldn't even recognize a specimen."[74]

Darkfield services were offered with increasing frequency by the mid 1960s, and in 1964 the VD branch initiated a darkfield school for state, local, and federal VD investigators to be sure that physicians would have assistance if needed during what was then the national effort to eliminate syphilis. Although the service was widespread geographically, it was not offered as frequently by the mid 1960s because physicians and health departments developed the capacity. With the nationwide syphilis eradication effort in full swing, it was necessary to be sure investigators did not lose their skills in darkfield microscopy.

Last July it was decided that training and retraining of VD field personnel in darkfield microscopy should be handled by the State laboratories, since it was evident that personnel who do not perform darkfield tests with reasonable frequency tend to lose their skill in this technique. To date 70 individuals from New Jersey, the District of Columbia, North Carolina, and Florida have completed darkfield microscopy training in the States.

Dr. William J. Dougherty, Director, Division of Preventable Diseases, New Jersey Department of Health, reports that since the completion of their last darkfield microscopy training course there have been 190 darkfields performed by individuals who took the course. Of this total, 83 darkfields were found to be positive. Through epidemiologic exploitation of these cases, 53 new primary and secondary cases were brought to treatment.

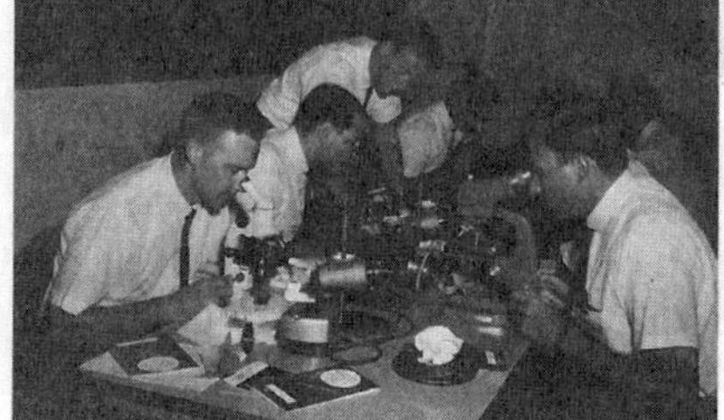

The accompanying picture is of a successful two-day darkfield course recently completed in Jacksonville, Florida.

Investigators participating in a two-day darkfield course held in Jacksonville, Florida, in 1964.
Source: Centers for Disease Control and Prevention, Contact newsletter, 1/22/65, p. 7.

Private physicians' reporting of syphilis diagnoses to health authorities was questionable even in the early 1960s, and the private medical community continued to show scant support for contact epidemiology. Yet both activities—reporting and contact epidemiology—were critical to syphilis control. In addition to basic VD education, the PHAs' work with private physicians was a job of marketing the importance of reporting and engagement with public health. In 1959 Jack Wroten found that his effort with physicians resulted in the identification of a syphilis epidemic among gay and bisexual men in Baltimore.

The epidemic was previously unknown because the physician would not report his positive cases to the health department for follow-up. The irony was that this particular physician was under contract with the Baltimore Health Department. Jack Wroten's engagement with this physician and the outcome of an identified epidemic among his patients and their contacts was enough to convince the physician and his staff of the importance of reporting and contact epidemiology, and of the PHA's value on the public health team.[75] The importance of Jack's work was heightened because he and four others were the first PHAs ever to be assigned to Baltimore, and this was one of the first times that gay or bisexual men were named as contacts in an outbreak investigation in that city—a significant achievement of trust in the 1950s. Prior to this success, Jack and his colleagues had trouble getting accepted by the local health department because the nurses who ran the VD program did not trust these "male investigators" and therefore kept the PHA role circumscribed. Wroten recalls that "they were selective in assigning cases to us. If they liked you, they would assign early syphilis cases. Otherwise, you would get low-priority stuff. Work was limited to working night clinics; no blood drawing in the field or talking to private physicians."[76] Jack's success was a big win for PHAs and for public health in Baltimore:

> I got lucky and was assigned to the Moore clinic at Johns Hopkins Hospital. One day as I was walking through the clinic, I noticed the physician in charge was using the microscope. I asked him what he was doing and he said "I am doing a darkfield." I said, "If it's positive, may I interview the patient?" He replied, "Well, I don't know." I talked to him more and convinced him that I could handle the case with care and confidentiality… He agreed for me to interview the patient. The initial interview at the Moore Clinic with the patient, a homosexual male, resulted in a large number of sex contacts named, mostly professional people… I approached this case as not only an opportunity to find and bring to treatment syphilis cases in Baltimore, but [an opportunity] to give credibility to the role of the PHA. I worked this case night and day for months, and I must say after all these years I still recall the people involved, well-educated professional men whose sexual orientation was hidden in those days. They were thankful and appreciative of the Health Department's handling of their cases.[77]

By the early 1960s PHAs would visit physicians in their assigned communities to increase their awareness of syphilis, their reporting of cases to health authorities, and their support of contact epidemiology. Visits to private physicians helped to ensure that VD control efforts could involve patients seen by these physicians. Bob Kingon remembers initiating physician visits in 1964 in Michigan. The purpose was to establish a relationship with doctors, provide information, and hope that they would recognize syphilis and call upon public health for support. At the time it was not clear whether physicians were intentionally avoiding the reporting of cases or were just not diagnosing them. The effort was developed to sensitize physicians and say, "Look, I'm here working in Grand Rapids with the health department, and we are ready to serve you. This is how we do business. We conduct our interviews in this way and we follow-up contacts that way, and please trust us to deal carefully with the sensitivities involved." Bob continues:

> The whole idea was to heighten their sensitivity so that if they saw something they would think syphilis. We also wanted them to know that the state laboratory was here and fully accessible to them including darkfield capabilities... It worked so well that the state laboratory began complaining about performing too many negative darkfield exams. Within two years, all syphilis cases in Grand Rapids were traced to sources outside the city.[78]

The effort was extremely effective because PHAs began to receive several referrals from physicians with whom they had made contact. Frank Berry remembers his experience with physician visits as a new co-op in 1960. The work resembled that of pharmaceutical representatives. He visited primarily dermatologists and internists to share information from the "White Book,"[79] a manual developed to educate physicians about syphilis signs, symptoms, and treatment:

> We would sit in the waiting room, get in, and pull out the book and some disease report cards. We'd tell them we were there to represent the health department... After a doctor flipped through it and read it, he said, "Hmm. Pretty interesting. It looks like some pretty good stuff here. But I don't see anything there about sulfa or bismuth." And that is how old his information was.[80]

The "White Book" would later become the "Green Book,"[81] which eventually would be transformed into other materials that are now electronically available to clinicians worldwide. In the 1950s and 1960s, however, physician education in syphilis was due largely to the PHAs' efforts, given the paucity of medical education for physicians in syphilology and VD generally. The endeavor would prove to increase physicians' knowledge, change their reporting behaviors, and strengthen their relationships with local public health. Once the program's success became clear, steps were taken to broaden the educational outreach to physicians more efficiently, using the PHA network. Larry Posey, hired as a PHA in 1959, directed the Physician Visitation Program, and would initiate the first "blitz" of New York City physicians to try to reach more clinicians who might see people with syphilis. He recalls:

> I arranged for guys to be transferred from all over the country to form a team of ten experienced PHAs. We set up a program to visit

4,033 PMD's to be visited in New York City . . .

Nineteen working days and 4,033 private physicians to be visited. That was the assignment given to the New York City Private Physician Visitation staff and 12 program representatives who arrived in New York City on temporary duty April 1st. The 4,000 doctors responded to a "direct mail" offer of professional and patient literature on VD, sent to 18,900 physicians registered in the city. The group was welcomed and briefed by Dr. W. D. Mortimer Harris, Chief, Division of Social Hygiene, New York City Department of Health, and Ferdinand D. Tedesco, Senior Health Program Representative (left).

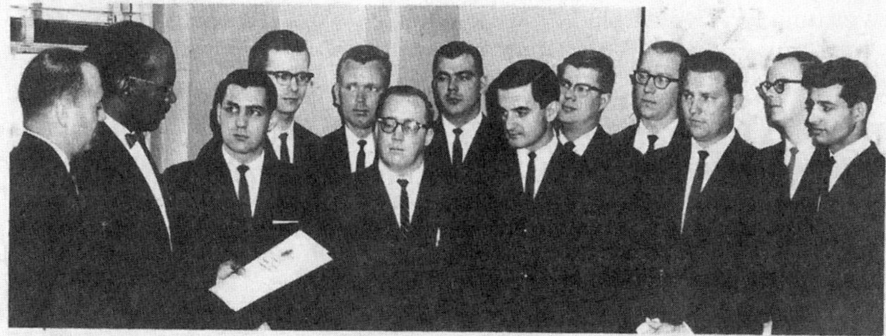

From left to right, 1st row – Philip Namy, Pittsburgh, Pa.; John J. Uffelman, Buffalo, N.Y.; Manuel Diaz, Jr., Philadelphia, Pa.; Jack W. Snowden, Miami, Fla.; Joe Vetro, Newark, N. J.; 2nd row – Walter D. Willihnganz, Chicago, Ill.; Charles W. Walker, Richmond, Va.; George M. Byrne, Washington, D.C.; Richard Bohn, Detroit, Mich.; Fred Fleagle, Jr., Charlotte, N. C.; and Jerry Ault, Chicago, Ill. The 12th program representative, Robert Mann, Albany, Ga., was not available for photo.

Photo and excerpt from Centers for Disease Control and Prevention, Contact newsletter, May 15, 1963, p. 2. This was another example of PMD (Private Medical Doctor) visitation via "blitz."

> private practitioners, internists, OB/GYN physicians, proctologists, and urologists. We visited around eleven hundred in ten days... These PHAs provided information about the clinic schedules in New York City, information about symptoms, laboratory services, information about reporting, and about consultation should they need to call one of our health department physicians to get help with diagnosis.[82]

The human resource capacity PHAs brought to local public health would be a tremendous contribution to syphilis control, and, eventually, to many other public health programs and efforts. In the case of VD in the late 1940s, the human resource capacity was brought in because local health departments did not have sufficient resources to conduct contact epidemiology and other methods of syphilis case finding. PHAs made their impact with local VD control programs through training, epidemiology, program development, and management, and they contributed significantly to the development of local public health career ladders and resources. Ultimately, though, PHAs could not control the way local and state governments invested in public health programs. The contrast between direct capacity provided by the federal government and the lack of local health capacity due to limited local spending in public health would remain part of the challenge that PHAs faced as they served local areas throughout the U.S. However, even as local and state VD programs developed their own capacity, they welcomed PHAs, and later PHAs would be welcomed by state and local tuberculosis (TB) and immunization programs. The use of PHAs in immunization and TB efforts would come following one of the largest program changes: the proud old VD Division's move to the small Atlanta operation called the Communicable Disease Center. As with every change, there was great opportunity for Public Health Advisors to contribute broadly to public health.

Chapter 5

The Expansion

In the spring of 1957, Surgeon General Leroy Burney determined that the VD Division of the Public Health Service should be moved to the Communicable Disease Center in Atlanta.[1] About ten percent of the Washington staff made the move. The rest, which included Lida Usilton and Johannes Stuart, resigned from the VD Division rather than go to Atlanta. Usilton left the VD Division around this time, or just prior, and worked in HEW until her retirement.[2] Johannes Stuart remained in Washington working for Surgeon General Burney, and eventually functioned as CDC's first congressional liaison until his retirement.[3]

Although the move to Atlanta did not concern too many PHAs in the field, it was a huge issue for the scientific and senior management staff in Washington. Atlanta would be a tremendous cultural change for the program and the staff. Cosmopolitan and "connected" Washington viewed Atlanta as a backwater town with little racial equality. As it turns out, the staff was rightly concerned about this last point. In 1962, as the VD program began to recruit more African American PHAs, a newly-hired PHA in Atlanta for training had difficulty getting served at local establishments. He and two of his colleagues resigned in protest.[24]

At the time of the move, Bill Watson had risen through the ranks and was serving as the deputy of the VD Division to Chief Dr. Clarence (Larry) Smith. Watson recalls the perception of the move at the time:

> Here was this proud old program that had been the largest thing in the PHS not too many years before that, now being subsumed into that upstart young outfit in Atlanta that nobody had ever really heard much about at that point.[25]

The VD Division's move to Atlanta would forever change the CDC. CDC was about the same size as the transferring VD Division in terms of budget and personnel, because the VD Division brought with it about six million dollars, a program of grants to states, personnel in the Public Health Service Regional Offices, and a large cohort of PHAs throughout the country. Bill made the move to Atlanta with his chief, and remained his assistant as Larry assumed his new role as CDC's Deputy Director.[6]

Although some mourned the Division's move to the Communicable Disease Center in Atlanta, others saw it as an opportunity to reinvigorate the VD program.[7] The program's regional office structure would benefit CDC, and CDC's direct relationship with states would enhance those the PHAs already had. The move also would provide an opportunity for PHAs to be introduced to the entirety of CDC. As new programs moved to Atlanta, PHAs would be called to assist their continued development. In 1960 the Tuberculosis Program would leave PHS for Atlanta.[8] At about that time CDC also would begin an effort to ensure childhood immunizations in the U.S. and abroad. These years saw significant growth in the number of Public Health Advisors and an expansion of their assignments throughout CDC. PHAs were in demand primarily by the VD, TB, and Immunization Programs,[9] though by 1961 PHAs were transferring in small numbers to Chronic Disease and to the Division of Dental Public Health and Resources.[10] By 1968, transfers from the VD Program expanded to include Health Mobilization and Injury Control.[11] Throughout all of these changes, the VD Program would continue to be the source of PHAs for all programs at CDC.[12]

The first use of PHAs outside the VD Program occurred in 1961 as a temporary detail to increase polio immunizations. A pilot effort in mass immunizations, called "Babies and Breadwinners," was initiated in Columbus, Georgia. This campaign would be an opportunity for CDC leadership to recognize PHAs' potential contributions.[13] Columbus was chosen because the local health department—the Muscogee County Health Department—was supportive of an effort to see whether a community-based mass immunization initiative would achieve higher immunization rates, and it was "big enough to prove something."[14] Larry Smith, by then the CDC director, asked his deputy Bill Watson to direct this local campaign. Bill brought in PHAs to assist:

> Boy, did we have a campaign. We got the Goodyear blimp, we had skydivers jumping down to the stations where people were getting their immunizations, we had clowns, we had everything! Talk about

> a mass campaign. Public Health Advisors knew what to do and helped get it done.[15]

Jack Benson was one of the PHAs asked to assist the Columbus effort. He recalled the massive effort and tremendous press coverage: "We were on the front page of the newspaper down there with pictures and articles every day except the day Sputnik went up. That's when we were knocked off the front page."[16] Jack coordinated the clerks, nurses, and the PHAs who were working on the effort. He organized three separate campaigns, each lasting eight days, because people needed to receive all three doses of polio vaccine between April and June. Vaccination teams were located on busy street corners, using, for the first time, the jet injector to deliver vaccine. According to Jack, "it seemed like we did about eighty thousand shots."[17]

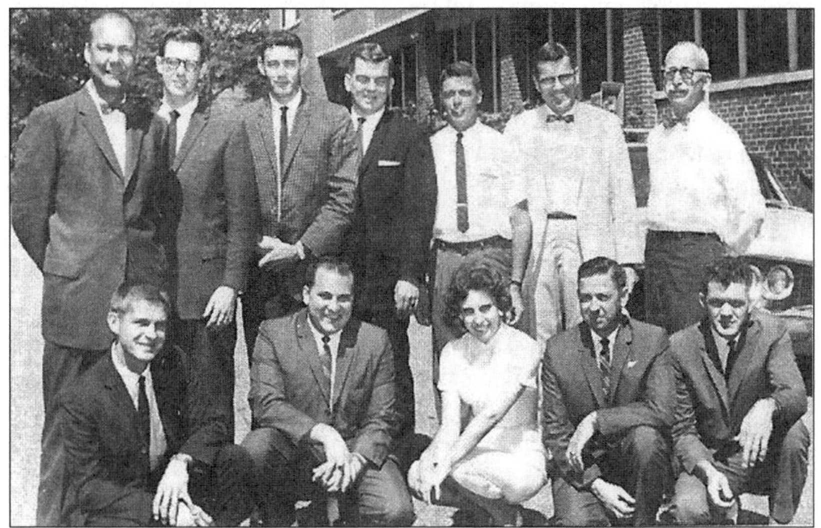

The Group from the Columbus Georgia polio campaign. Top row, left to right: Norman Bredesen (PHA, Arkansas), Dr. James Molloy (CDC Epidemiology Branch), Charles Munn (PHA, North Carolina), Bob Curry (PHA, New Jersey), Ray Shirling (PHA, Georgia), Dr. George Sciple (Technical Development Laboratories, Savannah), Dr. Terrence Billings (Atlanta). Bottom row, left to right: James Fowler (PHA, North Carolina), Ralph Burke (PHA, Georgia), Evelyn Elliott (CDC Secretary), Jack Benson (PHA, Missouri), George Morell (PHA, Georgia).
Centers for Disease Control and Prevention ***Contact*** *newsletter, June 22, 1961, p. 2.*

Jim Fowler was one of the co-ops detailed to work in the Columbus campaign. He recently had been hired as a VD investigator in Fayetteville, North Carolina, when he was detailed for six weeks to Georgia: "It wasn't bad duty, being single at the time and working with the Columbus School of Nursing at the hospital." The experience in polio immunization introduced Jim to many aspects of public health:

> We did a lot of driving through neighborhoods with loudspeakers on top of cars hawking the location of various outdoor sites for providing these immunizations. We also learned how to give the shots so that some of the EIS officers could take breaks every now and then.[18]

Despite the massive community effort, the Columbus project did not result in the expected polio immunization rate increase. However, the campaign did help demonstrate that a more sustained, planned, and national effort would ensure protection against not only polio, but also other childhood diseases. Bill Watson recalls that "Larry Smith used this to go to Washington and sell a national immunization campaign. We proved in Columbus that periodic mass campaigns were not good enough. Larry sold it to the Surgeon General and the Health Lobbyist at the time."[19]

Larry Smith sold Washington a national Immunization Program. It would be a grant program just like the VD Program, with financial and human resources provided to states. The "people" component would be PHAs placed as assignees in state and local health departments to help establish and develop a national system of childhood immunization. The use of PHAs had worked well for the VD Program, so when Bill Watson and Dr. David Sencer sat down to develop the proposal for the Immunization Program, they patterned it after the VD model.[20]

Things moved quickly. The proposal became The Vaccine Assistance Act of 1962. PHAs began to transfer into the Immunization Program by 1963. Dave Sencer arrived at CDC with the TB Program and soon after became agency's deputy director. He took on an additional role as the chief of the Immunization Program and functioned in this capacity until Dr. Robert Freckleton was hired to direct it.[21] Dave remembers that initially, the Immunization Program consisted of himself, Bob, Jim Bloom as administrative officer,[22] and a group of Public Health Advisors: "Actually, we only had me and Freckleton, and that was it. The rest were the Public Health Advisors, and we got it going."[23]

The Immunization Program was not the first program to enlist the help of PHAs outside of VD. PHAs were being considered for the TB Program just after the polio campaign concluded in Columbus, Georgia. The TB Program had arrived in Atlanta during the fall of 1960 after having been part of the Public Health Service since 1942. It had strong relationships with states through PHS physicians, nurses, social workers, statisticians, and some health communications specialists who provided consultation to states on every aspect of TB control.[24] States themselves had their own TB workers, though these professionals did not use the sophisticated methods of patient interviewing and contact epidemiology now firmly established in the VD Division. There was a lot of work to be done. By the early 1960s, new drugs were on the market for TB, and CDC planned to reduce the number of TB infections and deaths. The goal was to reduce the TB case rate from 31 per 100,000 population in 1960 to 10 per 100,000 by 1970.[25]

The TB Program's arrival in Atlanta coincided with a cultural shift taking place at CDC, and provided an opportunity to further the agency's organizational metamorphosis. It had been three years since the VD Division joined CDC, and several VD staff had been given important roles at the agency. Over time, the VD "way of doing business" became standard at CDC. According to Bill Watson, "VD had people assigned to states, and CDC didn't. It was a very different way of operating that we brought in. Gradually CDC came into our way of doing business. The first was with the TB grant program."[26] The value of PHAs to CDC programs and as part of the CDC management backbone was symbolized by Bill Watson's meteoric rise through the CDC ranks. According to Dave Sencer, who became the CDC director in 1966, PHAs were needed to manage program operations and to "come along behind the doctors to make sure that something happens more than just studies."[27]

The infusion of PHAs into the CDC's TB and Immunization Programs was not without challenge, because PHAs carried baggage from the 1957 arrival of the VD Program at CDC. Integrating the big VD Program into the small Communicable Disease Center was not smooth because the VD Program was a bit of a gorilla crashing the small club at CDC.[28] The VD Program came from Washington, D.C., and brought with it a Beltway attitude and a perception that the "backwater" program in Atlanta did not know what it was doing when it came to management or getting things done with Congress. Hard feelings in Atlanta complicated the TB Program's initial acceptance of PHAs. Even though the TB and VD Programs had coexisted previously in Washington, TB program leadership and staff had to be convinced that PHAs would assist their effort. According to Dave Sencer, "we had a hell of a time getting Public Health Advisors initially accepted there." As it turned out, the core issue was that the TB program staff were not used to working with PHAs. In time they accepted their new PHA colleagues and found them to be good contributors.[29]

By the end of the 1960s, PHAs were well integrated into the VD, Immunization, and TB Programs. Most of the state coordinators of VD, Immunization, and Tuberculosis Control Programs were PHAs. Virtually all of the PHAs working in TB and Immunization efforts had been recruited away from the VD Program.[30] John Shimmens was an early transfer from the VD to the TB Program. He was hired as a VD investigator in 1959 to work in Detroit and had just converted from co-op to a position level of GS-7, or PHA status, when he learned about an opportunity in the TB Program. It was standard VD Program practice to transfer those who were newly promoted in order to ensure broad geographic experience. John was slated to move to Flint, Michigan, but gladly considered staying in Detroit for an opportunity with the TB Program. John found that the work in TB was similar to VD. He followed patients, conducted screening, interviewed contacts, and went into the field to identify people who had been exposed or who had to complete their TB treatment. The primary difference for John was that he had to prove himself in the TB Program. By 1962, PHAs were an established part of VD programs after several years of proving their value. By the time John was hired as a co-op, he did not need to prove himself in VD, but he did have to convince his TB Program hosts in Detroit of his value as a public health worker in the TB effort. PHAs were a new concept, and public health nurses in TB programs were understandably threatened. As with VD, the TB Program staff came to appreciate the PHAs' contribution. John found his experience with TB highly gratifying, as it would prepare him for a public health career that included the emergence of AIDS. The devastating experiences that PHAs and others in public health faced with AIDS were presaged by tuberculosis in the 1960s:

> The people with tuberculosis were very sick. Every morning when we came to a hospital we would get a roster, and there would always be at least three or four who had died from tuberculosis. They hadn't taken their drugs. You've got to remember this is back in

1962. We didn't have a lot of drugs like we have now. We had INH (isonicotinyl hydrazine or isoniazid). We had a few of the other drugs. These people were sick and they were dying. As bad as some of the places were in STD, with tuberculosis it was a younger group. A lot of children involved, a lot of women involved, a lot of alcoholics who were on their last days. And when winter came and the flu hit, it just decimated our caseload.[31]

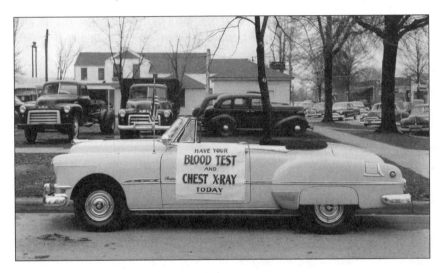

Tuberculosis and syphilis screening announcement, Arkansas. Circa 1950s. Courtesy Centers for Disease Control and Prevention, Global Health Odyssey.

PHAs helped TB programs ramp up to handle the ever-increasing case numbers in the mid 1960s, and they deployed in response to outbreaks. In 1965 John Seggerson was working in Wilkes-Barre, Pennsylvania, as a regional TB rep. His role was administrative and supervisory, but like any PHA, he was prepared to assist with the fieldwork:

> I was responsible for managing TB activities, working with the TB programs, and the nursing supervisors who ran all the Public Health Programs. I covered all of northeastern Pennsylvania, though there was a tremendous amount of TB in Lackawanna and Luzerne Counties. Sometimes I would go out in the field when there was difficulty with a patient. Generally, I was on the road

> trying to provide technical assistance to get folks established, to use TB registers, and to review those registers to increase the percent of patients on therapy.[32]

John's career would lead him to the role of TB field services chief at CDC headquarters. In 1977 he was in this role when called to work the first community-wide drug-resistant TB outbreak occurring in Alcorn, Mississippi. The outbreak demonstrated the challenge facing TB programs in the previous decade, as it was later linked to an ongoing community outbreak dating back to 1964.[33] Dr. J. Donald "Don" Millar was leading the Bureau of state services at CDC and needed help with the epidemic.[34] He had a great deal of respect for PHAs from his smallpox service (See Chapter 7). In 1977 he sat down with John to discuss the continuing outbreak in Alcorn, Mississippi which had begun a year earlier. CDC thought it had been controlled; however, by then it was clear the outbreak was still going strong. Don needed help from PHAs, and he expected that John could help him. Don's unabashed confidence in PHAs was not news to John who been a PHA since 1963 and had been part of the national effort to eradicate syphilis prior to his work in TB. When Don Millar learned that the Alcorn County TB outbreak was not under control, he called on the problem solvers to deal with it. John was among a unique cohort of public health workers who were viewed by others at CDC as problem solvers. Don bluntly stated the value of PHAs which by then was becoming well understood in Atlanta:

> You know how we fix problems? We implement what you guys recommend. You know how we fix problems at CDC, don't you? We throw a PHA at it. So I want you to get the best damn PHAs you can get your hands on and send them to Mississippi![35]

PHAs were detailed to help stop the Mississippi TB epidemic, and they would go on to contribute significantly to Mississippi TB, immunization, and STD programs generally. Dr. Ed Thompson worked with PHAs throughout his career, but never more closely than during the period from 1982 to 2000, when he served as the Mississippi state epidemiologist and later as state health director. PHA contributions in immunization, STD, and TB were innumerable, according to Thompson. They included the drop in syphilis rates, the increase in immunization rates, the drop in TB rates, and the establishment of program operations in all three public health efforts. Thompson recalled his experience with PHAs in TB while serving in Mississippi:

> We had a number of Public Health Advisors, but the one that I remember the most was Larry Sabrero... Through his efforts and later through the efforts of state health department employees—some of whom Larry helped to teach and train—we brought Mississippi's TB case rate below the national average for the first time in thirty-two years. It was a conscious effort. We set a target of bringing that case rate below the national average and did it through directly-observed therapy.[36]

The role of PHAs in TB programs was primarily managerial, unless the area was resource-poor and required them to work in the field. Generally, PHAs were assigned to state and local health department TB programs as their coordinators. These assignees would help to ensure that the TB programs' core elements were accomplished: surveillance, targeted clinical education, coordinated medical care and follow-up, and employee development and training. PHAs who were assigned to state TB programs through the 1980s tended to be in a "solo assignment," or working as the lone federal employee in a state or local health department. This difference was more than likely due to the lack of federal funds for TB as compared with resources for Immunization and VD Programs.[37]

In the 1960s and during the time that the TB Program was recruiting several PHAs from VD, the Immunization Program effort was ramping up and recruiting several of them as well. Harold Mauldin initially directed field operations for the newly-formed Immunization Program and soon become the program's deputy director, eventually recruiting, training and supervising over one hundred PHAs that were assigned to every state, major city and U.S. territory to run Immunization programs.[38] In 1963 he arrived in Atlanta to find a nascent program that desperately needed someone to get things going. To succeed, the program would need to use existing relationships with the states. As a Public Health Advisor, Harold brought with him both operational skill and strong local relationships. Knowing how to integrate the Immunization Program into state health department operations was critical to the program's success. Initial CDC efforts to find a home for the Immunization Program in state health departments put the success of vaccination outcomes at risk. CDC was trying to sell the new immunization effort to states as a Maternal Child Health (MCH) program. Harold knew from experience that

MCH program culture was different than epidemiologically-inclined programs, and therefore would imperil the achievement of Vaccine Assistance Act objectives. He quickly reoriented CDC's approach upon his arrival in Atlanta:

> They came to North Carolina trying to sell this program. I told them they were going to the wrong people. They were going to [get] MCH people to run the thing. MCH did not have the aggressive kind of approach. So when I did in fact come down [to CDC] I went back to North Carolina and met with [division director] Doc Ford. He said, "Harold, can you give me somebody to run the program?" And I said, "Yep." He said, "It's all yours." In less than an hour, that program got started... We in fact sold the program state by state that way.[39]

PHAs began to arrive in the states that accepted what Harold Mauldin and colleagues sold: a state immunization program funded under the Vaccination Assistance Act, managed by a PHA and staffed by state and federal personnel. The new Immunization Program had three goals: reach five million unimmunized children, provide booster shots to nine million children, and develop early immunization programs across the country.[40] Within two years, it became clear that if CDC were to make an impact on childhood illnesses, children who were difficult to reach would need to be the primary focus.[41] When the Vaccination Assistance Act was renewed in 1965, funding was added for measles, diphtheria, whooping cough, tetanus, and polio.[42] PHAs were in great demand, and the Immunization and TB Programs offered them opportunities to transfer out of the VD Program and broaden their public health experience. The Immunization Program also would serve as a career ladder for PHAs, because it recruited those above entry-level co-op and GS-7 levels. PHAs were hired in the Immunization Program at GS-9 or GS-11 levels with further promotion possible when placed in the states with increasing responsibility.[43]

John Shimmens was one of six PHAs called for an interview to be part of the initial Immunization Program. Like other PHAs in the program's early days, he called upon his community organization skills from VD, organizing screening on a county-by-county basis for VD and, by this time, for TB as well. John called on the same skill for an early measles campaign. He recalls working county-by-county:

> Early in 1963, I had a chance to go with a brand new program called immunization. Then the first big program came in. It was measles. That was another huge statewide coordination project. We were trying to do mass immunization. We had jet injector guns back in those days. It was mostly a school-based program, so we were setting up programs throughout the state, county after county after county. We'd move into a county usually on a Monday morning, start off with the schools, and do that whole county. Come back over the weekend, clean our guns, get everything ready, get new vaccine, and go out the next weekend. I was gone a lot back then.[44]

From 1963 to 1965, PHAs worked diligently to establish a national system of state-directed immunization efforts. As with efforts in VD, immunization funding would variously target particular conditions based on disease incidence and policy interest. By 1965, interest in the Vietnam War would put the renewal of the Vaccination Act at risk and redirect the policy focus to rubella, or German measles. As with the historical policy focus shifts from syphilis to gonorrhea and back to syphilis in a matter of fifteen years (1948–1963), federal policy focus in immunization shifted from polio to measles, to rubella, and back to measles following the reporting of forty thousand measles cases in 1970—a hundred percent increase over 1968.[45] This occurred even after a 1967 effort to eradicate measles. The campaign was a success, as demonstrated by a seventy percent reduction in reported cases of measles by 1968.[46] As with syphilis, however, when measles cases declined, so did the funding.

Steve Barid was assigned to a local Immunization Program in Nashville, Tennessee. Hired as a VD co-op in 1964 to work in Chicago, Barid joined the Immunization Program in 1967. Tennessee did not have a state program, so CDC worked with local city and county health departments to achieve the immunization goals. There was a flurry of activity in those days. Steve recalls that while he felt as though he and other local reps were "out there on our own," they would not have made it without support from Jack Benson in the Regional Office and from their PHA colleagues who were running the state TB and VD programs:

> Immunization had started doing a fair amount of recruiting in late 1963, and was expanding. Tennessee did not want a state program, so they had guys assigned in Memphis, Knoxville, Chattanooga and Nashville. Burt Russell, the state TB rep, and Ralph Burke, the state VD rep, would stop by and hold our hands on occasion

> and assure us that everything was really okay in spite of the way we were feeling. Jack Benson called us daily from the regional office to fill in whatever gaps Ralph and Burt hadn't... It was a local program, but actually a really good opportunity. At that time we had four full-time employees and a bunch of part-time employees because we were doing a lot of house-to-house canvassing.[47]

The efforts of PHAs in immunization programs would make a major contribution toward reducing childhood diseases in the United States. In 1977, PHAs would help to assure that ninety-five percent of the children entering school in the U.S. were immunized against the key childhood diseases. Former CDC director William Foege recalls how the effort emerged during the Carter Administration, and that PHAs helped to secure the success. The newly-elected President Carter, at the urging of Betty and Senator Dale Bumpers, told HEW Secretary Joseph Califano to improve immunizations among school children:

> Califano came to CDC, and he wanted to have a real initiative... I can recall Califano asking, "Could we reach ninety percent of all school children by the time they go to school?".... When that goal was achieved, it rested largely on Public Health Advisors in the states, [who] made this happen. Very quickly, none of us would settle for ninety percent. We got up to ninety-one, ninety-two, ninety-four, and ninety-five percent.[48]

The successes of U.S. immunization efforts stoked international confidence that they could be replicated elsewhere. In 1974, the United States committed to the World Health Organization's Expanded Program on Immunization. Three years later, CDC would play a major role by providing scientific and operational personnel for long-term assignments. Polio was a major focus, and by the late 1980s, the effort would have major funding from governments and private organizations, including Rotary International.[49] Tony Scardaci was among several Public Health Advisors who served the initial international efforts in immunization. His experience was with smallpox, and later with polio (see Chapter 7).

As with most PHAs of this era, Tony was hired in 1963 by the VD program as part of a national syphilis eradication effort. He worked in several California cities until he was picked in 1968 as one of the two PHAs (with Elvin Hilyer) to help set the newly-transferred quarantine program on track at CDC. The Foreign Quarantine Service had been a prestigious part of the Public Health Service since 1878, though in CDC's view it was "essentially bankrupt" and a waste of human resources. More than six hundred highly-paid Quarantine personnel—among them a few former assistant surgeons general—were located in ports throughout the world, in international airports, and at U.S. borders to give vaccinations, gather epidemiologic data, and conduct examinations of persons applying for entry into the U.S.[50] Tony and Elvin helped senior CDC and Quarantine Program officials reorganize the program, supervise the reduction of unnecessary personnel, and set the course for an early warning system that would help to target the use of personnel. Tony left his post as the chief of program operations for the Quarantine Program in 1974 to work in the CDC Washington Office. While working there, Tony got an unusual offer from Director Dave Sencer:

> Dave was up for an appropriations hearing.... We were going out to lunch before the hearing, and I felt a hand on my shoulder. We had not made up our mind where we were going. There was a place called The Deli, and what I heard was, "Do you want to go to The Deli?" I said, "Sure Dave, wherever you want to go to lunch is fine with me." He grabbed my shoulder and he turned me around and he said, "No. I said, do you want to go to New Delhi?"[51]

Sencer asked Tony to become the senior management staff member in India's Regional Office for Smallpox Eradication. Tony accepted the role. He and his family moved to New Delhi in June of 1975.

By the end of the 1960s, other domestic CDC efforts were using PHAs to manage and develop programs and to conduct some fieldwork. Health Mobilization, Urban Rat Control, and Chronic Disease Programs were among them, though their use of PHAs was either limited or brief. The Urban Rat Control Program was transferred to CDC after a federal reorganization in the early 1970s and had fewer than ten PHAs in the field for a job that was traditionally held by sanitarians.[52] Both the Rat Control and the Health Mobilization Programs were discontinued by the mid-1980s. Initially and through the mid-1990s, Diabetes Control Program field assignments for PHAs tended to be solo: one PHA would work with the state and local area (including Indian Health Service assignments) to coordinate the diabetes control efforts, identifying needed resources, providing surveillance systems, and evaluating the program.[53] By 1978, the Diabetes Program had eleven PHAs working in the field,[54] though they called in their field assignees in the mid

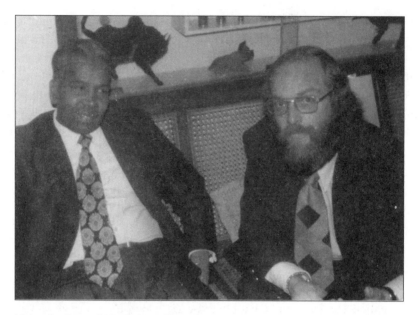

Mahendra Dutta, M.D. (left) and Tony Scardaci. According to Tony, "Dr. Dutta worked at the national level in India and was a significant force behind the success of smallpox eradication in India." Circa 1975.
Courtesy of Tony Scardaci

1990s.[55] By the late 1980s, there were Public Health Advisors in nearly all CDC programs, working in local assignments or at CDC headquarters, monitoring everything from environmental health to refugee health.[56] The growth of programs at CDC in the 1960s was mirrored by the growth in the number of Public Health Advisors working in them. In December of 1969, 605 PHAs were working in the VD, TB, and Immunization Programs. The majority (seventy-six percent) remained in VD, which reflected the national syphilis eradication efforts. At that time the TB Program had seventy-one PHAs working in Atlanta and placed in the field, and the Immunization Program had seventy-six PHAs working at CDC headquarters and placed in state and local health departments.[57]

An example of perhaps the more significant of recent contributions by PHAs to programs beyond VD is with HIV. While the story of HIV—its emergence and the U.S. government's response—often has been written, what is relatively unknown is the immediate response inside CDC when the early signs of HIV emerged, and when the agency needed "all hands on deck" to make a national

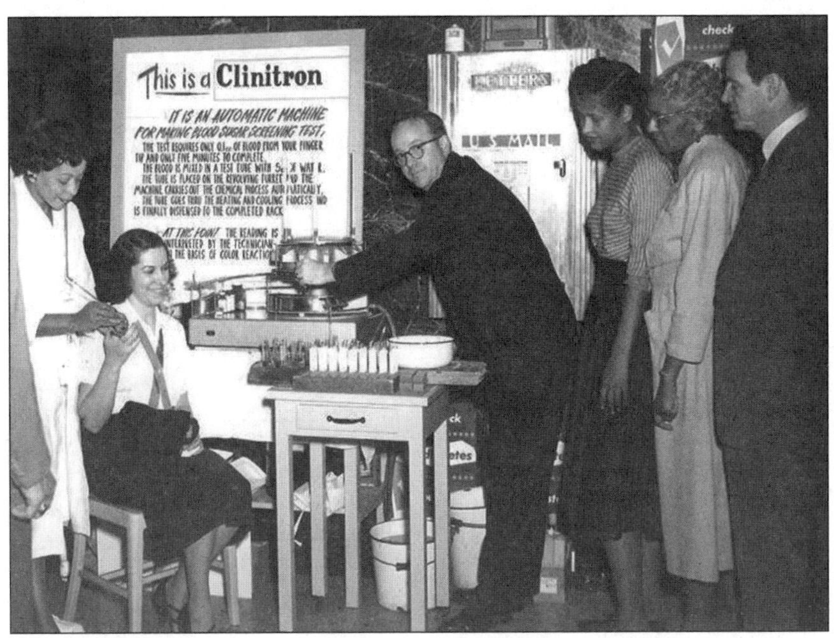

Jack Pendleton (center) and staff of the Washington, D.C. Northwest Health Care Center providing testing for Diabetes. Circa 1961.
Courtesy Jack Pendleton.

---

program of epidemiology, education, and testing occur. Dr. Bill Foege recalls that when HIV was emerging and before it was even called HIV, PHAs and others at CDC quickly shifted resources to make things happen. According to Bill, this history is "what gets lost or forgotten when people go back and look at budget lines and try to figure out whether the federal government put enough resources into this." The amazing story about CDC is that even in this recent time, the agency was sufficiently flexible to shift resources to help address the problem. Bill recalls:

> If you have a problem at CDC, you simply borrow people. And so immediately, Paul Weisner, who was the director of STD Division, put his own people toward trying to solve this problem. This included Public Health Advisors. They were involved right from the beginning. And I always think Paul doesn't get the credit that he deserves for the immediate decision on his part to divert resources to try to figure out what was happening.[58]

There was no budget for anything in HIV—clinical research, epidemiologic investigations, information development, program operations, or support. Windell Bradford was the deputy of the STD Division at the time. "There was no money," Windell recalls, "but we made it happen." Windell believes the STD Division was unfairly labeled an "ostrich" on the issue of HIV. It was this group that initiated the first information campaign about the new and fatal agent in 1983:

> Of course, it was during the Reagan Administration. Jim Mason was then the director of CDC. He was quite conservative and not, in my opinion, particularly interested in taking tough stands against Reagan and the other conservatives. We got nowhere agreeing on prevention messages that would be appropriate. But it was us, the "ostriches" who supposedly had their heads in the sand, who immediately came up with prevention messages that made sense for preventing a fatal, sexually transmitted disease. We soon found out that the government simply did not say those things.[59]

Dr. Jim Curran, now the dean of the Emory University School of Public Health, pulled together people from all over the agency with the help of PHA Wilmon Rushing. At that time, Jim was leading the clinical research section of the STD Division, when it was suggested that he get Wilmon's help. "They told Wilmon that I didn't know how to delegate,"[60] Jim said, continuing:

> Wilmon managed the AIDS activities with no money. We had people detailed from all over CDC and from the field, with little money for travel or other activities. So we struggled along and worked really hard and eventually got some resources. Then we were moved into the Center for Infectious Diseases where few PHAs had previously been assigned. We recruited over two hundred people; many of the best, and won the science awards, and even the HHS Equal Opportunity Achievement Award. The latter was easy because we merely hired a few top-notch women and minority supervisors. Many other great women and minorities wanted to work for them and work on HIV/AIDS. Responding to this epidemic was a group effort, working with good people and treating them right. A lot of it was that our effort was well-managed. Wilmon and his other PHA colleagues were key to that.[61]

Well-managed was an understatement. Wilmon was joined by another PHA,

Larry Zyla, who managed operations. Russ Havlak remembers that while "Jim Curran was attacking the scientific problems and stirring up the nation about AIDS, Wilmon and Larry took care of business and sweated the details."[62] What made the HIV effort work was an organizational design that would help this clearly cross-functioning group work in a traditionally siloed CDC organization. Wilmon knew he needed the help of a PHA who was famous for his organizational design skill and vision: Bob Kingon. Bob was glad to help out, and remembered the ninety-day effort in 1986:

> Wilmon Rushing helped me to get up and running and provided a lot of support. The question was how do we organize HIV, because it cuts across nearly all of the Centers and program offices (at CDC)? I spent three months interviewing everybody with a stake in the HIV program and came up with three proposals. We settled upon a matrix organization managed by an Office of the Associate Director for HIV in the Office of the Director of CDC. Dr. Gary Noble was the first person to take that spot, and Bill Parra was his Deputy. Bill did an outstanding job of getting the new structure functional and performing at a high level.[63]

CDC could contribute a valuable asset to the fight against AIDS: a national network of PHAs and grant relationships with states. PHAs at CDC headquarters and in the field stepped up to the plate, even though it was not clear just what was needed. Windell recalls that without PHAs in the field throughout the country, nothing would have been implemented quickly: "They played the same role they often played, and that was getting something off the ground, totally new, very quickly, and with the idea of trying to evaluate it as you went along."[65] Jim Curran recalls the strength and challenges of this national system grounded in STD experience and culture:

> The strength is that the STD Division had staff in the field, and they also had a mechanism of getting the money out and holding the people accountable for it. The weakness of it was that it was married to an STD approach, which was very clinical, not behavioral, and also was not at all community-based, and it had to learn. And I think it did a pretty good job of that.

The STD Division contributed its assets to the effort, and PHAs at CDC headquarters moved mountains to get things done in the midst of political barriers and lack of clarity from the federal government on AIDS. Russ Havlak remembers the incredible speed with which CDC was able to work. At the time he was directing the Training and Education Branch of the STD Division. He recalls that during this period things were spinning quickly and all attention was diverted away from anything related to STD and toward addressing this emerging entity, soon to be called HIV. In 1985, "HIV/AIDS became virtually all we were about":

> When FDA licensed the HIV antibody test that February, HIV/AIDS became operational at CDC. Our Center (it wasn't called that at the time) got that task. The STD Division was the obvious choice to take it on, and the TEC Section was Ground Zero for almost two years. HIV/AIDS consumed us, and while we continued a measured STD training schedule, most of our efforts focused on train-the-trainer activities for delivering a course on HIV-test counseling. As the rest of the 1980s saw, the entire STD Division became consumed with HIV/AIDS: it got to the point that the TEC Section was the only division entity doing anything with state/local STD programs. By that time, we had incorporated HIV-test counseling into the basic interview training because STD staffs all over were being called on to respond.[66]

In January of 1985 the FDA announced that it would license the first antibody test for AIDS within six weeks. "This meant that we were poised to abruptly transfer HIV/AIDS from an exclusively research and surveillance phenomenon to a full-blown operational issue," Russ said. Without a national network of PHAs, the large scale education efforts which were implemented in a stunningly short period of time throughout the country would have been impossible. Trainings were planned for all major U.S. cities focused on counseling those who would learn about their HIV status initially through blood donation because blood banks were the first and only locations selected to use the newly licensed test. This meant that donating blood would be the only opportunity to learn of one's HIV status. "Then something happened that shook us to the core," said Russ. Jim Curran heard from several contacts in the community that gay men would begin to use blood banks to learn of their HIV status since FDA limited access to the test. "Members of one of the highest known risk groups for HIV suddenly flooding blood banks would most certainly threaten the nation's blood supply rather than protect it," recalls Russ. CDC reacted quickly to plan alternate HIV testing sites throughout the country and to get a program of testing and counseling mobilized before the blood banks initiated HIV testing. The effort was swift. With the help of PHAs throughout CDC Russ' group was able to scrape together five million dollars, get HHS to match that amount, and initiate emergency grants to states. He remembers: "We gave states an unprecedented five working days to submit a grant application. They came in on Friday at the close of business. We pulled together every PHA in CDC and started reviewing them at 4:00 p.m., working through the night…until noon Sunday."[67]

The HIV-test counseling effort is one of the earliest and most widespread of the national responses to HIV. Even before much was known about the agent causing this unusual and deadly health condition, the country called upon CDC to provide information and techniques to help people understand their diagnosis and to think about behavior change even if they are found to be negative. State and local health departments, and specifically disease investigators, needed clear and accurate information to provide to their clients and the public. PHAs in the field witnessed the terrible outcomes of this devastating disease. John Miles recalled losing forty-seven of his staff members, "almost one a week," to HIV/AIDS. Phil Finley, who was working in Lauderhill, Florida, recalls how it felt to work with folks in the community during this very challenging time:

> I would say the most frightening thing at that time was that the choices of therapy were slim, and universal access to therapy meant that your HIV status may have to be revealed by a private doctor or healthcare facility in order to obtain medications. What I recall most about being a disease investigator in the 1980s was the uncertainty of life and how long an HIV infected individual would live. It was not uncommon for people to live only six months to a year after diagnosis.[68]

Bob Kohmescher was working in Raleigh, North Carolina when he was called in to do a series of presentations about the new FDA approved test. CDC was trying to help communities allay concerns about the test and deliver correct messages to those who tested for it. Communities were scared, overwhelmed, and also frustrated with what had seemed like slow or inappropriate effort. PHAs were often the targets of community frustration because they represented the federal, state, and local governments. Bob recalls being booed for the first time in his life:

> This was my first experience at actually being booed and having people in the audience yelling and screaming and that sort of thing, because AIDS activists were very skeptical about the tests... This was in February of 1985 shortly before the FDA's approval of the HTLV-III/LAV antibody test. We sent people out and covered the entire country to give presentations in every large city.[69]

Bob was among a team of four whom Russ Havlak chose to join him to conduct "train the trainer" sessions focused on counseling people who were testing for HIV, and those who tested positive. Fred Martich was one of the four PHAs chosen to help the effort. He remembers Russ' contributions:

> Russ gets loads of credit for developing the first pre-and post-test HIV counseling sessions. He was extremely sensitive to the needs of infected persons. At the time, many folks in the community, especially the gay community, were very concerned about government intrusion with counseling. The general public saw HIV/AIDS at the time as a death notice, so identifying someone through counseling was not too well-accepted.[70]

The PHA contribution in HIV/AIDS also extended to other CDC areas. Jim Curran argues that although a few PHAs were functioning as deputies in the 1980s and early 1990s, Wilmon Rushing's example opened up the rest of CDC to PHAs as high-level deputies:

> Wilmon Rushing was a brilliant guy. He became deputy director for the Center for Infectious Disease before he retired and was recognized as one of the best people at CDC. In this role, he moved out of TB, showing people that his skills were translatable. This helped to open [up roles for] PHAs throughout CDC.[71]

The 1960s and early 1970s were a time of program expansion for Public Health Advisors. This period also would be the time when CDC committed to hiring women and minorities. In contrast with the PHAs' rapid expansion into other CDC programs, the gender, race and ethnic diversification of the PHA cohort took a long time and was not without difficulty. Two men are thought to be the first African American Public Health Advisors. Although Public Health Service records for the VD Division are no longer in existence, PHA interviews permit one to estimate that Albert "Al" Billingslea was hired as a co-op in

Philadelphia around 1954,[72] and that around this time George Love was hired in the VD program as a co-op, though the location is not known.[73] Al Billingslea worked with Bill Doyle in Chicago in 1955 and earned his GS-9 and GS-11 promotions there.[74] In the late 1950s Al transferred to California as the state rep for the VD program,[75] returning in the early 1960s to Chicago to work in the Immunization Program. He resigned from CDC around 1966 to work in the Appalachian Regional Commission's Appalachian Program, which was initiated at that time to build capacity to sustain economic development in the region's most distressed counties.[76]

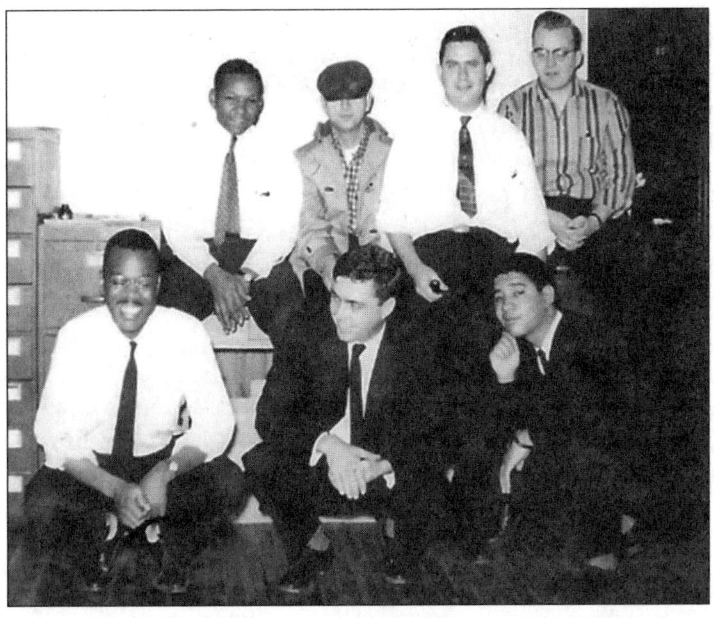

Chicago VD program staff in 1957. Front left to right: Bob Nelson (city), Lee Schuck (PHA), Al Billingslea (PHA). Back left to right: (unidentified, city), Jules Bednoe (PHA), Bill Doyle (PHA), Don Underwood (PHA).
Courtesy Bill Doyle.

Less is known about George Love. Frank Miller recalls George as his first supervisor in the Detroit VD Program in 1964. George later was transferred to Denver, and then he transferred to the Family Planning Program, leaving CDC by the end of the 1960s. Frank inquired about other African American PHAs early in his PHA tenure, and was told that the first African American PHA was serving in California. This may have been Al Billingslea.[77] Frank believes he was the third or fourth African American PHA hired, which means that the process of hiring racially and ethnically diverse staff was slow. In 1970, as CDC's equal employment official, Frank would have to push the agency to diversify its workforce. Despite the challenges, he considered it one of the top three assignments in his career:

> Keep in mind that 1970 was only two and a half years after the colored and white signs had been removed from the doors of CDC restrooms. The highest-graded official at CDC of African American descent was a GS-13 section chief named Norman Hayes. He was head of the Research Animal Section of the Animal Resources Branch of CDC at the time.[78]

Frank Miller's observations reflect the staff's slow diversification, despite the purported effort to recruit African American men as PHAs in the late 1950s.[79] By the 1960s, however, a major program was in place to recruit African American men. This effort eventually yielded a greater racial and ethnic diversity among the PHA cohort. Recruiter John Narkunas remembers:

> Although we were not able to recruit female candidates, we accelerated our efforts to attract African American male candidates. The competition for such candidates was fierce on college campuses, but we were able to recruit some top-notch people despite the handicap of a low starting salary.[80]

Despite the recruitment efforts of the 1960s, African American PHAs were not necessarily welcomed with open arms when it came to working in particular communities. A system was in place to limit their assignments to particular cities through what was called a "closed offer." John Heath left a job at the Internal Revenue Service to become a PHA in 1968. He was surprised to be given limited placement choices at a time when syphilis clearly was requiring widespread and national efforts:

> Even though it was a national program, I was offered assignments in Baltimore, D.C., NYC, Chicago, and L.A. The closed offer meant that based on my race and ethnicity, those were the only areas that they would assign me. At the time I couldn't be assigned to the other

> states because of political considerations. This was also a time when CDC had just begun hiring minorities. They did not have that many minorities in the program, so to some extent I was a part of the pioneer effort, if you will, in terms of minority recruitment.[81]

Four years prior to John's hiring, Frank Miller received a similar closed offer. He did not realize that his choices were being circumscribed until years later, when he became an EEO Officer. It was then that he learned there were no African American PHAs in professional positions in the South. Frank recalls his hiring experience and what lay behind the closed offer. Like every new hire, he was asked to identify his top few choices for co-op locations:

> I listed South Carolina, but was told "you can't go to your home state." So I said Georgia, Alabama, Tennessee, and Florida. I'm from the South. Do you know what assignments were offered to me? Detroit, New York, Chicago, and L.A. State and local health departments throughout the South, from Texas over to Kentucky up to Virginia, would not accept minorities of color, particularly African Americans, in professional positions in their state and local health departments.[81]

In 1965, Charles Watkins was hired as a TB rep and placed in New York City. He was given credit for the co-op experience because of his prior work in TB on a CDC contract in Hudson County, New Jersey. One year later he was transferred to St. Louis, Missouri. Charles went to St. Louis with "much trepidation, a little bit of apprehension, and plain old fear," not because he was a relatively new type of worker in the TB program, but because he had not been west of the Mississippi. This self-described "New Jersey kid" recalls the internal conversation and his surprise with the new assignment:

> Being an Afro-American to start with, you think, "What am I going to face here, what kind of doctor, who is this person I'm going to meet?" I knew nothing about Dr. Bill Banton, who was the sitting TB Control Officer in St. Louis… is he prejudiced against black guys? How am I going to be perceived? ... I walk into the City Health Department, meet the Commissioner, who was Dr. Jay Earl Smith, well-known in the Middle West as a big city health commissioner; he was a tough old cookie… Right away I'm scared to

> death. He marches me down the hall to meet Dr. William C. Banton, who turns out to be black and also a fraternity brother.[83]

By 1972 African American men were making their way into the CDC leadership, and the experiences of John Heath, Frank Miller, and Charles Watkins reflected it. John was promoted steadily throughout his career as a PHA and now is leading the STD Program in Washington, D.C. Although he has been given many opportunities to go elsewhere, he favors the unique aspects of working in the Beltway and credits his success with years of compounded experience as a PHA. In 1971 Charles Watkins was promoted to a GS-13 to work in the Southern Regional Office, located in Atlanta. This was a time when it was unusual to see an African American in the Regional Office, and Charles felt that he was well-accepted in his role because of the tremendous reputation of PHAs and of CDC. In 1971 the Regional Office was "made up of a bunch of old white men, and there weren't many persons of color in any department except for Joe Carter."[84] Charles Watkins would spend the next twenty years in the Regional Office system, and his last position with CDC would be as the director of regional operations. He would oversee the historic closing of CDC's Regional Office system in 1994. Charles retired two years later, in 1996, and continues to work periodically for CDC in various projects, including preparedness, HIV/AIDS, and workforce development. In 2004 he reflected on the particular challenge facing African American Public Health Advisors:

> One thing that many black Public Health Advisors have had to do is be "super reps." We've had to be able to live in a white culture and belong to a black culture, and cross over one to another and to tie them together in order to progress.[85]

Progress definitely was occurring for African American men, as evidenced by those in senior leadership positions today. Joseph Carter was the first African American PHA among the Regional Office leadership, preceding Charles Watkins by a matter of months. Like Frank Miller, Joe began as a co-op in Detroit's VD program in 1964. Throughout his stellar career, Joe had multiple leadership opportunities. He retired in 2004 as the director for Management and Operations for CDC—the first African American to hold this senior executive position. Joe calls this the "crowning point of his career" because in this position, he served the first African American CDC director—Dr. David

Satcher—and the first woman CDC director—Dr. Julie Gerberding. Joe retired, and is now the President and CEO of Carter Consulting, Inc., a firm that supplies CDC with executive management expertise (see Chapter 8).

During the 1970s, another type of expansion among Public Health Advisors occurred: the gender diversification of the PHA cadre. From 1948 until at least the late 1950s, Public Health Advisors tended to be white and male. When the early co-ops were hired in the late 1940s, women showed little interest in joining this new cohort of public health worker. Women certainly were working in the local-level public health field and specifically in VD programs as nurses, social workers, and clerical workers. By the mid-1950s there was some talk that women would make good disease investigators. Women's effectiveness as investigators was witnessed by PHAs at the local level and by Johannes Stuart. By this time, a few women had been working as local health department VD investigators, and a successful World War II effort had used female prostitutes as interviewers in Rapid Treatment Centers.[86] According to Bill Watson, in 1955 Johannes Stuart decided that he wanted to add women to the co-op experiment, and hired six female co-ops in Chicago. Unlike the original experiment, these women left the job within a year. Bill is the only person to recall this effort and its outcome; yet it seems likely that Johannes Stuart would have attempted such a strategy, given his sense of equity and his vision for public health. Bill remembers when Stuart decided to hire women:

> He decided we ought to have some Public Health Advisors who were women, so he selected Chicago as the place to do it. He worked it out with the Health Department and went there and did the recruiting of people who were graduating from colleges in the Chicago area. He hired six, as I remember... They were co-ops. They were doing the same kind of work as everybody else... Well, in that kind of work, it was not something that they liked to do, and it was scary. The failure in Chicago really kept us from getting back into hiring women and delayed that unduly.[87]

By the 1960s there was increasing talk about hiring female co-ops as part of the federal complement, because by that time women had demonstrated that they were successful VD investigators as employees of local and state VD programs. The barrier to women's acceptance as co-ops and PHAs lay with the VD Program at CDC, whose prevailing stance was that this was no job for a woman. The federal job appeared to be constructed for a man, and primarily a white man at that. A comparison of a 1968 recruitment brochure with that of the (circa) 1980s indicates the evolution of thinking about the recruitment audience (below and opposite):

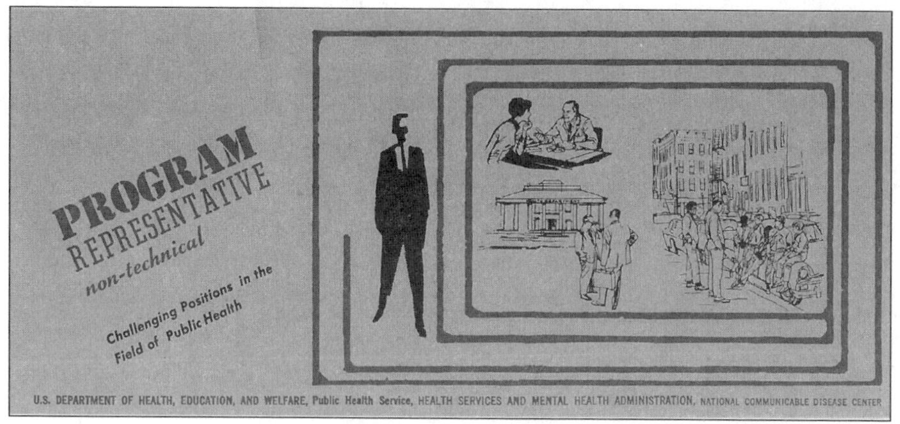

U.S. Department of Health, Education, and Welfare recruitment brochure for Public Health Advisors or "Program Representative," 1968.
Courtesy of Ken Latimer.

John Narkunas was a PHA recruiter for the VD Program at CDC from 1965 to 1967. He worked in New York City and recruited future co-ops throughout the Northeast U.S. During this period John met, interviewed, and sent forth the applications of several female candidates; however, headquarters never considered these women because the leadership believed that "the job was too dangerous for women to be working in high-crime urban areas."[88] Potential danger in a PHA's job was not to be taken lightly, even for the men John recruited. Despite the danger, plenty of female applicants were interested and able to do the work. The local VD investigators faced no less dangerous conditions, and women were among their ranks.

When John became the chief recruiter for the VD branch in 1967, he and others decided to push for change by unilaterally forwarding the names of successful women applicants. For the next three years, John and the other recruiters—Dave Puckett, Rick Crankshaw, Bob Baldwin, Roger Bernier, Orlando Blancato, and Joe Smith—offered to the VD Program the names of successful women candidates. The recruiters knew they were crossing a boundary defined by an unwrit-

Career Development

CDC greatly emphasizes developing the full potential of all staff in the agency and has devised many mechanisms for assuring that staff are fully trained for the job to be performed and that opportunities are provided for career-enhancing experiences. These aids include annual surveys of training needs, preparation of individual career development plans, agency-sponsored training and educational courses, opportunities for long-term academic training, short-term assignments in different programs, and special programs such as the management/leadership development program.

Other Benefits

Public Health Associates are entitled to most federal Civil Service benefits as Public Health Advisors in the regular Civil Service, for example, retirement, health and life insurance, thrift savings plan, and vacation and sick leave. New employees without previous federal or military service are entitled to 13 days of vacation leave; employees with more than 3 years of service receive 20 days of vacation leave; and employees with more than 15 years of service receive 26 days of vacation leave. All employees are also entitled to 13 days of sick leave each year.

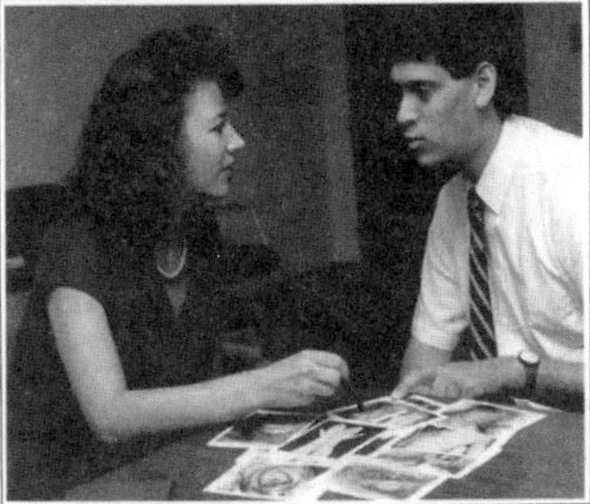

Counseling patient to accept difficult nature of his communicable disease

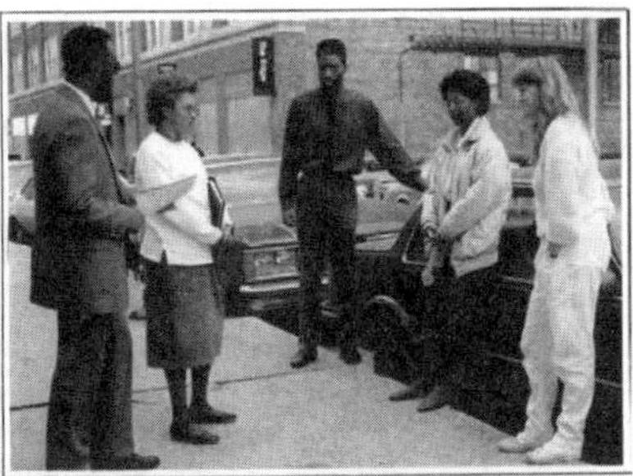

Getting information to control Legionnaire's disease outbreak. Work included blood testing, circulating "at risk" questionnaire, locating and sampling air conditioning reservoirs where people were believed to be infected.

Qualification Requirements

General

Applicants must be citizens of the United States and must possess or obtain a valid driver's license within 30 days of employment.

Because the field staff provides assistance to State and local health departments throughout the United States and its territories, all candidates must be willing to accept initial assignment anywhere in the United States and to travel and relocate as required for program needs and career development. Initial training takes place at a limited number of sites around the country. Travel to the initial assignment must be at the appointee's own expense. All other travel and relocation expenses are covered by CDC within the limitations of federal travel regulations.

Portion of a CDC recruitment brochure for Public Health Advisors, circa 1980s. Courtesy of Jack Benson.

ten rule not to hire women PHAs, a rule that was "frequently reinforced by incidents in the field where reps had experienced physical or mental trauma."[89] Despite the challenges, these recruiters strongly believed that times had to change, so they continued to force the issue for the VD Program. John Narkunas recalls that hiring policy changes followed the passage of the landmark Title IX and efforts to pass the Equal Rights Amendment in 1972:

> The recruitment of female candidates changed shortly after I left recruiting in 1970. The passage of Title IX in 1972 improved the status of women, and I heard that the STD program was aggressively recruiting female case finders in the early seventies. It was

> something long overdue, and it certainly upgraded the quality of our field staff and managers, as exemplified by the many outstanding female managers that have since moved from the 685 series into other programs at CDC… It was a long time coming, but eventually the VD/STD Program and CDC got it right![90]

The first female PHAs are believed to be Penny Friedberg, Susan Bass, and Janella Apodaca.[91] They were hired first by the New York City Health Department in the spring of 1970 to work side-by-side with PHAs. Bob Baldwin, a recruiter working in the Northeast U.S., was trying to solve a problem for Norman "Norm" Scherzer, who was the lead PHA, or "city rep," for New York City's VD program. Bob remembers that the federal hiring freeze was "dragging on interminably, with no relief in sight":

> Meanwhile, the federal complement assigned to VD in the City was dwindling. Norm came to me one day and said, "We have got to do something to shore up the ranks." He challenged me to think along non-traditional lines—how about hiring some different categories of staff and let them be New York City Health Department employees? So I came up with a scheme… [to hire] folks who had degrees and who I thought could do this job regardless of gender, or ethnic background, or college major. Penny and Susan fell into this category and turned out to be the first female VD investigators working side by side with feds in New York City.[92]

Bob, Norm, and all the recruiters were pushing for more women candidates. They believed the archaic and undocumented hiring barrier for women was ridiculous and unfair; not to mention a waste of resources because recruiters were still instructed to interview women but not to hire them.[93] After recruiting Penny and Susan, Bob left for temporary assignment in Cameroon working with the smallpox eradication effort. He later would hear that Penny was hired by CDC, but he did not know the trouble Norm Scherzer would go through to make it happen. When the freeze lifted, Norm offered Penny, Susan, and Janella jobs as co-ops—federal employees—in September 1970. The irony was that when they were initially offered jobs with the city, these women were in fact not city employees but project employees – paid by the federal government via grant resource. Despite the "almost federal" status of a project employee, the CDC did not want to accept women as PHAs and sent a representative to meet with Norm to strong-arm him into firing these women. Norm stormed out of the meeting, refusing to do as CDC directed. This forced CDC into a corner: if the agency did not want female PHAs, someone from headquarters would have to fire them. The agency did not want to make another move because times had clearly changed and women were accepted among the PHA ranks. Norm recalls that they "created a fait accompli."[94] He continues:

> When the federal freeze ended and we made job offers as federal Public Health Advisors, I was directed—and I use that term carefully—not to hire them as we did not recruit female Public Health Advisors as federal employees. I was flabbergasted... I was further told that if I proceeded with this recruitment that I would be fired. I replied that I did not want to be fired and left the office. Not too long after that someone in the federal government decided to count females as minorities, and the New York City transgression became an accomplishment.[95]

Change did not come quickly, even with the hiring of the first female PHAs, because the "old boy" mindset was embedded in the CDC hierarchy. Women already within the CDC system were caught between a rock and a hard place. On the one hand, the prevailing attitude circumscribed the role of women, while on the other hand, PHA field experience was so increasingly valuable that it became a requirement for senior operations managers at CDC. Anyone without it would not be seriously considered for these roles. Women who were currently in the system could not get access to greater responsibility because they had not passed the "litmus test" of field experience. Even those who were willing to leave headquarters and go back to the field to gain experience could not get it because CDC was not pushing to hire female PHAs in the early 1970s. Virginia "Ginny" Bales Harris had a tremendous career as a CDC leader, though it would not be the result of being a "traditional"—field-trained—PHA. Ginny began in the TB Control Division in 1970. Before her retirement in 2005, she had served as the deputy director of the Chronic Disease Center. Prior to that, she was the deputy director for management under CDC Director Jeffrey Koplan. Although these two positions can be counted among the highest roles the CDC gave to PHAs, Ginny recalls that early on, she and other women were limited as they tried to gain field experience. She remembers the very early 1970s when she was first at CDC:

> As I looked around in the very early 1970s, I saw who was doing the kind of work that I enjoyed doing and liked to do or aspired to do. I kept saying, "How did you get there, and how did that work?" I found out pretty quickly that you needed to start in the field. I was young and flexible back then, and I said, "Well, I'd like to do that." But the answer was, "We don't put women in the field. It's dangerous."[96]

It was apparent to Ginny that the jobs she wanted and the experiences she wished to have were out of reach, at least for a period of time. She started at CDC as a Public Health Analyst because women were not given roles as PHAs. Ginny eventually would become a PHA, but would always consider herself "not quite" a PHA because she missed the crucial set of compounding experiences in the field. The lack of field experience would prevent her from getting jobs reserved for PHAs for several years and until the system realized that she and other women could not in fact create experiences denied them in the first place: "I had applied for a lot of Public Health Advisor jobs and could never even make it to the panel because I didn't have the field experience. I guess that was always the litmus test of being a real Public Health Advisor." Ginny's experience would mirror that of other women moving up through the ranks at CDC, particularly women scientists. As she moved up the CDC ladder, Ginny often would find herself the only woman in the room.[97]

With the change in federal hiring policy and continued pushing by PHA recruiters, the VD Program hired several women in the 1970s and 1980s. Bob Baldwin would recruit two women in our interview cohort: Pam Chin and Wendy Wolf. Wendy began her work in New York City in 1974, and Pam began in Los Angeles. Pam remembered being in the "second wave" of hiring that followed another federal hiring freeze around 1972. The good news for the new recruits was that their male PHA colleagues were used to working with female investigators, and there would be few issues integrating them into the day-to-day operations. Today Pam is the deputy director for the Division of Violence Prevention and has served in similar capacities for the Division of Nutrition and Chronic Disease and the Division of Training for the Epidemiology Program Office. Throughout her career, she credits the development of the professional network that began when she was doing STD field work in Los Angeles and extends to her work at CDC headquarters today:

> The network that was created has benefited me. When I think about getting something done at CDC, I always know that I can call

> somebody... If you are tugging with somebody on an issue and you know [that a PHA] sits in that division or that branch, or remotely, you know you can get some insights.[98]

By 1992 the cadre of Public Health Advisors reflected the gender, racial, and ethnic diversity of the communities in which they worked. Recruitment and hiring analyses conducted by the National Center for Prevention Services at CDC in 1992—the most recent data available (see Chapter 8)—indicated that fifty-three percent of entry level PHAs were women, forty-three percent white, forty-eight percent African American, five percent Hispanic, two percent Asian, and two percent Native American. Only twenty-four percent of the entering PHA workforce in 1992 was white and male.[909] Despite the strides, the organizational transition occurred in fits and starts. Anne-Renee Heningburg recalls what it was like to witness and experience the raising of the glass ceilings as an African American female PHA. Hired in 1979, she got the message: "You're black and you're a woman. You're a woman, that means you can't go higher than an 11 (GS-11), and you're black, that means you can't go higher than an 11."[100] She remembers getting her "thirteen", GS-13, while working in Los Angeles in the early 1990s:

> I remember when I was in LA, I'd gotten my thirteen and this was still a big achievement for a black woman in this organization. There were still a few people around, guys who had been GS-11s for fifty-five years who thought they were never going to go anywhere else, and it was hard to distinguish whether that was because of skills and abilities or whether that was because of politics or other things. It was an interesting time in recruiting because when they started doing this massive recruiting of people...It was the first time that there were many more women being recruited into the PHA series than men. And they were much more diverse than they had been in the past. So this was really a changing time in terms of the series. It was a really interesting thing to be a part of even if peripherally. Still, after nine years in LA I can remember feeling "I've had enough of this. I need to do something."[101]

Anne-Renee did do something else. She went off to Harvard and earned her master's in public administration in 1995. She returned to a series of international assignments with polio eradication efforts. She found her niche as she worked to ensure a national immunization effort during Sudan's civil war (see Chapter 1).

Although PHAs initially were hired to provide contact epidemiology and patient interviewing in VD control, over time their value and potential contribution across public health efforts materialized. The initial cadre of 1948 co-ops blossomed into a field staff of hundreds who were experienced at several levels of public health and across many different public health programs. These men and women became valuable to other Public Health Service agencies in and outside the U.S. federal government. By the 1970s, the PHAs' value to other federal agencies was recognized, as evidenced by their frequent transfers from CDC programs to other federal agency positions. In 1974, CDC documented that 342 PHAs from CDC had taken jobs with other federal organizations, such as USAID and the Indian Health Service.

From the 1960s forward, PHAs became part of the CDC's management backbone. Their unique training of fieldwork—primarily in VD—frequent transfers across the U.S., and work in several different public health programs resulted in a tremendously valuable public health professional. Although many programs hired PHAs, the VD Program continued to serve as the portal for most newly hired co-ops. Even today, most of the Public Health Advisors in the CDC system were trained initially in the STD Program at the entry level of public health. This experience has remained with the men and women who serve in increasingly responsible capacities throughout the public health system.

The 1950s were formative years for the Public Health Advisors. They became established as part of the VD Division, were introduced to state and local public health departments, and became proven successes in field epidemiology, program development, and management. The move to Atlanta allowed other public health programs to take advantage of this specialized type of worker—one who had a "can-do" attitude, worked hard, understood field epidemiology, and could provide an important link with state and local health departments. This type of public health worker became part of the CDC management system almost immediately, as symbolized by Bill Watson's leadership at CDC. The 1960s and 1970s would serve as a growth and development period, and the PHA cadre would become diverse both from a programmatic standpoint and from the standpoint of gender, racial, and ethnic diversity. Throughout all the growth and development, a core set of characteristics typified these professionals. Was this type of worker a product of the person hired, or of training and field experience?

The answer was that they were created by a winnowing process: an important mixture of employee selection, coaching, and training, with several years of field experience and a grounding in PHA culture.

Chapter 6

Winnowing

Many people weeded themselves out because you had to interview patients for at least one year. However, precisely because of that requirement, those who stayed were the most committed, they actually liked helping people, and they saw a rewarding future working in public health. Later, even when they had advanced far in their careers, they could remember what it's like to talk to someone with an STD who is just scared.[1]

Gary West, senior vice president for operations
Institute for Family Health, Family Health International
Public Health Advisor (ret.)

It has been said that the ones who stay are either committed or crazy. The job of an entry-level PHA is grunt work by definition: long hours, challenging and fluid working conditions, intense and even sometimes shocking immersion into health realities that the average person knows nothing about. All in a day's work for a PHA - though not everyone is suited for it.

There is no documentation found about weeding out those who did not fit the PHA mold. Yet, over the decades, there appeared to be a process of self-selection whereby new recruits gained a sense of the job and decided for themselves whether it was a "fit" for them. A review of PHA entry-level hiring data from the 1940s until 1996 revealed a dropout rate of forty-three percent within the first two calendar years on the job.[2] Other analyses indicated that around thirty-eight percent dropped out by the end of the *first* year.[3] Certainly, by the end of the first two years, people had had a good hard look at the job, the required relocation, and the type of work, and they could come to the realization that things were not likely to change any time soon. Some PHAs argued that this was in fact a system of weeding out. When he entered the interview school in

Chicago in 1964, Steve Barid saw that the way things were set up engendered a "survival-of-the-fittest attitude." Today, he takes pride in the fact that he and his colleague Kevin Murphy are the only co-ops from his interview school class to retire from CDC:

> I'm convinced they hired many more people than they ever thought would stay. They were right, and the people who stayed were pretty interesting people who wanted to get stuff done and were pretty good at it.[4]

Victor Tomlinson's 1972 co-op experience in Washington, DC made him think long and hard about whether he wanted to be a VD investigator. Vic was no stranger to public health. He was recruited by CDC from a local health department tuberculosis program, and his father had worked in public health for years. Despite this history, Vic had no idea that "learning the ropes" of fieldwork meant dodging bullets:

> My supervisor took me to the field to teach me the ropes in field investigation. We made several visits to people who he was trying to find. We were riding along making these turns up these different streets, and all of a sudden I heard "POW!" I said, "What's that?" He said, "I think it was a gunshot." And then we heard it again, and he said, "Hit the floor!" And so I literally rolled out of the seat of that old van and hit the floor as he was making a sharp turn around the corner because we thought somebody had been shooting at us. Later on… we went and looked at the rear of the van, and it looked like there were a couple of holes in the van.[5]

Vic admits to questioning his return to the program after this experience. He stuck it out for about a year and then left CDC to join the state Immunization Program in Virginia because he wanted to remain in the area. Vic was newly married, and the prospect of raising a family while balancing the job expectation to relocate every few years was what helped him decide to leave federal service. His contributions as a Public Health Advisor did not end at that time, however. Vic joined CDC again as a PHA and worked in the STD, Immunization, and Tuberculosis programs across the country. He is now the deputy chief for the Clinical and Health Systems Research Branch in the Division of Tuberculosis Elimination at CDC.

This is a rare job, although no one else wants to do it.[6]

Tracy Ford, PHA
Field Operations Manager
Houston, Texas

Recruiting people with college educations to serve as VD investigators increased in difficulty when the 1950s became the 1960s and other opportunities for non-medically-trained personnel emerged in public health. The challenge heightened once recruits learned more about the job and its hardships. The work was gritty, the pay was not terrific; but those who stayed with it contributed tremendously to public health and were very interesting people. Recruiters knew that this was the case, so they spent their time looking for people who might just make it through the initial training experience. Recruiters like Mike Cassell were PHAs themselves and knew the job. Mike currently is stationed in North Carolina, as a rapid response team leader for CDC's Syphilis Elimination Effort. He worked as a recruiter of PHAs from 1985 to 1987 and contends that "the average person can't do this job." The challenge that faced him and other recruiters was finding good prospects and hoping that they'd make it through the training and the initial year in the field. When Mike was trained as a recruiter, he was told to look in the mirror and find that person—not someone who "looked like" Mike, but someone who had his characteristics as a PHA. According to Mike, a recruiter wants to hire people who have interpersonal skills, street sense, intelligence, and a strong work ethic, but if he had to prioritize, the top two characteristics would be work ethic and interpersonal skills:

> I always look for two things: give me work ethic, give me interpersonal skills, and we'll do the rest of it... The average person won't get a job with me because the average person is not going to go out at six in the morning or ten at night. They won't give up a Saturday or a Sunday to go into a drug-infested, dirty, high-crime area and do this job. There's something about the character of all good PHAs which is a little different than the average person. There is some uniqueness there. Your personality is just a little different in the way you probably click and think and do things. And you just hope you find those people when you've got a job opening.[7]

Like many recruiters, Mike believed that once a candidate is found with the basic building blocks of interpersonal skills and work ethic, CDC will "do the rest of it." The rest of it means initial training, job preparation and mentoring, "pounding in the learning," immersion in PHA culture, and years of accrued field and operations experience in several geographic locations. For most PHAs, the initial experience was in sexually transmitted diseases—with all the associated interpersonal aspects. Although other programs hired PHAs after 1960 (see Chapter 5), they did not train them for entry-level work. A recent exception is the Tuberculosis Elimination Program, which hired twenty-five entry-level PHAs in 1994. As most Public Health Advisors were trained for entry-level work in STDs, this chapter will focus on that kind of training.

Training for entry-level PHAs historically involved the development of interviewing and investigation skills; the imparting of information about syphilis and other sexually transmitted diseases; the development of clinical skills, such as darkfield microscopy and phlebotomy; and years of on-the-job training to sharpen a PHA's street sense and problem-solving skill. Although training content and format has adjusted to reflect evolving times and CDC hiring patterns, the general building blocks have remained the same. In the 1940s and 1950s the training took two or three weeks. By the late 1980s and early 1990s, the training process extended to months, with many learning modules. Over several decades, training was delivered variously in centralized and decentralized manners, reflecting the hiring situation at the time. During periods of mass hiring in the late 1940s, mid-1960s, mid-1970s, and late 1980s, CDC organized training regionally or in select locations with high numbers of syphilis, gonorrhea, or HIV cases (depending upon the era). This was done so that trainees could immediately apply newly-learned interview and investigation skills. During periods with little hiring, a centralized training location would be used, such as in Atlanta. Training courses were not exclusively for PHAs; they also were open to state and local public health personnel who were preparing for entry-level work in STDs. One might argue that with such training open to all types of public health workers (local, state and federal), the PHA is really not that unique among its public health peers. But although the didactic training and supervision are shared, the PHA culture itself, paired with the accrual of experiences over several different transfers and placements, makes the PHA what she or he is in a public health context.

Since the beginning of the series, training for PHAs combined immersion in the field, didactic training in case finding and patient interviewing, and on-the-job training, which ideally involved solid mentoring and coaching by supervisors or experienced PHAs. The supervision quality waxed and waned over the years, and CDC conducted several program reviews to improve the quality of training, supervision, and mentoring, particularly in the 1980s.[8] Formal training and coaching was augmented over the years by a strong and emerging PHA culture which reinforced hard work, a thirst for challenges and problems to solve, competition among peers to achieve excellence in the field, loyalty to CDC, and a bawdy sense of humor. Together, the didactic and experiential training methods, paired with enculturation, helped shape the PHAs in their early years, so that when they became managers or moved to other CDC programs, these men and women were equipped with strong interpersonal skills, a solid understanding of epidemiology, and the ability to work in a variety of challenging environments. The training in STDs prepared PHAs for the range of work experiences they could have throughout their careers. Fieldwork and patient interviewing techniques were applicable across public health programs, and helpful in the PHAs' new environments. Kathy Cahill is the deputy director for Integrated Health Solutions and Development at the Bill and Melinda Gates Foundation. She is a retired PHA who credits training and the accrual of interview experience with the development of interpersonal skills that she has used throughout her career:

> I think one of the advantages of interview training is the development of interpersonal skills. In order to get a patient to spill his or her beans you have to use one of two tactics: either the fear tactic or the interpersonal tactic. I was more prone to do the interpersonal approach than the fear approach. That constant building up early in your career of interviewing people, talking to people, trying to figure out where they're coming from, is helpful when you get into senior policy positions, because most of my day is spent talking to people about a difficult situation.[9]

The basic building blocks of training—immersion in the realities of STDs, interview training, epidemiology, and related skills development—have not changed much over the years. Central to the training was interviewing skill, a skill that has been called "the mother's milk" for anyone who began in STD.[10] For PHAs who were hired between 1948 and the mid 1960s, the name Bob Swank is synonymous with patient interviewing. He developed the syphilis interviewing method and was a major influence in PHA training efforts, even after his death in 1966.[11] In the early 1940s, Bob opened and directed the first Public Health Service-sponsored contact interviewing training school for local and state VD workers, and later became the director of the National Personnel Training School at Alto, Georgia from 1950–1951.[12] He believed that the interview, and thus the interviewer, was the "key figure in determining the success or failure of syphilis control programs." Then, just as today, epidemiology involved identifying the unknown and unreported cases of disease. Its success rested (and rests) upon the interview. Bob emphasized the importance of the interview in a 1962 speech at the World Forum on Syphilis and other Treponematoses:

> The contact and suspect interview must be performed so effectively that the information obtained will result in finding and bringing to examination all contacts within the period of infectivity of the patient being interviewed.[13]

Jack Wroten remembers Bob Swank. The two rode together in Georgia when Jack worked for Fulton County as a co-op and Bob worked with the VD program there. Jack recalls Bob underscoring the importance of interviewing as a primary method of syphilis control. At the time, the VD program emphasized blood testing or screening; however, Bob thought these efforts were not going to lead to elimination of syphilis. Jack recalls him saying, "I'll tell you one thing. You can take all your needles out there and blood test all the people you want, but I'll go out there and I'll find more syphilis than you can with your needles."[14] Swank's perspective became the core belief of VD programs across the country and became embedded in PHA culture. Retired PHA Russ Havlak recounts the "truths" about syphilis interviewing that have been passed down from one PHA generation to the next:

> The uncomfortable truth is that the syphilis interview is an intense adversarial proceeding. For lots of reasons, the syphilis patient instinctively wants to protect his [sic] privacy, while a total stranger wants him to bare it all to a degree he's probably never done for anybody... Depending on the evolved skill of the PHA, the syphilis interview can be a productive personal, professional, and public health event, or an embarrassing, palm-sweaty bust. Every PHA begins to get a grip on this tension about halfway through the second day of Interview School. We learn three incontrovertible truths about this job. One: every syphilis patient has at least one sex contact. Two: every syphilis patient has a contact who gave

> him the disease, and three: every syphilis patient probably will lie about, or refuse to name, or omit naming, one or more of his contacts, and possibly every one of them.[15]

Interviewing takes a unique set of skills, and several years of observed practice. This fact was slow to dawn on physicians in public health and private practice who believed that their ability to take patient history prepared them to conduct a patient interview about sex contacts. One interviewing experience was enough to persuade Dr. David Sencer that perhaps someone else should do the interviewing of STD patients. Dave was first introduced to the outcomes of interviewing while working in the TB Program in Columbus, Georgia, in the early 1950s. The VD doctor was not available that day, so PHA Harold Coleman asked Dave to examine a patient he thought had secondary syphilis—the second stage of the most contagious phase of syphilis. It was immediately apparent that Harold possessed a skill that Dave did not:

> The patient had classic secondary, so I talked to her for half an hour and I got one contact: her husband. Harold went in and came back in half an hour with thirteen! So I said, "You know, that's not my business. Somebody else can do it better than I can."[16]

Dr. Willard "Ward" Cates, the president of research for Family Health International, was the director of the Division of STD Prevention at CDC in 1982. That year, he went into the field to get a "real field experience of what the Public Health Advisor is really doing." He went to the Durham County Public Health Department in North Carolina during an outbreak of penicillin-resistant gonorrhea, a major public health issue that required excellence in contact epidemiology and patient interviewing. PHA Jim Fowler took him to the health department to demonstrate the patient interview and its outcome: named sexual contacts which establish a pattern of sexual behavior congruent with the patient diagnosis. As a physician, Ward thought he could talk with a patient about anything, so he wanted to give it a try. He confidently went into the examination room saying, "Hi. I am Ward Cates, and I want to talk to you about a controversial topic." He got nowhere:

> After about twenty minutes, sweat is pouring off my brow, and I am asking about all of these sensitive things. This was really tough

> stuff. I came out and I had one partner and no locating information at all. I was so proud of myself. I walk out and say "Jim, I got a contact. Her name was Martha at the wall." And Jim says, "Oh, Dr. Cates, just give me about a minute with this person." So Jim goes in for a few minutes. He returns and says, "Well I just got a few more." He had four more names from this guy and locating information on the one that I had, and in four minutes! I walked away in awe of what a well-trained, talented individual could do and what people possessing the sort of skill learned in this school of reality of the streets could do.[17]

Through developed interviewing skills, PHAs were trained to elicit all sexual contacts of an STD patient within a critical infection period. For syphilis, this meant that on average, each interview should identify at least three to five contacts. Successful interviewers would gain information that identified the source of the infection, and would bring to treatment or identify one or more persons who were credited with spreading the infection in thirty to fifty percent of patients who were interviewed. Such an overall success rate was to be maintained for a minimum of eighty-five percent of the interviews.[18] The interview is a primary way of gathering information to understand the spread of syphilis and other communicable diseases among contacts over a period of infectivity. Patient health history, including history of symptoms, when paired with laboratory data, helps to identify the stage of illness and to set the timeline for infectiousness among partners. In the case of syphilis, the naming of contacts is important but not sufficient. A competent interviewer must know syphilis epidemiology well enough to document the timeline of patients' sexual contacts and behaviors so as to understand whether they have full and complete information. For example, if a person with early syphilis is interviewed and provides the names and information for about five contacts, a pattern of sexual behavior emerges. If there are gaps in the pattern, the interviewer must be savvy enough to identify them during the interview and press for additional information about contacts. Without such knowledge, the interviewer will lose the chance of identifying others who need treatment.[19] Throughout the series' history, PHAs have had to learn the various methods of interviewing and become comfortable with exploring sexual history.

Louis Salinas was a tuberculosis worker for the State of Texas when he was hired as a co-op in the VD program and transferred to Miami in 1974. Coming from TB work, Louis thought he would have no trouble making the transition to

VD—"Oh sure, I can do that"—until he went to interview school. There he realized the uniqueness of working in VD control and the accompanying cultural education he would have to acquire in order to become an effective public health interviewer. This Hispanic man from south Texas had to step out of the comfort of his respectful culture, which prevented asking about someone's "business," and become accustomed to talking about sex in all its forms. He had to go even further to work comfortably in the gay male culture of 1970s Miami. He admitted to being "so green" that he did not know about the sex clubs in Miami: "There was a gay club in Miami, and I'd asked what they did there....the class and the instructor began laughing so hard we had to take a break."[20] Louis remembers the moment in interview school when he realized that he was working in "a whole new disease entity":

> We get to the part where we're doing the interview, and the next question is, "Who is the last guy you've had sex with?" And I looked at my trainer, and I said, "Wait a minute. They don't do things like that in Texas." It was a whole new disease entity. Asking a lot of personal questions that I had always thought were none of my business... It was a major challenge asking really invasive questions to patients who really didn't care. The shocking thing for me was that people were having sex with about the same frequency as I shook hands.[21]

Over the decades, PHAs were trained to face myriad challenges inherent in patient interviewing. First, a patient receives news about their diagnosis of syphilis or possibly gonorrhea or HIV. This may be shocking news. The patient may have been monogamous and now is faced with the likelihood that his or her partner or spouse has been unfaithful. The diagnosis might cause feelings of shame, sadness, or anger. Following the diagnosis, a stranger approaches and wants to discuss behaviors that might embarrass them, cause harm to them, place them in danger or in jail, cause them to lose status, or leave them open to blackmail.[22] To handle the challenges, PHAs and their local colleagues were taught ways of expressing sincerity, and emphasizing confidentiality and the patient's human dignity. They also were trained to use a complex interviewing method pioneered by Bob Swank with the help of his colleagues and sexologists Alfred Kinsey, William Masters, and Virginia Johnson. Ken Latimer worked closely with Bob Swank in the early 1960s as the interview method was undergoing enhancement:

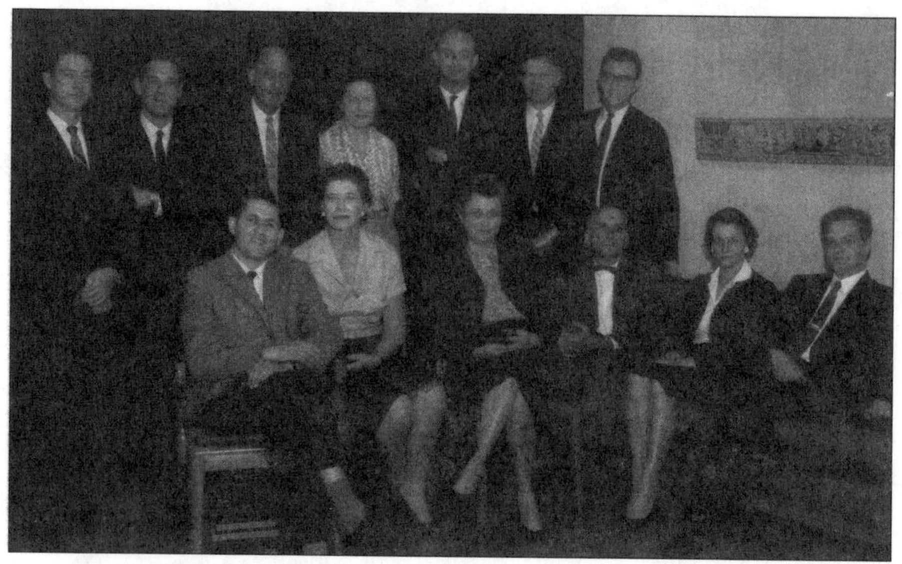

Conference at the Institute for Sex Research (ISR), Indiana University May 18, 1960. Top L-R: Ken Latimer (PHA), Clyde Martin (ISR), Bob Swank (CDC), Margaret Bright (Johns Hopkins University), Fredrick "Stu" Kingma (PHA), Bill Watson (PHA), John Gagnon (ISR). Bottom L-R: Fred Ederer (National Cancer Institute), Hilda Nivala (CDC, nurse consultant), Cornelia Christenson (ISR), William Masters (Washington University), Virginia Johnson (Washington University), Wardell Pomeroy (ISR).
Courtesy of Ken Latimer.

> Bob Swank had developed a relationship with Dr. Kinsey and his staff early in his career, and we continued discussions over the years. The Kinsey Institute staff all complimented the interview techniques we developed. They pointed out that they only had to establish rapport and obtain information. We did that, plus we obtained detailed personal information about sexual contacts; locating and bringing to exam those contacts; and maintaining the medical confidential demands of our ongoing program.[23]

Through the years interview training offered various opportunities for PHAs to study the method and practice the skills with coaching from instructors. The use of two-way mirrors was initiated in the 1950s to allow trainees to observe actual interviews with their classmates and instructor. Those who were trained with this method found it to be a tremendously useful tool for teaching and coaching. Paul Burlack recalls his training experience at the Chelsea Clinic in New York City in 1972:

> We had a two-way mirror at the time, before it was outlawed. We had our in-class training and then our interview training, where the rest of the class was able to view the interview sessions with the patients. I think for all who were new to this job, it was a learning situation.'[24]

In October 1972 PHA Bill Doyle became chief of program services in the CDC's VD Branch. In this role, he was responsible for the entire field staff and training facilities. By early 1973 all training facilities stopped the use of the two-way mirror in light of the Tuskegee experiment (see Chapter 7). Bill recalls that there was some pushback from the field: "My decision did not sit well with some of the trainers."[25] Despite the value of having the opportunity to observe an interview in this manner, the lesson of Tuskegee was that patient privacy outweighed the need for this training method. Following this decision, new trainees were offered interview practice through role-play and observation. This would be followed by field shadowing, where a new trainee would accompany an experienced interviewer in the field to see how the job was done. Ideally, and after awhile, the roles would switch, and the trainee would conduct interviews and receive feedback from the experienced colleague. Observation and feedback from an experienced interviewer is critical to the new PHA and his or her skills development, because the interview method is not a "turnkey type of tool." Russ Havlak, who served as the chief of the CDC's Training Education and Consultation Section from 1983 to 1994, believes that Interviewing School "never did turn out a polished syphilis interviewer."[26] It requires experienced observation and feedback to help the new PHA identify mistakes in applying the interview method and to correct them. During periods where CDC did not have sufficient numbers of supervisory PHAs in the field, new PHAs would have to hone the skill on their own, through practice and self-reflection. Russ believes that practice is necessary but not sufficient: "Yes, it takes practice, but introspection has its limits because you are one-half of an interview process. You really need to thoroughly evaluate it." He continues:

> Keep in mind that the syphilis interview of the 1950s and 1960s was not a rushed affair. Done right, it would take at least an hour, just to work the "pattern" [of questions] and to get the patient mo-

> tivated to cooperate. An interview could take several hours if the interviewer ended up eliciting detailed locating and identifying information on a sizable number of sex contacts.[27]

The original "pattern" was the Modified Direct Approach developed by Bob Swank. Although it was modified further over the years, the Swank iteration was in use in the early 1960s when CDC hired a large numbers of co-ops as part of a nationwide syphilis eradication effort called "Operation Pursuit." In 1961 Surgeon General Luther Terry called for a syphilis task force to make recommendations regarding the elimination of syphilis. The task force, chaired by New York City Health Commissioner Dr. Leona Baumgartner, outlined several recommendations necessary for syphilis eradication and in 1962 published a report calling for the eradication of syphilis by 1972.[28] That same year the CDC VD Program field staff—PHAs assigned to local and state health departments—would reach 486 due to the addition of 178 new co-ops during the previous three months for the eradication effort.[29] Every new case of syphilis was treated as having the highest priority. The words of Dr. William Brown, chief of the VD Branch, echoed: "Until further notice, the eradication of syphilis is the sole mission of this Branch."[30] U.S. cases of primary and secondary syphilis in 1962 numbered 21,143—the greatest number of cases reported since 1950,[31] and syphilis interviewing was at the heart of the intervention.

By 1963, the number of PHAs serving state and local health departments had grown to more than six hundred, putting stress on the training and supervisory system for new recruits and relatively inexperienced co-ops.[32] The science of interviewing and epidemiology was in continuous development, and there was a need to improve and standardize the training offered to new co-ops and to PHAs who were working in the field. By the early 1960s, the interviewing schools had decentralized to accommodate the number of new hires,[34] and were supplemented with regional meetings and seminars providing additional training opportunities for co-ops and PHAs. In 1963 the VD Program established the Epidemiologic Consultation and Training Unit to standardize and enhance all training with a deeper understanding of syphilis epidemiology.[35] Ken Latimer was appointed as the director of the program in 1964. "It would no longer be just about who you were having sex with," he recalled.[36] A national review of syphilis case finding records identified a wide variety of interview approaches and weak outcomes. This was of particular concern if CDC was going to eradicate syphilis by 1972. The Epidemiologic Consultation and Training Unit would initiate a "new era and new philosophy" in syphilis epidemiology. Ken recalls:

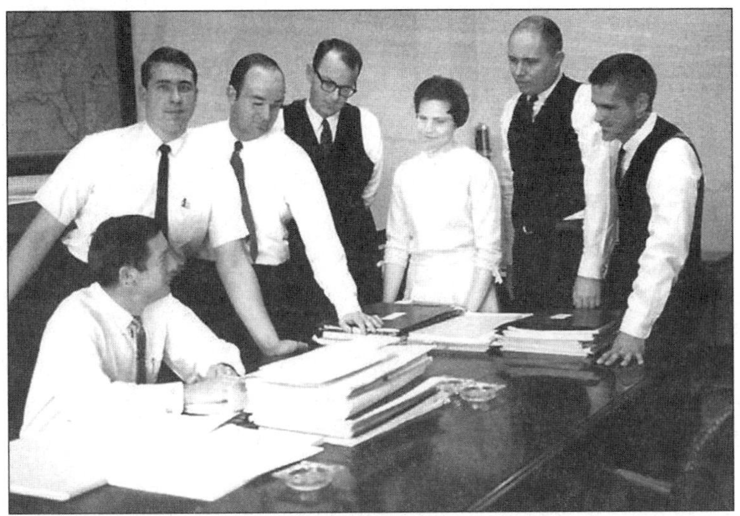

Epidemiologic Consultation and Training Unit, CDC 1968. Standing L-R: Russ Havlak, Bill Parra, Bob Kingon, Carolyn Short (Administrative Assistant), Dr. Richard Thatcher, Jim Fowler. Seated: Ken Latimer.
Courtesy of Ken Latimer.

> There was considerable variation among the areas where we had assignees. And while our federal program had responsibility for the basic training, assignment of staff to the state and local areas, and their "care and feeding" as feds; there was not much in the way of technical support in the area of our specialty... This was the beginning of a new era, and a new philosophy. We were still "VD Investigators"; however, there was a desperate need for trained and experienced field supervisors, program specialists, and managers at the local and state levels.[37]

Ken Latimer asked Windell Bradford and Jim Fowler to join this nascent endeavor. Windell was a relatively new PHA, having been a co-op since 1962. Jim Fowler was then a trainer at the Chicago interview school. The unit would provide training to PHAs and health departments and would offer epidemic consultation.[38] A major contribution of the epi training unit was the case management system. Windell recalls:

> Ken Latimer had moved to headquarters and was trying to improve the training of the field staff. It had been, other than this interviewing school, a pretty hit-or-miss thing. He also was trying to improve the scientific epidemiological basis for what we were doing to improve the understanding of it so that people could do a better job by understanding the purpose of all this interviewing and contact tracing and clustering.[39]

The case management concept involved an analysis of the relationships among sexual contacts and their social circles to identify whether there were gaps in the information as it compared with the patient clinical symptoms and disease staging. The objective was to refocus the effort of PHAs (and others) away from mere case finding and toward the prevention of new cases. The shift would enhance the PHAs' analytical skills. Windell recalls the theory of case management:

> Without intervention it can be assumed that a person who progresses through all stages of early syphilis (primary, secondary, and early latency) will spread the disease to others and thus continue to fuel the epidemic... If you quickly find and treat those "spread" contacts who are still in their primary or secondary stage, you shorten the period when they are capable of infecting others. The real payoff in prevention comes from identifying recent contacts and treating them prophylactically—before they enter into the infectious stages of the disease. Their opportunity to spread the diseases to others is eliminated, not just truncated.[40]

The concept of case management signaled a major shift in the way syphilis was handled. Up until this point the emphasis was on case finding. If syphilis were ever to be eradicated, cases had to be prevented, not just found. Bob Swank knew this, and before he died, he and Ken Latimer worked on the idea of a case management system. Ken was its ultimate designer. According to Russ Havlak, a member of Ken's staff, the syphilis case management system was "nothing short of turning the nation's entire approach to syphilis eradication on its head":

> The case management concept was conceived in the early 1960s by Ken Latimer and Joe Blount, with input from Bob Swank be-

> fore he died. Joe cranked out the stats behind the concept. The case management chart, plus the case management course, which used these implements to teach the concept, were the creations of Windell Bradford and Jim Fowler... It was clear from the first couple years of the syphilis eradication effort that the campaign was surely going to fail if all we did was "find" cases rather than prevent them from ever occurring.[41]

Russ believes that although the case management method was a major contribution to syphilis control and eradication, it was never fully implemented because the system of PHA promotion had been developed on the indices that were artifacts of the case finding system: "This is where case management hit a brick wall." As long as the VD Program continued to demand and value the indices of the past—the "brought to treatment" index, the "lesion to lesion" index, etc.—public health behavior and program practice would never change. Russ recalled that because the VD Program did not try to identify prevention-oriented measures which could be related to program performance, "people in the field always knew where the gold was to be mined. They talked the case management talk, but mostly walked the case finding walk."[42] The failure to implement the case management innovation would not be the last innovation failure to be experienced by the VD Program due to incongruity with the PHA culture and incentives system. Within a decade, Bill Parra, one of Ken Latimer's staff members, would go on to lead the effort to augment patient interviewing techniques. This effort, though it reflected the changing times, also would meet with significant field resistance.

Changes in interview approaches reflected the spirit of Bob Swank, who believed that "no successful interviewer can ever cease to study the resistance of patients to the interview."[43] Even in 1961, Swank was concerned about interview practices, method elements, and even interviewer attributes that might serve as deterrents in the interview process.[44] Over time, the interviewing techniques evolved, and the location and means of delivering training would change. Change did not come easily. Bill Parra believed that interview techniques needed to reflect changes in the times and patient circumstances. He was among the early staff of the Epi Consultation and Training Unit, joining in 1967. After three years, Bill left CDC headquarters to return to the field as the epidemiologic specialist for the Los Angeles VD Program. He then helped USAID implement a nutrition program, and went on to direct the VD program in Puerto Rico. After such varied experiences, Bill returned in 1976 to the STD Training Education and Consultation Section, or "TEC." He became TEC section chief in 1978. In the ensuing four years, the approach to patient counseling and interviewing would go through tremendous change and development to emphasize behavior change theory.[45] Bill recalls the advent of the change, which was brought about through the nexus of training, clinical, and communications expertise:

> It actually started in about 1978... The VD Division was bringing together the components of education and training and clinical consultation... That was a very powerful mixture of people.... We began to develop some theories about how clinics and patients should be handled, and that spilled over into our training programs, it spilled over into our clinical training programs, and it spilled over into our health communication efforts. We were really into behavior change.[46]

Up until the late 1970s, the syphilis interview had the goal of contact elicitation. But after 1972, PHAs in the field were under significant pressure to implement a new Gonorrhea Control Program while at the same time striving to address syphilis. Notably, despite the national eradication program called "Operation Pursuit," VD Control efforts were flat-funded each year from 1962 until 1972, and this period saw several federal hiring freezes. With the Gonorrhea Control Program came resources to hire new PHAs, but the program's implementation would prove to be rife with complications and would eat up the time of a declining complement of managerial PHAs in the field. Who suffered? New co-ops in the field and the patient interview.

With the Gonorrhea Control Program, the VD Program at CDC once again would expand its focus to accommodate something more than syphilis (see Chapter 4). This involved, among other things, interviewing newly-diagnosed male gonorrhea patients as one means of locating and treating persons presumed to have asymptomatic disease. But a serious logistical problem arose. Local VD clinics typically lacked the confidential space for their new PHAs to interview many gonorrhea (or syphilis) patients at the same time. When PHAs tried using the gonorrhea interview method taught to them in interviewing school, they tied up the few available interview rooms for at least thirty minutes per patient, thereby creating a tremendous backlog of diagnosed male patients who were increasingly distressed to be waiting so long for an interview. "With the national mandate to interview a hundred percent of male gonorrhea patients, the situation quickly became intolerable," Russ Havlak said.[47] As a result, the gonorrhea interview became considerably condensed. This also affected the syphilis interview. It too was shortened. What was an elaborate interview process designed by renowned sexologists and refined over years by the VD Program had become a "fast and furious process which produced no usable public health results." Russ Havlak, director of the TEC group from 1983 to 1994, reflects on the change:

> Every STD interview became a cursory five-minute affair. "Hi, I'm so and so, I work here at the clinic, you have gonorrhea, and we need to discuss your contacts. Who was the last person you had sex with?" That's an exaggeration, but only a slight one. The process was rushed, rote, and lacking in much if any semblance of skill or finesse... Many experienced PHAs told me that this mind-numbing, assembly line, five- to ten-minute "interviewing" process made it very difficult to switch gears when suddenly presented with a syphilis patient. This form of interviewing of male gonorrhea patients produced some results in terms of named female or gay male contacts during the prior one to two weeks. But when a syphilis patient came along, PHAs were finding themselves unable to step back and refocus on this different sort of interviewing challenge. For syphilis, with its longer and critical periods depending on disease stage at diagnosis, this rushed "interview" rapidly became a concern. And the tools needed to fix it simply weren't available at the time. With supervisory attention focused on other issues at the time, being concerned was the extent of remedial action in many places, and in 1972, as the development of syphilis interviewing skills became a hopeless cause, major syphilis outbreaks began to occur all across the country.[48]

Russ believes that syphilis interviewing "never recovered from the depletion of basic skills that occurred among an entire generation of the STD field staff."[49] He also cites an overarching problem for PHAs that began in 1972 and was to influence much of what followed for more than a decade. Gonorrhea had replaced syphilis as the top priority. This cultural shift for PHAs should not be overlooked. Syphilis traditionally had been seen as the priority for PHAs. Even in the Peppy Epi days, PHAs were to follow early syphilis without delay, and when possible, gonorrhea would be left to local health departments. Russ clarifies the cultural value of syphilis to PHAs:

> We were taught from the get-go that gonorrhea was a simple disease to work with and that public health nurses and local VDIs [in-

> terviewed these patients]. It was considered an inferior challenge compared to the more complex, difficult, and more serious disease that PHAs, from the beginning of the 685 series, were exclusively trained to handle.[50]

Dr. Jim Curran, dean of the Emory University School of Public Health, directed the clinical research unit that addressed gonorrhea in the Division of STD at the time. He calls this the "lingering love affair with syphilis." During these years, he said, it was becoming clear that "most syphilis was not having a devastating effect anymore."[51] The shift away from syphilis was difficult for PHAs and was accompanied by what seemed like an onslaught of multiple program priorities. Russ Havlak recalls:

> CDC added one new activity after another requiring PHA attention, i.e., gonorrhea screening, gonorrhea interviewing, PID screening, PID interviewing and, profoundly, beginning in the mid-1980s, HIV testing and counseling in STD clinics. Yet veteran PHAs, whether in denial or just longing for the clearer one-disease "STD" Program of bygone times, often raised the question, "What is the order of STD Program priorities?" As the STD mission creep expanded, the most common complaint heard from older PHAs was "Everything is a priority, therefore nothing is a priority."[52]

The erosion of interviewing skills continued through the 1970s, and by 1978, when Bill Parra took the helm of TEC, skills had deteriorated throughout the country. Bill and his colleagues witnessed the decreasing public health productivity when conducting a nationwide review:

> We reviewed the performance metrics over the last four or five years and saw that there had been a decline in productivity in interviewing. It was our view that the productivity was related to the way we were approaching the patient, in a kind of 1950s Southern style that really wasn't applicable. I had worked in Los Angeles. I had worked in West Hollywood with gay, middle-class patients. The system that I had been taught, which was in the South dealing with more rural types of patients, simply didn't work in the sophisticated city.[53]

The TEC group believed the decline in public health results was caused not by the erosion of traditional syphilis interview skills and the dismantling of a carefully crafted process, but instead by a changing relationship between patient and public health system. They felt the time had come for the CDC Interviewing School curriculum to accurately reflect the STD Program's gonorrhea priority. The school could only do this by refocusing course time and attention on working effectively with gonorrhea patients at the expense of time and attention that up until then had been given to syphilis interviewing. A new interview approach needed to emerge, and it had to embody an evolving view of the patient. The interview no longer had to be adversarial. The patient could or would want to do certain things for his or her health and the health of his or her partners, the TEC group reasoned. Russ recalls that interview instructors from the TEC group "led a training staff revolt" because they were struck by some of the harsh, confrontational interviewing methods which they observed in the field. "They insisted on change," he said.

Change was already afoot because the traditional interviewing method was not what was being observed in the field. TEC colleagues were seeing a watered-down, rushed, and inappropriate method that resulted from the pressures of patient load and lack of proper field supervision. Many priorities were entering into the interview task, including medication counseling. By this time, gonorrhea treatment required a seven-day regimen of oral tetracycline, which was a necessary departure from the previous injection of penicillin due to the emergence of drug-resistant gonorrhea. As such, patients would need to be motivated to complete their treatment. Further, the emerging hope to apply behavior change theory in public health gave rise to a strong belief among the STD Program leadership that the time had come for behavioral interventions that focused on prevention. This translated into integrating condom use motivation and education into the process of working with all STD patients, but mainly gonorrhea patients. The task of motivation would fall to the interviewer. Russ recalls that "this element added to the pressure from instructors for an interviewing approach that discouraged 'browbeating' confrontations over contacts,"[54] so that the patient would not become alienated and refuse to take his/her medication or to integrate condom use or other behavior change messages.

A change with patient interviewing had to come, in view of the dismal epidemiologic outcomes from the interviews, dissolving syphilis interview skills, changing views of the patient-interviewer relationship, and staff pressure. Bill recalls that the patient interview, and therefore the interviewer, would need to be reoriented. "We were moving into an age where the patients were much more educated; they had a better concept of what they needed to do. And they should participate essentially in the solution of their own problems."[55] Patient interviews were reoriented to emphasize behavioral outcomes such as patient referral of sexual contacts for testing/evaluation, condom use, and compliance with oral medication, all of which were intended to focus mainly on patients with gonorrhea rather than syphilis. The change was embodied linguistically, as the "interview" became the "counseling session." Contact elicitation would still occur as part of the patient encounter; however, it was no longer the interview's central activity.

As with the case management concept ten years before, the emphasis on behavior change was a major shift in the way things operated in the field. The change, according to Bill, "created a clash within the STD Division at CDC. There were people who were called old-timers, and there were people who agreed with this change."[56] Russ Havlak recalls that the "old-timers" at CDC and in the field who rebelled at the change were really the remnant of properly-trained syphilis interviewers, and in that context, they rightly could call the change "heretical":

> Calling it "counseling" and making contact elicitation anything other than the sole objective of the syphilis interview, or any interview, was widely viewed as heretical. From the perspective of many "old timers," it debased the very process.[57]

These PHA "remnants" fought the change from their senior positions at CDC. They believed the change would forever reduce the kind of public health outcomes possible in the field of STD. They were hired and trained in an era of syphilis eradication and held to a belief that both the methods they were trained to use and the disease on which they honed their skills made the best platform for developing new PHAs. Although Bill Parra was also from this era, he and his TEC colleagues understood that there was a need to strengthen other approaches to STDs because, perhaps, eradication was no longer a reasonable objective. History teaches, for example, that although syphilis rates declined in the late 1940s and early 1950s, due primarily to the PHAs' work, resource constraints and the challenges of handling multiple STDs confounded the effort. The change led by the TEC group was nothing short of a clash of eras, and a fundamental challenge to the developed PHA culture of the time. PHAs were interviewers, not "counselors," and they marked their success by the outcomes of interviews, even if the results had become paltry by the late 1970s. A cultural shift gradually occurred within the STD Division at CDC and out in the field, but not without a fight. As with the case management concept, the way things were done was in stark contrast with the recommended changes. Bill Parra recalls that "people were trained; they would go back to their program bases and then their supervisors would say to them, 'You've learned something in Interviewing School. Forget about it. You're going to learn the real way now.'"[58]

Although the process was incredibly difficult, the STD Division and the field staff made the shift toward a model of encouraging behavior change. Interview outcomes remained terrible throughout the country; syphilis re-emerged with a vengeance, fueled by crack cocaine; and HIV entered the scene as a dominating new priority. In 1983 Russ Havlak took over the TEC group (later called the Training and Education Branch, or TEB), and had the challenge of following in Bill Parra's footsteps to "find a harmonious middle ground" so that strides made by the TEC group could be integrated with a reinvigorated focus on STD patients' sexual contacts. He asked PHA veteran Bob Emerson, then the chief of the Training Section within TEB, to modernize the Swank approach. Russ calls Bob "the most skilled syphilis interview I have ever known."[59] Bob created an interview methodology that was so successful it was taught in advanced interview courses, and was used both to educate the large number of field staff brought on between 1988 and 1993 and to retool the "lost generation" of PHAs who never had been trained properly in syphilis interviewing in the first place. Bob went on to lead TEB and retired in 1995.

FIELDWORK

> *I went down to try to find this guy who lived under the overpass in a box. He was a contact to a syphilis case, and we tested him for HIV at the time. He tested positive. So I went to tell him his results, but he didn't want to hear his results. He pulled out a machete, and he chased me from under the bridge. When he pulled that knife out, guys came from everywhere. I couldn't believe it. There were probably five guys who jumped this guy, pushed him aside and told me to get out.*[60]
>
> Kathryn Koski, PHA
> Deputy Chief
> Health Services Research and Evaluation Branch
> Division of STD Prevention, CDC

Although approaches to epidemiology and interviewing have changed, the basic elements of fieldwork have remained the same. The gritty and challenging experiences with fieldwork help to define the PHA, teaching problem solving and relationship building as no other training experiences could. Fieldwork for the PHA involves locating the sexual contacts that are named during a patient interview and developing and maintaining relationships with people in communities who might help the process. Fieldwork has been called "shoe leather epidemiology" because it involves a lot of walking around in the community, knocking on doors and basically interrupting the lives of people to follow the chain of infection. This element of the PHA job is not easily learned, and often requires time to get used to. While PHAs are selected in part for their street sense, many share that they have to get over the initial shock of fieldwork. Bassam Jarrar is the deputy director for the Division of Global Public Health Capacity Development of the Coordinating Office for Global Health at CDC. In 1990, he was hired as a PHA and trained in Los Angeles. During his first month of training, Bassam observed fieldwork by accompanying experienced STD and HIV investigators in the field. While the chance to shadow a field investigator helped, the observation did not mitigate the transition he and others had to make when they began working in the field alone. Bassam recalls that it took time to overcome concerns for his own safety and become accustomed to the work:

> Well, the first thing is overcoming fear. A lot of the places we went to are places I would have never gone on my own. So there is that element of that kind of safety, security and not knowing when you knock at someone's door what to expect.[61]

New PHAs must overcome their fear of working in community situations that may appear risky. They also must learn to recognize risk and know when to exit the situation. Laura Shelby spent most of her career training other PHAs. She is now with the Program and Training Branch in the Division of STD Prevention at CDC. As she worked with new recruits, Laura often told the story of how in Philadelphia she lost her sense of personal safety. She tells new PHAs this story to demonstrate just how fragile safety really is; and while it is important to find a way to work comfortably in communities, one must never lose the sense of the potential risk inherent in the job. It was in 1991 during a time when there were several carjackings in Philadelphia. Laura was conducting an interview in her car when an unknown car pulled up beside them:

> I saw out of the corner of my eye this car pulling up beside us. And I thought, "Well, that's strange. I wonder why he's doing

> that." Then the car pulled out in front of us and this guy came around to my side door, my door, and then just opened the door! As it turns out the guy was a police officer in an unmarked car. He was interested in the person I was interviewing. I felt bad for this poor guy I was interviewing because I got very upset. It was really the only time I lost my sense of safety.[61]

The process of becoming accustomed to working in the field and closely in communities is so significant that it remains with PHAs long after they leave the field. Today Louise Galaska is the chief management officer of the Coordinating Center for Environmental Health and Injury Prevention at CDC. Even though her career has been filled with many and various work experiences, Louise calls her early fieldwork the defining experience of her life. "It changed me as a person. I saw things I didn't know existed. I met all kinds of people from all over." Louise was hired in 1978 and began in Chicago at the STD clinic called "The Little Red School House," located at 26th and Wabash next to the "L" train track. The building was literally a condemned school house. "There were roaches everywhere. When you opened your desk drawer, you'd have to wait for a moment before putting your hand in to get a pencil." The prospect of working alone in the field scared Louise more than the roaches, but she got used to it:

> For the first couple of weeks I was scared to death. I went out because that's what I was supposed to do. I was terrified but I did it because that was the job. Then around the third week the weather was nice and I was sitting at a stoplight with the car windows rolled down. I looked around me and suddenly realized I wasn't afraid anymore. My fear just somehow evaporated over the course of having good experiences. I'd gone out in the field for two or three weeks and nothing bad had happened to me. I was in communities, I was in neighborhoods, there were little old ladies, there were young people and old, there were women with children, people were living their lives.[63]

Getting over one's shock of being in the field is soon replaced with the need to perform. Field investigators in STD control have very specific measures for success. New investigators are placed in areas with high STD and HIV incidence so that they can experience the challenge of handling the caseload as they introduce themselves to the community. Part of becoming a PHA is learning that you can in fact get the job done, even in the face of huge caseloads and challenging community situations. Figuring out how to do this is the first lesson of problem solving in the PHA career. When he began in Chicago in 1967, John Miles used ingenuity to solve his burgeoning caseload. He was hired in Chicago at the height of the syphilis eradication program. Like Louise Galaska, John was trained at the famous Little Red School House. The scene there was astounding: "I just couldn't believe it. The place was filled with people. Five hundred or so people in the waiting room. Staff are screaming out the numbers "forty-eight, forty-nine, fifty; this way." It was in Chicago that John learned the basics of disease investigation. He spent one week shadowing other more experienced investigators to learn how things worked on the streets. Then he quickly learned how difficult it was to manage his massive caseload. When John's supervisor reviewed his fieldwork outcomes, he told John that he was doing an average job, and that average was not acceptable. He then pushed John in a way that changed how John handled this caseload: "He put the fear of God in me and that set me about doing something that nobody at the time had done." John continues:

> My supervisor looked at my interviews, my contact indices, my brought-to-treatment indices, my cluster index...How many reactors did I follow in the field, how many bloods did I really draw? He said "You know, this is just not good enough. We are going to need more." ...I then proceeded to kick myself in the butt, so I was closing in the neighborhood of 150 - 200 good closures a month...That's when I realized I could work smarter instead of harder. I got it down to a science. I grouped things, I made sure I wasn't crisscrossing the city, and I got to the point that I would get home in the evening and would make about twenty phone calls to patients and contacts. And I did something most people probably won't do now—I went out on Saturday and Sunday mornings. I wasn't getting paid for it, but I was bound and determined that I was going to make this successful because I was motivated.[64]

Classroom and interview training takes a new PHA only so far. Unless one has field experience, paired with solid supervision and coaching, he or she does not excel as a PHA and the public health effort suffers. Good supervisors knew how to motivate PHAs as they went through culture shock and adjustment in the field. They knew how to encourage them to solve problems so that they could handle their caseloads, and they demonstrated that they, too, understood the field. Jack Spencer is a retired PHA who spent years in STD prevention and ended his career serving in Cambodia with the Global AIDS Program at CDC. His first experience as a "first-line supervisor," a manager of PHAs who exclusively worked in the clinic and the field, was in Trenton, New Jersey in 1970. He had to win over several jaded staff members who had been managed previously by someone who loved to stay in the office and "do paperwork." Jack knew that to establish credibility with his field staff and improve their outcomes as investigators, he would need to work alongside them in the field. This came as a surprise to his staff. This was a "hands on, make or break kind of entrance." Jack recalls saying at his first staff meeting:

> I want to be out in the field with you guys. The best way I know to do this is not just to come out with you, but to take your tough interviews. Anybody that you've interviewed with unproductive results, let me come and talk to them.[65]

The staff gladly handed over the tough interviews to Jack in order to test his mettle as a supervisor. Employee Bill Davenport called with a syphilis patient he and one other employee had already interviewed without any success: a man they presumed to be gay. It was assumed that Jack would not want a case like this. Instead, he reveled in the chance to demonstrate relationship-building and successful interviewing. Jack recalled that the success also helped him shape his Trenton staff into better interviewers and investigators:

> I made an appointment, I met this guy, and we sat on a park bench in Asbury Park, New Jersey. I looked at him and I said, "How long have you been gay?" He said, "I'm not gay." I said, "I apologize. How long have you been bisexual?" He said, "Oh, about ten years." And we started talking. By the end of the interview he had provided the name and locating information for eight contacts. Since it was only about 6:00 p.m., I worked all eight of them that night. The next morning I provided all the documents for Bill to follow-up.[66]

Strong supervisors were remembered as teachers as well as coaches. They used many tools to instruct new PHAs and to redirect those who needed improvement. An example of such a tool, particularly in the 1960s and early 1970s, was "chalk talks." Dean Mason, a former PHA who served as the president and CEO of the Sabin Vaccine Institute until 2006, recalls them:

> A chalk talk was a discussion of syphilis cases—successful and unsuccessful interviews. What did you miss, what could you analyze about the case? Why do you think there would be more contacts to the case or why do you think it would be brought to closure? It's like going over your basketball plays before a game, and it was intense.[67]

Chalk talks were opportunities to present difficult cases to the VD or STD staff so that solutions might be identified and information shared among staff. "Chalk" referred to the chalkboard used to record the data presented for discussion. Each investigator brought a problem case for consideration by the staff group. Highly confidential information was exchanged in an effort to find a contact or make a breakthrough on a case. For some, these talks were legendary. For others, they were a terrible waste of time. By the late 1960s, chalk talks were so prevalent that there was an effort to standardize them across the country to ensure consistency and quality.[68] Gary Conrad recalls his experience with chalk talks as a new co-op in the 1960s:

> There would be a presentation of select syphilis interview information, where it might be a difficult case or it might be a classic example of how we found the source of the infection and prevented disease. The investigator would put certain information on the chalk board, and we would discuss those situations where we were not able to find the source of the infection or whatever. The other people in the room would offer suggestions on how to approach that difficult case. So a chalk talk really was a way to look at exemplary investigations, investigations on people that couldn't be located or were difficult, and to provide good investigative feedback.[69]

Successful fieldwork relies on initial training and continual opportunities to build problem-solving skills. It also depends centrally on a PHA's ability to build trust and establish rapport with patients, potential contacts, and community gatekeepers. If a PHA cannot build trust and maintain confidentiality, the public health outcomes will be poor. Over the years, recruiters have selected people to become PHAs in part because they appear to have a special personal characteristic that allows them to gain trust, paired with a willingness to risk their own safety while doing so. Tracy Ford is a PHA working as the field operations manager for the Houston Department of Health. She has these special characteristics, and says that her work in STD has helped her gain sensitivities necessary for the job:

> Everybody has sex at some point in time, so you understand the privacy of it, you understand where they're coming from, and you see the person at their most vulnerable state. It is here that you learn to talk to them and explain and teach them things so they can be a better person overall.[70]

The training and the realities of working in a health program where issues are centrally sexual provides PHAs with a sense of what is most private, and yet more than likely universally experienced. Tracy feels that the central component of her success is the ability to establish trust with a client. She has been willing to do this in any situation. In 1991, Tracy was working as the jail coordinator in Long Beach, California. There she worked with inmates who tested positive for sexually transmitted diseases, including HIV. In the jail situation, people are often inmates for short periods of time, so Tracy developed relationships that she hoped would extend into the community. She would "chit chat" with her clients: "I'm the type who asks, 'Well, what are you in here for, girl? You did that? Now you know better, girl!'" Tracy established rapport during initial conversations in the jail setting, but often needed to reestablish rapport on the street with the same client. One of Tracy's clients in Long Beach was in jail because she had stabbed her husband with a fork for eating her chicken. "Wouldn't you know," Tracy said, "this is the woman who would test positive for HIV, and I would need to find her in the streets." She found the woman easily enough, but did not recognize her at first. The woman did not identify herself in order to see whether Tracy would break her confidentiality just to find her in the street. This client put Tracy though more than a few tests. The first one began in a crack house. Tracy learned from talking with folks in the community that this woman was probably at a particular crack house. She went there and found a few women in an upstairs room smoking crack, but they denied seeing her client:

> "Nah, we ain't seen her, she not out [of jail]." I said, "I know she out, 'cause I was just over there talking to her the other day, so where is she, what's going on?" And I had to sit up there and wait

> while they finished smoking a crack rock, and I'm thinking now, "Where is the police when you need them?" When they finished, I said, "You all finished? Now where is she?" They say, "Well, so and so gonna show you where she is down the street; we think she's over there." I said okay... We get in the car, we go around the corner to this apartment, duplex-type style place that was huge and abandoned. We walk in, and I'm yelling "Health Department, it's Tracy, Health Department!" We go down to an apartment where this guy's asleep. I'm banging on the door, he go, "What!" I say, "You seen so and so?" "No." I'm banging on the door again. "When she gonna get back?" I mean this is like four or five times of knocking. He finally tells me she's not here, she'll be back later. So I said, "I'm leaving a note on the door. Don't open it. Tell her to call me." We get back in the car, and I take the girl back to the crack house. I'll be daggone because the next day this woman comes to the clinic. She was one of the girls smoking drugs, but I didn't recognize her anymore. She said, "I saw you out there, but I just wanted to make sure you weren't going to break my confidentiality. Thank you so much; now I'm coming on in to the clinic."[71]

Maintaining client confidentiality at all costs is central to the job of any disease investigator, and Public Health Advisors learn this early and through difficult experiences. The outsider might think that issues of confidentiality are cut-and-dried, black and white; however, confidentiality in health situations is often in a gray area—which is where the PHA stands. Lisa Speissegger is a policy analyst in the Office of Policy, Planning, and Evaluation at the CDC's National Center on Birth Defects and Developmental Disabilities. She learned about the more difficult side of maintaining patient confidentiality when she was working as a PHA in San Francisco. In that role, Lisa followed up on reports from San Francisco General Hospital and from the local STD clinic. At this intersection she saw the stark realities of confidentiality:

> I was working with San Francisco General Hospital, and I'd pick up patient reports of positive GC [gonorrhea] and chlamydia tests. One of them was for a four- or five-year-old girl who tested positive for chlamydia. We often had reports of children with STDs, but we never did the follow-up on these cases—that was left up to the cops and social services. Within hours of receiving this report, the mother of the child came in to the city clinic because she found

> something in her partner's possessions with our information on it. She came in demanding, "What is this? Why is he getting this? My daughter has chlamydia. Does it have anything to do with that?" It was really frustrating, because I wanted to scream, "Yes, the bastard came in here, he had chlamydia, he got treated for it. Here's his medical record—get him!" But we couldn't do that. We couldn't even be subpoenaed—the city lawyer was called in, the staff was counseled... it was a bleak time for all staff involved. I often think that this situation might have been one worth losing my job over.[72]

Interview skills, interpersonal relationship building, and contact epidemiology are a PHA's core skills. In addition, PHAs possess the technical skills of performing phlebotomy and darkfield microscopy to aid in epidemiology. Since the time of the second PHA class, all new hires have been required to learn how to draw blood in the field. In the early years, blood screening was a significant part of the VD Division's effort to combat syphilis (see Chapter 4). Although blood testing en masse is not commonly practiced outside of outbreak situations today, the skill to perform phlebotomy remains a critical component of epidemiology because the PHA can obtain a sample for examination anywhere, at any time. Because of the job's 24/7 nature, sometimes the boundaries of the PHA's work and home life become blurred. Gary Conrad was a PHA in New York City during the syphilis eradication efforts in the 1960s. He and his colleagues drew a lot of blood at all times of day and night, and had to store it at home:

> In New York City we would draw blood from people in the streets, in the back of cars, in bars. These are some of the experiences that we didn't talk about... When I worked in New York City and we drew blood, we used to go out to bars at night, gay bath houses and street corners, and we did these syphilis blitzes. Collected blood by sometimes the hundreds. What I would do is package the blood up. We would have the label filled out, and the blood would get all over the tubes. We would put it in brown bags, which had blood all over the brown bags. I would take it home and put it in my refrigerator. You wanted to keep (the blood samples) refrigerated so you could turn them in Monday morning at the laboratory. My wife didn't like seeing blood and that sort of thing, but that was okay. We did that throughout several assignments, where I would take home infected blood and put it next to the milk and think that was perfectly normal.[73]

Although PHAs came to think that drawing blood and storing it in a home refrigerator was "perfectly normal," they did not easily gain comfort with the task. Every PHA had to become proficient at phlebotomy, but some tried to avoid it for as long as possible. Bob Keegan was hired in 1974 and spent his first two weeks in Newark, New Jersey, "studying up" for interviewing school. He was a history major, which meant that he was not prepared in any way for his technical training as a phlebotomist. Though he passed the course and received his certificate, Bob spent the first year of his work as a co-op avoiding blood drawing:

> I didn't want to draw anybody's blood. I didn't want to touch that needle. And at the end of the two weeks it came down to it. The instructors brought in those dummy arms, and had somebody from the Health Department give us the formal training. They let you stab the dummy about five or ten times until you think you have the hang of it; then you start drawing bloods from other people in the class. I'm just petrified. I [tried], and there was no blood. I'm thinking, 'Oh, shoot. Here comes the end of the job right now. I couldn't get it.' The training school instructor took the needle from me and jiggled it around and got the blood to come out. They gave it back to me as if I did it myself. Well, I hadn't done anything. I didn't have a clue what was done to get the blood to come out. They said, "Alright; you did it. Way to go!" and gave me a certificate like I'd actually done it. So of course I'm thinking, 'Well, I passed the next part of the class, but Lord, I don't want to go back to Newark and try this on a real patient.' And so I didn't. I spent the next year avoiding a blood test.[74]

The fear of drawing blood is natural, particularly when one thinks about the potential for exposure to blood-borne diseases. Even in the days prior to HIV, the concern was hepatitis. The kind of equipment used in the 1950s and 1960s increased the potential for exposure, and the fact that PHAs often took samples in less than clinical conditions enhanced the risk. Gary Conrad remembers his experience from the 1960s:

> To identify syphilis, we used what we called Sheppard tubes, which had a rubber neck with a glass capillary inside it. You would insert the needle to see the blood in the capillary, and then snap the capillary between your fingers to release the blood into the

> tube. Often the broken capillary would cut your fingers, and so the infected blood would run onto your blood.[75]

Becoming comfortable with performing phlebotomy was as important as becoming comfortable with interviewing. Although some were able to avoid drawing blood for a period of time, all PHAs eventually had to do it. Their job in STD investigation required it, as did many other assignments. Phil Talboy did not anticipate that he would be drawing blood from rats to investigate hantavirus (see Chapter 1), though this skill was critical to the job. No one in the Florida Health Department was willing to do this at the time, and since Phil was a trained phlebotomist and a PHA, he was willing to do the job. Facing the fear of blood drawing was an important part of training for PHAs. Phil remembers one particular PHA, Kim Do, who worked overtime to become an effective phlebotomist. He trained Kim in 1989 in Florida:

> When Kim came to the training center, we told him he had to draw bloods. He turned white, saying, "I cannot draw bloods. I cannot draw bloods." At that particular time we were practicing either on each other or on an orange. Somewhere I found a dummy arm to practice on. It had red dye for the blood and rubber tubing as the veins, but it looked like an actual arm.... Kim finally, very tentatively started to draw bloods on the arm. I later found out that after everybody else had gone home, Kim was staying late to practice on the arm. Kim was in Palm Beach County, so he would stay after hours to practice and then drive fifty miles to get home. In January 2004 he called to thank me for teaching him how to draw bloods. He was on a big project in California that needed somebody to draw blood at the jails, and he was chosen because he was such a good phlebotomist – so good that he was now known as Dracula.[76]

Gritty field experiences, long hours and intense realities are shared across generations of PHAs, and help to make each PHA a part of the PHA culture. However, willingness to serve and loyalty to CDC define this culture more than any other qualities. PHAs from across the decades talk about the cohort's culture of service. When Louise Galaska reflects on her field experiences, she says they "made me a better American because I really began to appreciate people and all their differences, no matter how challenging." Early in her career she also learned that her job was different than those of her friends. She remembers rooming with several college friends in Chicago. One worked for the Federal Reserve Bank, one was in sales—and then there was Louise. "No one thought I'd make it," she said. But make it she did, and she protected the health of a lot of people. Louise recounts "a day from hell" when she worked diligently to get a pregnant woman to the clinic for gonorrhea treatment. Once at the clinic, the patient learned she also had syphilis; a situation that was much more serious for the unborn baby. The effort to get this woman to the clinic was colossal. She did not want to get treatment; she wanted Louise to leave her alone. At the end of a long and arduous day, Louise was tired, but proud of her service—even if it was not appreciated by the woman she sought to assist. Louise told her friends that while they thought they were doing important things in their "power jobs," she was making a more meaningful difference:

> I was asked to follow a pregnant woman who had a positive test for gonorrhea. I went out to the woman's house. She had a young child there, about two years old, and she didn't want me to come in. It was hotter than hell out. I'm talking, talking, talking, trying to get this woman to the clinic. Finally got her in the car, but then she insisted I drive her past the street corner, where her boyfriend was hanging out. I drove her past, and of course her boyfriend was belligerent, wanted to know who I was, where was I taking her. I told him it was to a clinic for her prenatal checkup. Got out of there as fast as I could and got her to the clinic. Long wait at the clinic, had to babysit this woman's child so the mother could go in and get treated. I thought she was hungry so I bought the kid lunch which she didn't eat. The kid wailed, snot coming out of her nose. I'm telling you, it was the day from hell. I spent all day on this woman. I dropped her off at four o'clock, she gets out of the car. I think I also interviewed her because of course she gave me a hassle about her sex partners and did not even say thank you. She just walked away in a huff. It was not a good day. Got home that day, and we're sitting around with my girlfriends talking about what we did today, and I thought for a moment and said, "I saved a baby today".[77]

Even as work values change in the United States and the thinking about overtime and working conditions evolves, PHAs learn that their jobs are a bit different than those of the "average person." PHA culture helps to instill and reinforce values of working early and late, and around the clock, because of the importance to the public's health. Ray Bly recalls coaching and modeling the job for new co-ops in the early 1960s. He thinks this initial modeling was reinforced by the work culture that PHAs throughout the decades hold dear:

> We wanted to set the tone for work, so we got up early and plowed late, as the old saying goes. I was seldom home before ten o'clock at night. Oftentimes left real early in the morning and hardly saw our two sons.[78]

Motivational leadership by people like Frank Miller and the late Joe Moore hammered in the importance of the PHA job. Joe was the "iron-fisted" director of the VD program in St. Louis from 1973 to 1983. He is remembered mostly for his intensity as he strove for standards of excellence among the workforce. Bob Kohmescher, who once spent time in a tree in order to flag down someone who needed treatment for syphilis, worked with Joe from 1974 to 1976. He said that working for Joe was like "going back to graduate school." It prepared Bob and others for successful careers in public health.

> The two things that Joe conveyed was the sense of urgency in the importance of what we were doing, and the need to have broad program experience. You were accountable for knowing everything there was to know, and they would quiz us constantly, making sure that we knew that information backwards and forward. And then we had Joe Moore hammering on us with a sense of urgency to get your work done immediately. Last thing in the world you wanted to tell Joe was that "I called them Sunday night because I didn't want to ruin their weekend or leave them upset all weekend." He wanted us to call them Friday night and find a clinic to get them treated over the weekend.[79]

Russ Havlak recalls that Joe Moore turned the St. Louis STD program around from a disrespected and dysfunctional program to one of the strongest in the country. Joe was an innovator. He was the first to develop a computerized means of tracking syphilis, using his home computer and enlisting the help of a colleague at McDonnell Douglas. The result was a model for the country and the precursor of the first national version of the STD management information system.[80] His determination would reverberate throughout the staff.

Russ recalls:

> In five years Joe could proudly point to one of the finest STD clinics in the country and certainly the most effective syphilis prevention program anywhere. The most amazing fact was that more than eighty percent of the syphilis cases in St. Louis were considered at the time to be the most logistically difficult to succeed with—gay and bisexual men who frequented bathhouses. Joe Moore accomplished this renaissance through a combination of his forceful personality and his fierce determination to "make it happen." Joe's path to this success was anything but smooth; it was pockmarked with firings of a number of incompetent tenured local employees, suffering through indignities in consequent hearings and even lawsuits, and rebuilding the reputation of a previously disrespected arm of the Department of Health. No price was too dear for Joe to pay, and he achieved his dream of having the best STD program in the country.[81]

The supervisory education provided by Joe Moore and others like him was often delivered in a way that left no questions about their expectations. Those who served in St. Louis with Joe Moore recall that he "left an indelible impression on you that stayed with you through your entire Public Health career." Bob Kohmescher remembers one staff meeting:

> I can remember one of our weekly staff meetings [in] which Joe told an employee that if he didn't quickly finish his work and get his reports in on time and follow up with the paper [cases] that he had open, that he would be sitting on the seashore of North Carolina watching seagulls shit. Ironically, that's exactly what happened. He ended up returning to North Carolina, where he was located on the seashore of North Carolina.[82]

Excellence was reinforced through supervision and coaching, and through an enduring spirit of competition between and among co-ops themselves. PHA stories from as early as the 1940s told of competitions in blood drawing, patient interviewing, and contact identification. Pat McConnon, the executive director of the Council of State and Territorial Epidemiologists, recalls the culture of competition as an initiation of sorts. Co-ops would be sent out into the community to look for a contact by the name of "UNK" (unknown first name) "UNK" (unknown last name):

> If there wasn't some way to get the experience for somebody who worked for you, people would contrive situations. "Don't come back until you find every one of these contacts." They sent you out on larks looking for UNK UNK. There were some initiation sorts of things, gallows humor, pressure, all kinds of good stuff.[83]

Dick Conlon recalls working in Cleveland for "the master motivator," Frank Miller, from 1968 to 1971. Frank knew the challenges of investigation and spurred his PHAs toward excellence through friendly competition. The strategy worked, because it pushed Frank's staff to succeed with fieldwork's challenges. They, like John Miles, learned to be problem-solvers. Dick Conlon recalls:

> Frank Miller really knew how to motivate people. I can remember an instance where Deane Johnson had worked this case, and he couldn't find the guy. He lived on the southeast side, and he was a plumber. Frank called Deane in and says, "Are you done with this? Is there nothing else you can do?" And Dean said, "I've done everything." Frank said, "I bet Conlon can find this guy in fifteen minutes." Deane said, "I'll bet you two to one odds for a Coke," something like that. So Frank Miller calls me and he says, "Here, Conlon, can you find this guy?" I remember the man's name, he's forty-seven years old, he was a plumber, he lived at [cross streets].84 And I said, "Yeah, I can probably find this guy. Take me about ten minutes." And so he said, "You're on." Five minutes later I had the guy on the phone, and he was headed to the clinic. We had these crisscross directories for the City of Cleveland. I found the guy as a plumber, called him up, asked him where he lived. I didn't tell him what I had, he told me where he lived. I said, "Well, I have some information for you, and you need to come in and see me right away," and he was there.[85]

The initial training and early field experiences provided new recruits with the opportunity to see the PHA's job, and helped to shape them in their future public health roles and careers. After two years in the field, only about half of the co-ops remained because the work was arduous. Those who remained became part of the cohort upon which CDC relies when they need trained and experienced public health personnel in assignments throughout the world, in major public health efforts, and in times of public health crisis. The PHAs would take on these challenges in their daily work assignments and through special temporary duty assignments. In each case, the accrual of training and experiences prepared the PHA to be "ready to go."

Chapter 7

Ready To Go

On March 28, 1979, the Three Mile Island 2 nuclear reactor near Middletown, Pennsylvania, suffered a severe core meltdown.[1] Nuclear Regulatory Commission authorities underestimated the severity of the situation as unsubstantiated reports about releases of radioactive material increased public concern. Pennsylvania Governor Dick Thornburgh advised all school children and pregnant women within five miles of the plant to evacuate. Public health officials urged swift and massive production of a potassium iodide solution for distribution to the public in the event of a widespread radiation release. If taken in time, a few drops would prevent the thyroid gland from absorbing radioactive iodine.[2] Pennsylvania health authorities were unprepared for an emergency of this magnitude, so they called the CDC to help.

Joe Carter was working in the Philadelphia Regional Office when he got the call. CDC was asked to mobilize to distribute potassium iodide and to help with evacuation if necessary. The work would be dangerous. With the deluge of confusing information at the time, anyone taking the assignment would understand it to be life-threatening. Joe recalls:

> I was called by CDC, since it was in my state of Pennsylvania, outside of Harrisburg. They wanted to know if I could get together a workforce, and they told me about the dangers. They wanted to know if I would care to do it or whether I would want to opt out. I said no, I would want to help and that I would call around to see if I could get a team together to go up and do it, knowing the dangers. I called all of the senior reps I had in the state and two others. They all said they would help any way they could. They said they'd first need twenty-four hours to tell their families. They would be there: "Just tell me where and when."[3]

PHAs are "ready to go" by training and by constitution, reinforced by a

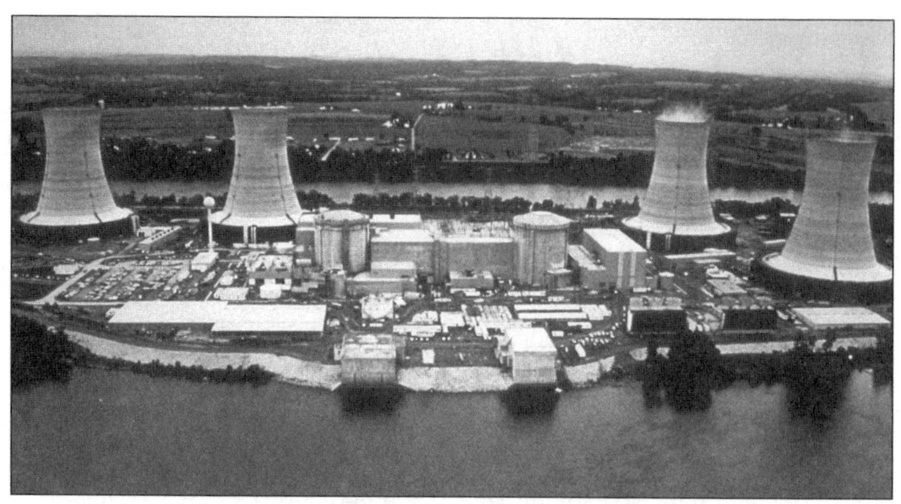

Three Mile Island nuclear power plant near Middletown, Pennsylvania.
Courtesy Centers for Disease Control and Prevention, Public Health Image Library.

culture of service. Their training and skill sets allow for quick study of issues and awareness of diverse geographic and cultural terrain. Their initial, singular experiences working on the ground in sexually transmitted disease programs provides a flexibility that is not found in other fields. This kind of worker is not hired, but made over many years of experiences in different communities and across several public health programs; bolstered by a PHA culture that values this kind of service.

Public Health Advisors were not the first type of public health worker to be deployed in times of health emergency. Since the 1870s, the Public Health Service commissioned physicians to provide medical infrastructure and emergency assistance throughout the U.S.[4] In 1957, when PHAs moved with the VD Division to CDC in Atlanta, they were joining an agency that had an established reputation for emergency response. They soon would work alongside a sibling cadre of professionals—EIS officers—who likewise were poised for deployment.[5] It was not until 1961 that PHAs were used for anything other than VD control deployments. In that year, CDC wanted to increase the number of persons immunized by the Salk vaccine for polio, and targeted their efforts to "Babies and Breadwinners"—those surmised to be undervaccinated. A group of PHAs was detailed to Columbus, Georgia, to help provide mass vaccination and to assist with publicity (see Chapter 5)[6]. After this effort, PHAs were called on for deployments outside VD because of their field training, their logistical acumen, and their ability to draw blood and vaccinate.

The term "TDY" is a military acronym for "temporary duty assignment." PHAs over the decades have come to know this term well, because it marks their experience with domestic and international short-term assignments. "Temporary" might be as short as a few weeks or as long as a few years. Anne-Renee Heningburg spent several years during the late 1990s working in India and Nigeria for the Global Immunization Program through a string of TDY assignments. Ken Latimer spent two years in Puerto Rico conducting mass blood screening for syphilis in the early 1950s. Kevin O'Connor spent months in Miami working a 1983 syphilis and PPNG (Penicillinase-Producing Neisseria Gonorrhea) outbreak on a TDY. In 1975 Dennis McDowell spent two intense weeks at a refugee camp set up at Camp Pendleton after the fall of Saigon. The time frame for deployment is based entirely on the situation of need.

Establishing a locally trained and geographically varied workforce has allowed CDC to have ready and deployable human resources in the field for emergencies or emerging needs anywhere in the world. PHAs are part of an inimitable, deployable team that can be credited with the eradication of smallpox, the identification of new strains of disease, and the halting of epidemics. PHAs think modestly about these deployments, because they are just part of the job. Prior to 1994, those recruited to be entry-level Public Health Advisors knew that they would start their career in STD programs in the field, and that they might be sent on a string of deployments based on public health need. These assignments would make use of their accruing field operations skills, yet might not have anything to do with their program placement or background. Joe Betros, a retired PHA who worked in sexually transmitted disease programs for most of his career, recalls his many and varied TDYs as if he is reading a laundry list. Few of his deployments had to do with STDs:

> While I was in Cleveland, they sent a scientist to investigate children who were going into aplastic crisis due to sickle cell anemia and Fifth Disease.7 Two of us were assigned to assist the investigation. I went TDY to Toledo to run the STD program while they were looking for a new city program manager. Then I was sent to Albany, New York to assist a CDC Epidemiologist in the Eosinophilia-Myalgia Syndrome investigation. In 2003 they sent me to San Francisco In-

> ternational for fifty days to check inbound aircraft from specified Asian countries during the SARS problem. Then to Honolulu International for an additional twenty-six days.[8]

Bill Gimson, CDC's chief operating officer, recently was sent to Iraq as part of a federal reconstruction team focused on government, budget, business and economic issues.[9] In December 2007, he left his family and his job at CDC to work for six months in an undisclosed location in Iraq. Bill's situation is unusual, because those being deployed are typically already on the ground working in a public health program somewhere in the world so that they are ready in a moment's notice—what Bill calls "embedded." He believes that CDC's success with mobilization efforts is tied directly to the availability of highly trained PHAs in the field:

> If all of a sudden you've got stuff coming out of Vietnam, you've got people already embedded there working. It's the same thing here in the States. We probably could have been even more successful with SARS had we the field staff that we had in the past.[10]

Temporary duty for PHAs began in the 1950s and became widespread with CDC's effort to eradicate smallpox. PHA Billy Griggs was enlisted to help Dr. Donald "D.A." Henderson eradicate smallpox in 1965. He and D.A. functioned together as a management team—a PHA and an epidemiologist. This successful pairing of a scientist and a PHA not only cemented the management custom at CDC, it initiated the pattern of extensive use of PHAs for public health emergencies. Like Bill Gimson, Billy Griggs believes that having a ready cadre of trained PHAs in the field allowed CDC to be effective with smallpox: "What you need to be a successful response agency is the availability of trained, skilled people that you can pick up and throw in the breach."[11] He recalls several effective TDYs, including refugee resettlement following the fall of Saigon. "PHAs went to the stations overseas… they literally managed the administrative aspects of the stations in California, Pennsylvania, and Arkansas,"[12] he said. More than two hundred fifty people served in short-term assignments with smallpox. Many served recently with the response to the terrorist attacks on September 11, 2001. For Griggs, readiness depended on having between fifty and one hundred PHAs in the field ready for deployment. CDC can deploy a highly skilled workforce capable of working beyond their particular job description and able to hit the ground running. This justifies the resources invested in a PHA workforce, says Windell Bradford, a retired PHA who served in several senior leadership capacities at CDC and led a major review of PHA field staff in the 1990s: "PHAs responding to emergencies that had nothing to do with their particular job justifies every penny that's ever been put into this program."[13]

Having a ready force is one thing. Having a willing workforce is quite another. Over the years Public Health Advisors have established a professional culture that reflects their unique work experiences of being moved frequently, placed throughout the U.S. and abroad as part of their training, and being deployed in response to public health emergencies or disasters. This PHA culture values long hours, hard work, challenging assignments, and hardcore humor. It makes the more interesting assignments, such as smallpox eradication, highly coveted among PHA ranks. This is a problem that any response agency would love to have, because not every organization can claim a ready and willing workforce for rapid deployment into challenging situations. Phil Talboy's experience with hantavirus in Florida (see Chapter 1) is one example where the culture of Public Health Advisors reinforced his decision to do the dangerous job—the job that local health department staff were afraid to do.[14] The ease with which Joe Carter was able to pull together a team in response to the Three Mile Island nuclear disaster is another example.

Since the 1960s, PHAs have been given many types of rapid deployments and temporary duty assignments which have required a variety of skills honed over different types of experiences and in different communities: epidemiology and case finding, diplomacy and policy work, operations and logistics, vaccinating and teaching or training. PHAs have been called to respond to outbreaks of disease such as hantavirus, Lassa fever, monkeypox, encephalitis, tuberculosis, measles, AIDS, smallpox, polio, Legionnaires, Guillain-Barré syndrome, SARS, syphilis, PPNG, babesiosis, and cholera. PHAs were detailed for health campaigns such as Guinea worm, malaria, syphilis, diarrheal diseases, yellow fever, yaws, and swine flu. PHAs have been detailed in the wake of major events such as floods, hurricanes, volcanic eruptions, earthquakes, and the anthrax scare in the U.S.[15] They even were detailed as poll watchers in select Southern states during the 1972 and 1976 presidential elections.[16] Public Health Advisors have been detailed wherever the events occurred, in the United States and in every conceivable location elsewhere: throughout the African continent, in South and Central America, and throughout the Asian continent. The stories that follow are examples of the types of deployments PHAs have experienced since the 1960s. They highlight the PHAs' singular contributions to health situations here and abroad: those of highly skilled, street-savvy professionals willing to go rapidly into any crisis.

They're gonna ambush me down the road: Hospital Integration, 1964[17]

In the1960s access to the healthcare system in the South was often two-tiered, echoing Jim Crow. Segregation denied equal access to healthcare by racial and ethnic minority populations, particularly African Americans who often were diverted to separate and inferior hospitals or nursing homes, or were segregated to a section that was overcrowded and in poorer condition. The case of *Simkins v. Moses H. Cone Memorial Hospital* was the landmark decision that led to the elimination of segregated healthcare through Title VI of the 1964 Civil Rights Act. The Medicare program, enacted two years later, hastened the integration of healthcare facilities more quickly than other institutions providing public accommodations, because it prohibited healthcare providers receiving federal funds from discriminating based on race.[18] The hammer that would force institutional change was the threat of losing Medicare funding. Healthcare facilities would have to prove that they were compliant and did not discriminate on the basis of race, color, or national origin. By 1966 several hundred complaints had been filed with the Department of Health, Education, and Welfare (HEW), primarily against Southern healthcare facilities.[19] These complaints needed to be investigated quickly and efficiently in order to determine compliance with the law. In 1966 Dr. David Sencer, then CDC director, was attending a meeting of HEW officials that focused on how to handle the burgeoning number of claims. He recalls offering the help of PHAs and EIS officers:

> They were trying to figure out how to do the inspections necessary to enforce Title VI, which involved visiting and inspecting all the hospitals in the Southeast. I got tired of their worrying and lack of decision and said the CDC would train and launch inspectors from our PHAs and EIS. They jumped at the suggestion. [PHA] Stu Kingma organized a week-long training session and off they went.20 ... We pulled everybody out of the states. We had everyone under the sun. We put on a two-week training course, turned everybody loose, and got the job done.

CDC pulled inspectors primarily from its ranks of PHAs, though a few EIS officers also participated. PHAs later would be joined by staff from other federal agencies. The process to investigate hospitals and nursing homes was established by PHAs. In a brief training, PHAs reviewed the law, the complaints, and the methods to investigate health care facilities. Hospitals would be the focus of the first phase, and nursing homes would follow.[21] Teams of PHAs went to Georgia, Alabama, Mississippi, Tennessee, South Carolina, and Florida to investigate specific complaints. They met with the individual filing the complaint to gain complete information about the practices of the facilities involved, and then they visited the facility to interview staff and leadership, consult records, and observe. Before leaving, the inspectors briefed the facility management regarding their findings. A written report would follow, though as investigators they were to "avoid discussions of possible repercussions of our reports."[22] Windell Bradford was a PHA working in New York City's VD Program at the time of this charge:

> The team set up a base of operations in Atlanta, and rented cars against the insistence of CDC Financial Management Office staff that we use GSA cars… Having grown up in the South, I [felt] that our use of rental cars and normal business dress would let us pass off as normal salesmen traveling the back roads. Bill Marshman and I were buying gas somewhere in South Georgia. The proprietor said he didn't know who we were or what we were doing: "I thought at first you are FBI, but noticed that you aren't wearing brown shoes." He asked what we were up to, and we said we sold swimming pools.[23]

The assignment of PHAs to investigate hospital and nursing home integration was a tremendous success. Years of complaints were addressed in a matter of months.[24] Bob Longenecker, a PHA from the Immunization Program in Kansas, completed his assignment of visiting eighteen hospitals in thirty-three days. He recalls that only two of the eighteen were found to be in compliance:

> I visited one hospital in Orangeburg, South Carolina, and questioned one of the black patients as he was lying in his bed. I asked him how he liked his room. He replied that it was great. He said it was a lot better than the basement room he was originally in that morning. Apparently, the hospital had made some cosmetic changes just for my visit.[25]

CDC needed to use workers who were accustomed to careful investigations, because whatever was found would end up in litigation. A lot was at stake, and PHAs were a perfect fit for the job because they were shrewd investigators who could see beyond the quick or superficial changes meant to suggest hospital compliance.[26] Although "white" and "colored" signs were removed from the bathrooms, perhaps only whites would receive a key to the previously-labeled "whites-only" restroom.[27] PHAs interviewed patients, families of patients, staff, and health administrators. They requested records to get a sense of the staffing patterns, patient admissions, and rooming placements, data related to the catchment area served by each hospital or nursing home. They would tour the facilities and observe the subtleties of racial segregation. This job did not go unnoticed. Significant hostility was expressed toward the PHAs who were detailed for their assignment. Jim Fowler was working in the Chicago VD Program when he was assigned to investigate hospitals in Mississippi. He recalls the reaction:

> We were treated with rather a lot of hostility. I can remember being introduced while I came into the hospital. The hospital administrator said… "Where are you from originally?" I said, "Well, I grew up in North Carolina." And he said, "Well, then you'll understand our problems, right?" I said, "No, I don't know what that has to do with anything."[28]

Windell Bradford recalled that during the time of their assignment, Alabama Governor George Wallace made his first of many remarks about "those disgusting black-briefcase-carrying federal bureaucrats who had invaded the South."[29] This investigation was one of many symbols of change threatening white hegemony in the U.S. Threats both implied and actual were made against the PHA investigators. Bob Longenecker recalls being followed out of town after meeting with hospital officials in Beaufort, South Carolina. In the meeting, he was told that the hospital had no intention of integrating and that he should head out of town immediately.[30] Windell Bradford recalls hearing about a threat not to himself or other investigators, but to patients themselves. When investigating a complaint in a Southern capital city (which he would not name), he got a call at his hotel late one evening from an unidentified person asking him to go to a nearby payphone and call a number. Windell complied and spoke with a woman who told him that she heard he was "in town doing civil rights" and wanted to talk with him privately. This was a time when several efforts to improve civil rights occurred: voting rights, workers' rights, working conditions, and—with this investigation—healthcare. Windell did not know what he was getting himself into, but felt that his duty was to follow through. He was given directions to a place outside the city on an unlit dirt road:

> Occasionally I could see house lights to the right and left of the road and could read mailboxes in my headlights. Dogs barked as I avoided deep sand and bounced over ruts in the road. I found the mailbox and turned left onto a long, uphill driveway; typical PHA investigation so far. To my surprise I was greeted by a middle-aged white couple. They were both orderlies in the state's mental health hospital. They assured me in the vernacular of the time that they were not supporters of civil rights, but that something was about to happen that they thought was wrong. The hospital had been ordered to integrate, and black patients were soon to be moved to the "white" ward. Several white staff, they told me, were planning to convince white patients to smother these black patients with pillows while they slept. I asked if they would repeat this on my tape recorder, and they agreed. I waited until morning to call [CDC]....I heard no news reports in the following months to suggest that this threat was carried out.[31]

Jim Fowler recalls the harassment and his thinking that his "time had come" when investigating a hospital in Alabama. He was traveling on Route 80 when he noticed that he was being followed. This was no ordinary road. It was the same stretch of road on which civil rights worker Viola Liuzzo had been killed by members of the Ku Klux Klan the previous year.[32] He recalls leaving a complainant's house and being followed out of the neighborhood:

> They followed me. I made a number of different unnecessary turns, and they were always behind me. I got back on the road heading back to where I was spending the night... then all of a sudden they pull around, and they pull up beside me, and I tried not to look, and I thought, oh boy, my time has really come. Then all of a sudden they took off, and got out of sight, and my next thought was, "Oh, God, they're going to ambush me down the road."[33]

Hospital integration was not the only national need met by PHAs during the early 1960s. In 1962, every PHA was dispatched to collect thalidomide from all physician offices within their assignment areas[34] following the discovery that the widely-prescribed antiemetic caused severe deformities in children. Two years later, as PHAs were investigating hospitals for evidence of racial discrimination, outbreaks of St. Louis encephalitis (SLE) occurred in several locations throughout the U.S. The largest occurred in Houston, Texas, during the summer and fall of 1964. Two hundred forty-three people were infected, and twenty-seven died.[35] The epidemic's epicenter was downtown Houston, and the elderly were at greatest risk of death and complications from this mosquito-borne viral disease.[36] In this period Harris County, home to Houston, reported the highest SLE incidence in the country.[37] Prior to the advent of West Nile virus, SLE was the most common mosquito-transmitted human pathogen in the U.S., with a case fatality rate between five and fifteen percent. This was the first time that St. Louis encephalitis had been identified in Houston.

Don Eddins was working as an Epidemic Intelligence Service officer at CDC when he was called to work on the encephalitis outbreak. He joined several PHAs, other EIS officers, laboratorians, and mosquito experts from CDC after it was determined that the local health infrastructure could not handle the outbreak on its own.[38] The help needed was with control of the outbreak as well as surveillance of hospital units for suspected viral disease involving the central nervous system.[39] Don managed the field investigators, who were tasked with collecting blood samples from potentially infected people. This was 1964, and it was the first time that a computer was used in the field to do public health epidemiology. Don describes the type of assistance the PHAs provided:

> And by assist, I mean locating patients, following up on the patients that had been reported in, collecting acute sera, and two weeks later collecting covalence sera. I think in a few cases we collected a second round of covalence sera... The PHAs were brought in specifically to help with the data collection, to help with the patient management from the field perspective, and to draw the serum.[40]

The work on the 1964 SLE outbreak would foreshadow several others in the months and years to come. A similar outbreak occurred in Dallas and Corpus Christi two years later, as part of a widespread outbreak from Texas to the Delaware River Valley.[41] PHAs were called in to help and would continue to be busy with TDYs because meanwhile, CDC was gearing up to join forces with USAID to enhance efforts in malaria and smallpox control.

THEY VOLUNTEERED IN DROVES: SMALLPOX 1969–1977

The Biafran War was raging in Nigeria when Charles Watkins took the two-year assignment to work on smallpox in 1969. Over the next two years, Charles, his wife Judy, son Gordon, and soon-to-be-born son Terrence would become part of CDC's "smallpox club." This group served bravely during the smallpox eradication effort and would forever after share an esprit de corps. Their commitment to the effort was total. When practical, families accompanied PHAs on the African smallpox efforts, but they would face precarious security situations. Just as new PHAs experienced culture shock when beginning field work (see Chapter 6), Charles and his wife experienced culture shock when they arrived in 1970 Lagos, then the capital of Nigeria:

> The Biafran War was between the Igbo tribe of eastern Nigeria and mostly the rest of Nigeria being Lagos, the capitol, or the Yorubas. This was a tribal conflict… [W]here we were going, the war had just ended… We were going from the northern or western part of Nigeria into the eastern area of Igbo land, and this was where they had just been conquered. The federal troops were still in charge, and it was brutal. On the way in we were stopped every hundred miles for a passport check. They said, "Do you have arms? Are you carrying any type of contraband?" And this was our beginning of culture shock. Me, a kid coming from Milldale, New Jersey, and my wife from Montclair- somewhat of an upper-middle-class snobbish area for Afro-Americans in those days… so she was definitely in culture shock.[42]

Watkins worked by himself, as did the other PHAs who were assigned in many parts of Nigeria. The Watkins family would see the birth of their second child, Terrence, during this time, though he would not be born in Nigeria because of the need for good prenatal care. As was true for many who served in the 1960s with their families, these moments were part of the experience. After Terrence was born in West Germany, Charles brought the family back to Nigeria. Always the PHA, he immediately resumed the work: "When I got back, I put Judy, new baby Terrence, and Gordon back into the truck going back to Enugu, and I immediately took off for a conference of all of the operations officers, as we were called, in Danare."[43]

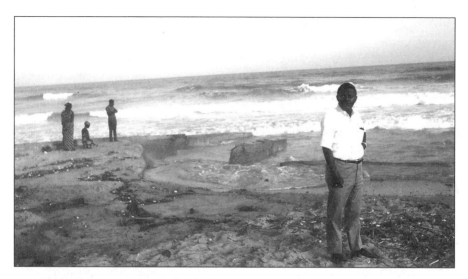

Charles Watkins, Lagos, Nigeria, circa 1970.
Courtesy of Charles Watkins.

In 1966, CDC and USAID initiated the combined Smallpox Eradication-Measles Control Program from the previous CDC smallpox unit and the USAID measles control program.[44] Efforts took place in twenty-one countries of West and Central Africa from 1966 to 1972,[45] and continued in India, Brazil, and Bangladesh.[46] Dr. D.A. Henderson directed the global effort from Geneva, and soon was assigned PHA Billy Griggs as his deputy. Billy ensured the availability of a cadre of PHAs for logistics and operations help to all scientists assigned.[47] Dr. Bill Foege led the efforts in India and initially was assisted by Bill Watson. Dr. Stan Foster led the efforts in Bangladesh, assisted by the late Andy Agle,[48] and Dr. Don Millar led the efforts in West Africa, assisted by PHA Jim Hicks. The EIS-PHA pairing was historic, and it became CDC's recipe for success with public health efforts in the U.S. and abroad.[49] Bill Watson and CDC director David Sencer were convinced that an infusion of PHAs to serve as operations officers would be just the element to ensure successful eradication efforts. In 1966, CDC began training teams of Medical (EIS) and Operations Officers (PHAs) for two-year tours of duty in twenty West African nations.[50] By the end of the smallpox crusade, more than two hundred twenty PHAs had served in the program.[51]

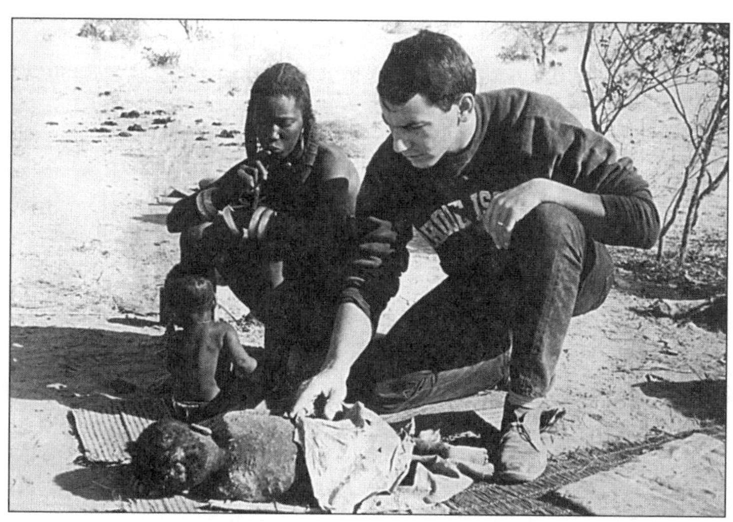

PHA Tony Masso examines a child with smallpox in Niger, late 1967.
Courtesy of Centers for Disease Control and Prevention, Public Health Image Library.

Dr. Mike Lane was a CDC physician working in the smallpox program before it became the combined CDC/USAID effort. He recalls that PHAs were brought into the smallpox eradication effort because CDC required several more epidemiologists than were available, willing, and trained from the EIS ranks: "There was no way that we'd get thirty-six epidemiologists who were good, young, healthy, and interested." PHAs on the other hand, particularly those at the mid-career level of GS-9 and GS-11, "volunteered in droves. Bill Griggs was brought in to be the associate director or the management director, and we hired Public Health Advisors for every one of the nineteen nations of West and West Central Africa."[52]

The massive effort to eradicate endemic smallpox involved the cooperation of governments, communities, and hundreds of healthcare workers to identify people with smallpox and to vaccinate those around them. The method, called surveillance containment,[53] shifted efforts away from mass immunization and toward those who were infected and their immediate contacts. PHAs made tremendous contributions using this approach, because it involved identifying and vaccinating those who were socializing with the person who was the smallpox case. The PHA skill set and the ability to work across cultures ensured success with the surveillance containment method. Mike Lane recalls:

> [You needed to] find out the social milieu of the smallpox patients and vaccinate… [anyone] who is likely to interact with these folks. And of course, the people who knew [the social network] were not the medical hierarchy, the French- and British-trained African physicians. They were the local tribal leaders. The people who really understood how to talk with those people were the PHAs, and they were good at it. They recognized that if you had eight cases of smallpox in a village of eighteen hundred, it was more sensible to vaccinate everybody than to try to make little diagrams and all that. But if there were two cases in a town of one million, you did contact tracing… At the same time there was a need for personal diplomacy… and the PHAs were good at that kind of stuff.[54]

The effort was a success as a result of the CDC's massive human resource infusion. The last case of endemic smallpox was found in Somalia on October 26, 1977.[55] PHAs made a tremendous contribution to the effort because of their skill in dealing with the myriad cultures and situations. Mike recalls being amazed at what PHAs had to offer:

> Flexibility and adaptability. I mean, just amazing. Every country was different. Different traditions—the huge difference between the old French colonies and the old British colonies in the way they did things. Obviously the language, the way they trained Africans, a tremendous amount of the job turned out to be training. But then other things that PHAs are not traditionally asked to do, which is take apart a Dodge truck engine and put it back together again. Or change axles and stuff like that.[56]

The effort was not without challenges. Initially, it was thought that Lagos, Nigeria, would be the central communications and operations point for the continent. This was soon found to be terribly wrong, and Atlanta became the central coordination point. Immediate efforts to reconfigure the operations, cable traffic, and emergency shipments occurred as a result of the leadership of Billy Griggs and Bob Hogan in Ghana and Jim Hicks in Nigeria. This was truly "emergency administrative and management stuff,"[57] and the PHAs were the only people who were skilled enough to accomplish it.

The work was often dangerous. In this same year, West Africa saw an estimated two hundred thousand to four hundred thousand smallpox cases.[58] It was a time of emerging independence for many of these nations. Transportation, communication, and medical systems posed challenges. Chad was in the midst of a civil war. In a recent interview celebrating the thirty-year anniversary of smallpox eradication, D.A. Henderson recalled that the work was tiring and often dangerous:

> There was civil war and insecurity. In Ethiopia the government would not allow any foreigners to go outside the capital city except those of us working in smallpox. We had their confidence. Still, workers were fired upon and sometimes kidnapped. UN officers would have to persuade the guerillas to release the public health workers.[59]

Smallpox eradication in Bangladesh proved very challenging. Monsoons in 1974 made surveillance difficult and prompted mass migration within the country, spreading additional disease. In addition, returning refugees from India imported smallpox following the war between East and West Pakistan.[60] Working in India and Bangladesh also raised challenges for PHAs because of differences in cultures of medical work. PHAs who worked in India and Bangladesh were assigned as World Health Organization consultants. Prior to this time, WHO was accustomed to health workers who possessed MDs, PhDs, or perhaps nursing degrees. A PHA was a different type of worker. Mike Lane recalled the PHA's initiation to the WHO culture. The field staff finally were integrated, though not twenty years later, Bill Parra would find that WHO still did not understand what a PHA was (see Chapter 1). Mike Lane recalls:

> WHO was a little nervous, and the absorbing countries sort of said, "Well, we need physicians. This is a medical program. Don't you have to be a doctor to do this?" And so the first couple of Public Health Advisors were very, very carefully chosen by Bill Foege. Bill Watson was seconded, went over voluntarily for six months, and they very carefully selected the first few PHAs. They did wonderfully in India, and finally WHO said "More, more, more."[61]

Smallpox efforts in India had come to a halt, and the relationship with the United States at the time was poor. The U.S. had been inconsistent in its relationship with India and Pakistan. In the mid-1970s, when smallpox efforts were to resume in India, the U.S. was politically pro-Pakistan and anti-India.[62] PHAs thrived in this challenging environment. Their skills in contact epidemiology and cross-cultural diplomacy proved their value beyond what any traditional med-epi could do for WHO. PHAs knew how to get information about potential smallpox cases because of their field training in the United States. A typical way of identifying cases was used by PHAs in West Africa. They would develop a relationship with the tribal leaders and sometimes the religious leaders. Mike recalls the method PHAs used:

> The way you contacted them was you knocked on their door and you paid respect and you said some nice things and then asked them about smallpox, and they would say, "Well, not in our village, but this next village over there. Or if you really want to know, tomorrow there'll be a marché, a market, and people from fifty villages around here will all be there." And we would go around, walking around with a picture of smallpox, and we may not know the local language because our guys all spoke good French… they'd just go around saying, "Anyone seen anything like this?" And someone would say, "Oh, yes."[64]

In 1975, PHAs Pat McConnon and Jerry Wheeler had a constant work load of thirty and forty outbreaks per week in Bangladesh. They would vaccinate everyone within a half-mile radius.[64] It would be the first of Pat's two TDYs for smallpox. The work was grueling and physically demanding. It was extraordinarily hot, and food in Bangladesh was limited because in 1975 the war had just ended with Pakistan. The self-described "big guy that required three squares a day" would lose about twenty percent of his body weight during the assignment, despite his efforts to buy and eat goat meat about once per week. Pat remembered his introduction to smallpox work:

> Smallpox was a difficult assignment, particularly in Bangladesh. They gave us three days' training. [At] the end of three days I think they said, "You are now one of the five hundred most experienced people in the world in smallpox diagnosis and control." And then we were given our assignments. My assignment was physically demanding and difficult. The area I was working in didn't have any roads, so it was just footpaths. Our whole team… myself and four Bengalis, had three motorcycles, and that was our conveyance.

> So we hauled our vaccines around and did all our supervision on that… when the sun went down you stayed where you were… We slept in a lot of places that were just where we ended up at the end of the day: little villages, no beds and stuff, and we just sacked out on the ground. You'd do that for four months, seven days a week. It was just exhausting. But it was really also the most personally rewarding sort of experience.[65]

The fieldwork and operations management tasks were a natural fit for Pat and other PHAs, though sometimes a bit burdensome because of the lack of infrastructure. Pat had to carry thousands of taka (the local currency) to pay more than four hundred people who were working as vaccinators, trainers, and twenty-four-hour guards for quarantine during the many smallpox outbreaks. Gary Conrad, a retired PHA who spent his career in communicable diseases and preventive health services, also worked in Bangladesh during this period. He was assigned to the local Bengali health structure. It was February 1975:

> If a suspected case of smallpox was reported, we would go out to the village. We would go out by Jeep, by walking, by motorcycle, or by riverboat. We would and look to see if this was chicken pox or smallpox. If it was smallpox, then we would do green containment, known as isolation. [We would] hire house guards within the village to stand guard so that nobody could enter the hut until they were vaccinated, and to insure that the infected person didn't leave or intermingle with the rest of the village. If there was a smallpox case we would go in with our vaccine and begin an inoculation program, and so we would start with the huts, the houses around that infected person. Oftentimes the number of infected sites would multiply, and we would begin vaccinating and recording… identifying information of every single person in that village, and then the team would fan out to the adjoining villages and would go hut-to-hut and vaccinate everybody; then they would go back and read the vaccination in ten days, or whatever it was at the time.[66]

Part of the PHA culture is a hearty humor about the difficulties of the work. Pat McConnon laughs when he recalls the remote aspects of the work. Telegraph communications would come in to the nearest town, which might be a day's bus ride away plus hours of walking in the bush. He would be easy to find, though, because he would be the only Westerner there asking, "Where are the goats? Does anyone have a goat for sale?" Humor aside, for PHAs who were away from their families for several months, the remoteness and lack of communication were challenging. Gary Conrad recalled his experience:

> I went to a place called Camilla on the Burmese border, and I was there by myself. After two days of orientation I was in this strange country and doing smallpox work with the Bengali physician, with the most meager food, no food source per se, you couldn't go to the grocery store. You just found your way. Without communication it was pretty lonely at times. Fortunately for me, I was glad I that I wasn't there during the monsoon season. You were not only alone and incommunicado, but when the monsoons came you were stranded, and so you might be sitting there for days wherever you were and not able to do anything or go anywhere.[67]

Smallpox also left its mark on PHAs, because everyone who returned to the United States had a new confidence in their ability to work effectively on intractable public health issues. Although they had learned a host of skills in their initial field assignments in the U.S., the smallpox experience, particularly in India, helped shape the next generation of PHA leaders and problem solvers. Dr. Bill Foege, CDC director from 1977 to 1983, recalls the two-way contribution of the experience:

> PHAs made the absolute difference, both in Africa and where I worked in India... In Africa, the Public Health Advisors were by and large stationed there for long periods of time, they got to know the culture, and they learned how to get things done. In India we had many of them come in on three-month TDYs. And it was amazing that you could give them three days' orientation in New Delhi, provide them with a driver and a vehicle and an interpreter, and then throw them into those places in India. Once a month, we would have a meeting in the capital city of each state. People would get together and report on what was working, what wasn't working, and we'd revise our tactics for the next month. But three months later, these people would come out having accomplished an unbelievable amount of work. I remember Don Millar, who was heading up the program in Atlanta, once sent me a note, and he said, "I don't know whether these ninety-day assignments are doing you any good for smallpox, but keep asking for them, because these people come back and they no longer are willing to

> put up with the barriers of the United States because they found that they can handle tougher problems in India." It just changes the way they work in this country.[68]

What Are They Doing to Undercut the Work That We're Doing? Righting the Wrong of Tuskegee[69]

It was 1966 in San Francisco when PHA Peter Buxtun learned that a physician who treated an elderly African American man in Alabama for syphilis was the recipient of a thrashing by public health authorities. "The man was plainly insane and his family did not know what to do," said Buxtun. The private physician examined his patient and tested his blood. It was clear that the man's insanity was a result of having neurosyphilis. The physician promptly treated his patient with penicillin, which was the standard treatment for syphilis:

> The doctor suddenly had the county medical society and the local medical society complaining, "See here, you've spoiled one of our subjects. How could you do this? Didn't you know about the Tuskegee study?" Eventually they forgave his terrible transgression of treating an elderly man with syphilitic insanity.[70]

Driven by a sense of fairness, Buxtun set out to find out why someone in the United States would be denied health care for an obvious condition that the U.S. government was trying to eradicate at the time.[71] Peter Buxtun was one of many VD investigators hired as part of Operation Pursuit, CDC's 1960s effort to eradicate syphilis by 1972 (see Chapter 6).[72] Buxtun quickly learned that there had been a study in Tuskegee, Alabama, since the 1930s, which recorded the evolution of untreated syphilis in the African American male. This study was initiated by the Public Health Service and was continued by the CDC after the VD Division transferred to CDC in 1957. It required that participants be denied the curative treatment for syphilis, which by 1966 had been on the market for decades. Although the study was not a secret—findings often were published in medical journals—the study participants did not know the study's purpose, and they believed they were receiving curative treatment for "bad blood." According to Bill Watson, "by the 1960s, the VD Division researchers assumed that study participants had been exposed at one time or another to penicillin."[73] Even so, there was no acceptable rationale for continuing the study. Times had changed in the United States since the study's initiation. What may have appeared appropriate for science in the 1940s was no longer so, or even ethical by the 1960s.

Peter Buxtun did what any PHA would do: he investigated the situation to solve the problem. This time, however, the problem was not a public health outbreak, but a government-sponsored study that had become entrenched in the VD research hierarchy. The VD Division leadership did not like that some upstart VD investigator from California was challenging the study's appropriateness. They were insulted by the implication that their study of syphilis in Tuskegee, Alabama, was racist. Buxtun continued to press for change because "there was a terrible injustice which had to be exposed and stopped":

> I was extremely troubled by what I read in the reports from CDC... And I thought, my God, I'm working for this outfit. What are they doing to undercut the work that we're doing? We're doing good work.[74]

It would be six years before Buxtun could get anyone from the press or the government to pay attention to his concerns. In July 1972 his friend, Edith Lederer, a recently-hired AP reporter, listened to his story and wanted to write about it. Her boss told her to give it to a more senior person, so Lederer sent copies of Peter's files to Jean Heller. The Associated Press covered the story. By that time, Peter had moved on from his role as VD investigator to finish his law degree at Hastings College of the Law. When the story broke and the government was forced to respond to public concern, an ad hoc advisory panel was convened in Washington, D.C., from August to October 1972 to review the study and to make recommendations.[75] The panel concluded that the study was "ethically unjustified" and should be stopped at once because its scientific gains did not outweigh the risks to participants. One of the three recommendations made by the advisory committee was to locate any surviving study members. According to study records, there were three hundred participants with syphilis and two hundred controls (patients without syphilis). The committee recommended that "arrangements be made with all speed for the immediate health assessment, treatment and care for persons included in the study in a suitably adequate facility easily accessible to the surviving patients."[76]

Franklin Miller was working at CDC headquarters in Atlanta when news of the Tuskegee study hit the press. He attended the ad hoc advisory committee meetings with great interest. Frank recalled that Dr. David Sencer, then CDC director, asked him to lead the effort to locate all surviving study participants because he had listened to the committee and "understood the letter and spirit of the recommendation that the panel was making."[77] Frank had one condition before accepting the assignment:

> I and I alone would handpick fourteen or fifteen PHAs to assist me... because they had the same background as I... The ones that I did select were the ones that I trusted, the ones that I perceived, rightly or wrongly, accurately or not, to have the sensitivities necessary... It was a very diverse group of folks.[78]

Frank Miller selected the best of the PHAs. Dick Conlon was working in Toledo when he got the call from Frank:

> There was a TV series at the time called Mission Impossible. One of the lines from that was, "Mr. Phelps, if anybody finds out about this, the Secretary [of State] will deny your existence." That's sort of how this call was from Frank Miller. He told me they had a very sensitive project to undertake, and his job was to recruit people that he felt capable of handling the sensitive issues.[71]

The handpicked group of PHAs first convened in Atlanta during a major ice storm in January 1973. At that time, Frank Miller, Bill Watson, and David Sencer laid out the task ahead, giving everyone a chance to opt out of the assignment. No one did. Dick recalled this first meeting:

> We were told what was going on with the Tuskegee follow-up, that it wasn't a cup of tea, that it could be dangerous, that it was necessary to contact all of these men, sometimes to contact their families, and we were offering them free medical care for the rest of their lives. People were going to be angry, they were going to be suspicious of CDC; but our job was to get the patients and the controls to sign off, to acknowledge that we'd made them the offer, and to make sure if they needed anything immediately—and that meant anything: dentures, eyeglasses, any kind of care at that time— to arrange for it. And so that was all laid out for us in January, and then we went back to our duty stations. They weren't yet ready to give us the assignments; they just wanted to lay out what was ahead of us and the risks. So we had a chance to commit to it or to withdraw. I accepted it and went back to Toledo doing my work, and in April everything started.[80]

On Easter weekend, 1973, seventeen PHAs converged in Atlanta to be trained by Frank Miller and David Sencer in their task to find survivors of the Tuskegee syphilis study. They reviewed the study's scientific and technical aspects, and they were trained in media relations in anticipation of media coverage. The fieldwork and the personal sensitivities came with the PHA field skill set. Pat McConnon found himself among this historic group of PHAs, along with Windell Bradford, Larry Burt, Pete Campassi, Joe Carter, Dick Conlon, Jim Fowler, Russ Havlak, Willie Green, Gorge Hurney, Jack Jackson, Bob Kingon, Ernie Montez, Casey Riley, John Supinski, Ron Thomas, and Dan Vander Meer.[81] Pat's Tuskegee follow-up team went to Phoenix City, Alabama, to find study survivors. Although the job represented a landmark in U.S. history, for this PHA it was a straightforward task of finding someone with only a little bit of locating information. The study had started in 1932, and these PHAs had to identify any surviving study members and their immediate kin. Just as his training in VD had taught him, Pat took the referral information and planned not to return until everyone was located. He was in the field for three weeks:

> Our job was to find the survivors of the Tuskegee study from the last known address that they had, the last information they had on them—some of which was like twenty to twenty-five years prior because all of this had been inactivated... It was basically detective work, trying to find out where people were, and subsequent to that, CDC set up a program that I think probably is still operating today.[82]

In 1974, a class action lawsuit was settled out of court on behalf of the study participants. Part of the settlement involved providing them lifetime medical benefits and burial expenses. The benefit was extended to spouses and offspring a year later. When Dick Conlon met with study participants and their families in Ohio and Pennsylvania, he would explain the study's purpose, and that lifetime medical benefits were available if the participant wished to have them. Dick had an eerie experience while visiting an eighty-six-year-old man in Youngstown, Ohio. His visit took place during the six o'clock news with Dan Rather:

> Tuskegee was all over the news at this time. And Bob Schiefer was doing this report from a cemetery in Tuskegee, Alabama. There's a gravestone, and the gravestone has the name of the man I'm sitting

> there talking to! And I said, "Excuse me, look at that." And he says, "Uh, huh." I said, "Well, how is it that you have a marker in the cemetery?" He says, "Well, that's a cousin of mine who died, and we didn't have enough money for a gravestone, but I had a gravestone, so I let him use mine."[83]

Russ Havlak visited with about two dozen study participants. Although he and others had been trained to expect a chilly reception, Russ found that people "could not have been more gracious":

> I can't cite for you a collection of people who were warmer or more down to earth. They had been used, abused, and deceived by the government I represented, but if any of them held a grudge, they sure declined to take it out on me. In fact, just the opposite: in place after place, I was received with unbelievable politeness and hospitality. I will never forget their example. They had so little—usually just a small plot of land and a tiny, distressed wooden shack sitting on concrete blocks. I was always invited inside, offered a seat and something to drink and eat, even though it probably would have stretched their means. What dignity they showed me and what a rewarding experience it was to help these folks, even in some small way.[84]

Although Peter Buxtun did not remain a PHA, he is pleased to know that his PHA colleagues worked to correct the historic wrong created by the Tuskegee syphilis study. Those who were detailed for the study follow-up served for several years as the contact people for study survivors and their families. Jim Fowler found this assignment one of the most rewarding of his PHA career:

> That was probably the hardest assignment in terms of emotion that I had to deal with, because obviously, the sons and daughters of guys who had died from that study, or after that study, were not real happy to see anybody. It was also rewarding in that you helped some of these people who really need some help.[85]

We Were Immediately Thrown into the Breach: Refugee Resettlement Following the Fall of Saigon[86]

Thousands of people fled in search of safe harbor when Saigon fell to the North Vietnamese Army in 1975. Within four years, approximately fifteen thousand people were arriving monthly in the U.S. from refugee camps throughout Southeast Asia.[87] Refugees were crowding into camps in Thailand, Malaysia, Indonesia, Singapore, and the Philippines. They awaited family or other sponsorships to come through before they could leave the refugee camps. CDC would have the responsibility of maintaining these refugees' health from the time their sponsorship came through to the time they entered the U.S., and the primary health concerns were tuberculosis, mental illnesses, sexually transmitted diseases, and anything that might emerge in the camps, such as cholera.[88] PHA Bob Keegan was the CDC's assistant coordinator for refugee services during this time. He worked directly with camps in Asia that were temporary homes for Vietnamese, Laotian, and Cambodian refugees. He recalls the conditions:

> While many of the refugee camps were run quite professionally, the conditions at some camps were quite awful, and the health of some refugees was very fragile. Occasionally, I would visit a patient sick with malaria or tuberculosis who was close to death. When I tried to visit the same patient the following morning, I would learn that they had died. There were very, very serious health situations, the likes of which I had never seen. And the conditions of a few of the refugee camps were just horrible. The camps in Thailand were under the control of the Thai government and UNHCR, and were fairly well run. But the camps in other places were much less suited for human life. Hong Kong was particularly notorious for cramming people into very small spaces.[89]

Jim Coan was working as a VD investigator in Baltimore when he was detailed to a refugee camp in Thailand. His primarily operations-oriented job soon was transformed into epidemiology when he had to investigate a cholera outbreak. Jim had to work quickly because cholera was spreading like wildfire in the crowded and unsanitary camp conditions. Fortunately, he was skilled in contact epidemiology, and as a PHA he was willing to take on the job. He recalls that tracking down the cholera sources was not easy:

> When cholera broke out we had to check every water source we could find, and there were multiple sources. People sold water and other products and devices. They sold sodas out of cans, and sometimes there was ice, and the ice would come packed in straw. We suspected that perhaps the ice might be a problem because of the

straw that was covering it, and then it would get on the bottle of soda, where they put it in a cup to make it cold, and so on. In the midst of this, the USAID office in Bangkok had meetings, and they were very concerned about it... They came to us and they said, "You've got to solve the problem." And I said, "You have to understand I'm not a sanitarian. This is kind of out of my range." They said, "Do the best you can. You're the only one we've got." I don't think you can be inspired to any higher degree than having that kind of confidence put in you.[90]

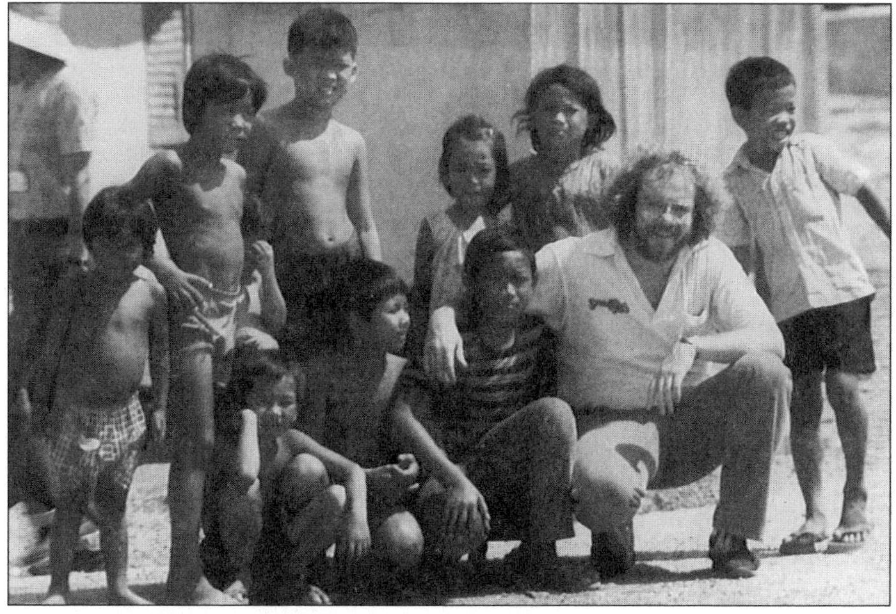

Jim Coan with children at a refugee camp in Thailand, 1975. Courtesy of Jim Coan.

The fall of Saigon put significant pressure on the U.S. government to quickly serve people who were fleeing Vietnam—practically overnight. People arrived from refugee camps in Asia to sites in Guam, California's Camp Pendleton, Florida, and sites scattered elsewhere in the U.S. CDC had to mobilize a team of people quickly to help conduct health screenings at the receiving camps in the U.S. Dennis McDowell was the assistant director of the STD control program in Birmingham, Alabama, in 1975. A Vietnam veteran who spoke Vietnamese, Dennis was a perfect candidate to be detailed to Camp Pendleton. The assignment was a two-week whirlwind. Dennis recalls that CDC asked him to go immediately: "We'd like you to go out to Camp Pendleton to-morrow and join a group of people that is going to be involved in the Refugee Resettlement." Dennis said that he and other PHAs were immediately flown to the West Coast and thrown into the breach.[91] They worked eighteen-hour days for fourteen days to get the job done. He recalled that the benefit of using PHAs in times of crisis is that "they don't know what eight-to-five means. I don't think I took a walking step for ten or twelve days in a row, maybe fifteen. I mean, we ran everywhere we went, we were that busy." Dennis continues:

> We had only a few hours to organize the screenings and figure out the logistics. Then we had to decide how and where to process the tests and how to evaluate and document the results. We had to figure out how to match the tests with people. This was all in an environment of a U.S. Marine-run hot, dry tent city, which was new to all and quite confusing... The people coming in were leaving their homes because of the collapse of the government and fleeing for their lives. So you can imagine that this is an environment of considerable tension, anxiety and confusion.[92]

People brought with them their most valuable possessions. Dennis saw these items through chest x-rays, as they were hung around the refugees' necks: "[t]he things that people thought most precious in their life, whether it was memories—the photographs and things—or whether it was money converted into precious stones." The environment was chaotic, but the PHAs performed well in it because of their training and experience. They were not "buffaloed by the magnitude of a challenge or the energy and emotions surrounding it, but stayed focused, really trying to be innovative, to be very, very aware and sensitive to the emotional distress that these people were in at the time and be respectful of it." Dennis believed this was due to the PHAs' intense and field-oriented training: "We remained in the lead role... because of PHA ingenuity and being able to quickly size up the situation and understand what it was going to take to deal with it, develop a solution, and implement it:"

> We were used to dealing with people that were in high emotional distress in the STD business, and somehow this was similar. We were used to getting blitzes organized, so we were experienced in getting a large number of people efficiently through a screening

> process. There were people there who knew TB, there were people there who knew immunization, there were people there who knew STDs, and there were people there like myself who had served in Vietnam. After our first day of really struggling to try to think about getting things set up, we had a little huddle, and because I spoke a small amount of Vietnamese, I had discovered there were a number of physicians and nurses in the population that was coming in. And so I recommended that we recruit these nurses and physicians to help us... We quickly organized medical teams from the refugee community and put them to work helping us calm down people, explain what was going on and what the processing was going to entail. Some of these volunteers even helped with various aspects of the processing.[93]

The situation at Camp Pendleton was "pretty impossible" because normal timelines and strategies weren't going to be sufficient. The goal was to help these refugees start a life in the United States as quickly as possible. To increase efficiency PHAs found themselves organizing the refugee screening efforts and using innovation to solve problems such as laboratory availability. They set up two hotel rooms to serve as public health laboratories. Dennis recalls what today would not be possible:

> We had as many as two hotel rooms, actually motel rooms, in San Clemente... There was a lot of blood testing going on, and the cleaning staff in the hotels were just absolutely shocked. In today's time you probably couldn't get away with that because we know more about the risks of and how to handle blood specimens... We were probably exposing ourselves... we were pretty careful, but it was not the degree of care that you would exercise today. It seemed like the driving force at the moment was to really get these people processed through Camp Pendleton so that they could move on with their lives. And that was what was at stake.[94]

The response effort was massive, and would be a good learning experience for the refugee situations that would follow in 1980: the Mariel boatlift from Cuba and refugees fleeing the Duvalier government in Haiti.[95] In 1980, more than one hundred twenty-five thousand Cubans arrived on U.S. shores.[96] They soon were followed by more than fifteen thousand Haitians. Although Haitians had been arriving on U.S. shores since about 1972, the early 1980s saw a steep increase in the number of refugees seeking asylum,[97] whose sheer numbers were overwhelming to the public health system.[98] PHAs were assigned to assist with both situations even as they assisted with Vietnam refugee resettlement and with other health emergencies and situations in the late 1970s and early 1980s.

Just as many PHAs were returning to their "day jobs" from smallpox, Tuskegee follow-up, and refugee resettlement details, eighteen-year-old Army recruit Private David Lewis collapsed during basic training at Fort Dix in January 1976. Within hours this young and healthy man was dead. The cause soon would be identified as "swine flu."[99] By the end of the month, more than three hundred recruits would be sickened by the same virus. Private Lewis's death would recall the 1918–1919 great influenza pandemic because its targets were healthy young adults and children.[100] Mounting evidence was pointing toward the potential of a major influenza outbreak in the general population. Health officials advised President Gerald Ford and Congress to proceed with a national vaccination program for swine flu. Although some historians might suggest that the immunization effort and resulting cases of Guillain-Barré syndrome were evidence of a disastrous effort, PHAs and others who deployed rapidly would disagree. If anything, swine flu was a test of the ability of public health to ramp up for a disaster—an ability that may not be present today. Dr. David Sencer recalls just what was demonstrated:

> The swine flu vaccination program demonstrated the possibility of organizing and managing an immunization program involving procurement, distribution, liability issues, and adverse event surveillance while vaccinating forty-three million persons in two months. Lessons learned by CDC during the 1976 swine flu vaccination program are being used to improve preparedness for pandemic influenza.[101]

The risk facing public health leaders was acting too quickly or too slowly.[102] John Shimmens, a retired PHA who ended his public health career as the deputy director of the Division of Environmental Health and Epidemiology with the State of Missouri, recalls the conundrum. Like other public health issues, it is difficult to prove that public health efforts prevent the catastrophes or outbreaks they target. Nonetheless, the efforts are important. John recalls with pride the swine flu mobilization:

> One of the jobs that I've always been very, very proud of is the swine flu program. It was fantastic. Now suppose we had done

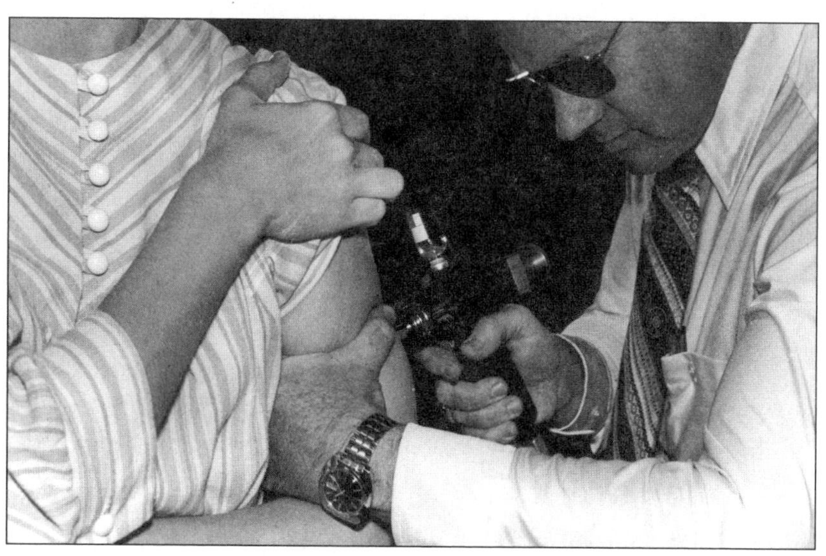

PHA Don Stenhouse giving an injection of flu vaccine during the 1976 swine flu immunization campaign.
Courtesy of Centers for Disease Control and Prevention, Public Health Image Library.

> nothing and swine flu hit? I mean, it was sort of damned if you did and damned if you didn't... Now, nothing happened... Public health is trying to prevent something, and it's awfully hard to prove effectiveness because illness never happens... As an example, in food sanitation, cold food should be kept cold and hot food should be kept hot. In this way, you will prevent foodborne outbreaks. This is the hardest thing about public health – proving something that never happens.[103]

PHAs and local health departments throughout the country mobilized to provide more than forty-three million doses of vaccine against swine flu in two months.[104] Bob Delaney was working with the Illinois Childhood Immunization Program when the ramp-up for swine flu began in 1976. Many public health professionals had to juggle current services with the added swine flu vaccination program. Bob recalled his experience:

> We had to continue with the childhood immunization program. We still had to run the clinics and manage the vaccines and do the

> education and work with the docs and all that. But then we also had the swine flu program, which was really managing huge quantities of vaccine being introduced... It really showed you could mobilize and really get things done and work throughout the state. We worked with many local health departments, public health nurses, and volunteers. How do we deal with the elderly? How do we deal with the different populations? Making sure the vaccine was shipped to the right place. It was an incredible experience.[105]

"Hush Up and Run the Paper:" The 1983 Syphilis and PPNG Blitz

Pete Moore, PHA
North Carolina STD/HIV Program
Senior Rep

Syphilis, with its cyclical reemergence, has eluded efforts to eradicate it dating back to World War I. Returning servicemen from World War I seeded syphilis in the U.S. civilian population, and the disease was a major public health priority from the time of Surgeon General Thomas Parran's effort to stamp it out in the late 1930s and 1940s. The infusion of PHAs in the late 1940s and early 1950s caused a significant reduction in syphilis, which was reversed when efforts were redirected away from syphilis programs in the 1950s. CDC's "Operation Pursuit," in the mid-1960s, redoubled efforts at contact epidemiology and caused a leveling off of syphilis by 1966.[106] In the 1970s, a major syphilis epidemic erupted among gay men.[107] When syphilis became prevalent again in the early 1980s, it was due to crack cocaine's emergence. Although other parts of the country were seeing reductions in syphilis by the mid-1980s, Miami, Florida, was struggling with sharp increases in syphilis and a recently-identified, treatment-resistant type of gonorrhea called PPNG, or Penicillinase-Producing Neisseria Gonorrhea. The antibiotic-resistant gonorrhea strain first was identified in the 1970s and would emerge in sixteen states by 1983.[108] Seventy percent of all new PPNG cases in 1983 were found in Palm Beach and in Dade and Broward Counties in Florida.[109]

In 1982 Jack Wroten was directing the Florida STD program. He had been serving the State of Florida since 1966. When syphilis increased in Florida during the 1970s, local and state public health staff were able to handle it. The situation was different in the 1980s, and Wroten found himself talking with PHA Don Ward, his project consultant at CDC, who was a former colleague from Florida. The local health infrastructure could not handle the epidemic. "Don and I talked and talked and talked. We finally decided that we were going to blitz Miami in September 1983,"[110] Jack said. CDC's decision to help Florida with a "blitz" reflected its concern to assist the Miami-Dade Health Department and to protect the country's health. The Miami outbreak had the potential to spread throughout the U.S. because Miami was temporary home to several transient populations and because tourism was a major economic element of southern Florida.[111] If syphilis and PPNG could not be controlled in Miami, a national epidemic could be ignited. In sexually transmitted disease parlance, the term "blitz" refers to a saturation of contact epidemiology—case finding and syphilis case management with the purpose of reducing new infections to manageable levels. Although "blitz" may have negative connotations today, it is an apt description of the bombardment of case finding and analysis that is carried out to reduce syphilis in a community. Russ Havlak recalls that PHA John Hill was the first to coin the term in rural Alabama in the early 1960s. His colleague PHA John Supinski adapted it in 1965 for the urban context in Newark, New Jersey, changing "blitz" to "Red Dog Program." The term "blitz" survived in both public health and football parlance. Russ recalls:

> Red Dog" and "blitz" were succeeding terms for the same basic defensive maneuver employed in the NFL, and their selection for the syphilis control effort was not a coincidence. Each term in its time brought instant recognition from most of a nearly all-male PHA staff, and evoked the image of an exceptional effort involving an intensity that was far greater than normal. John's term survived, probably because the term "blitz" survived. To this day "blitz" is an enduring part of [the] football lexicon at every level.[112]

When it was determined that early syphilis in a particular locale had reached levels above the epidemiologic threshold, the state health department, with encouragement from CDC, would request federal assistance to enable the local health department to deal with every aspect of disease control from surveillance, clinic operations and management, to case finding.[113] Mark Schrader, a retired PHA, who spent his career in STD/HIV Prevention efforts, explained what a syphilis blitz involved:

> We would gather the best people from around the country and pop them into these places and let them do what they did best. Syphilis blitzes were nearly always quite successful and the methodology was also applied to PPNG in the late '70s and the early '80s. Everyone worked incredibly long hours to get the job done in the best possible manner. When we became "too tired", we would go out and have a couple of beers and then go back to the hotel or the health department to discuss and analyze cases in preparation for the following day. Incredible thought and analysis went into the cases night after night and the supervisors and their team of casefinders were always prepared to begin the next day with a new set of instructions and priorities. These folks were innovative and imaginative beyond belief. People who worked on blitzes were always amazed about how much fun it was. I don't think in my experience anyone ever complained about the work and the hours—never. Working those eighteen hour days provided a tremendous amount of job satisfaction and people learned things that they would use for their entire career.

Jack Wroten knew that he needed to bring in a significant number of PHAs to control syphilis and PPNG in addition to redirecting the work of his local and state investigators. Sixty Public Health Advisors from around the country were detailed to work in Miami from September 1983 to February 1984.[115] Jack and his local staff continued the work until May or June of 1984. The effort was proving successful, and by late February, the ever-increasing rates of syphilis and PPNG had been reduced.[116] Success in blitzing or other increases in public health case finding efforts lies in the added workforce's ability to hunker down and do the case finding and epidemiology; or as Pete Moore would say, to "hush up and run the paper."

Kevin O'Connor arrived for his assignment with the Dade County Public Health Department's STD program just days after the blitz had begun. He was twenty-five years old at the time and was invigorated by the intense work: "Being a VDI is just about as encompassing an experience in this field as you could want."[117] Kevin and his colleague PHA Wendy Watkins tried to reduce patient barriers to seeking treatment for syphilis by reaching out to the com-

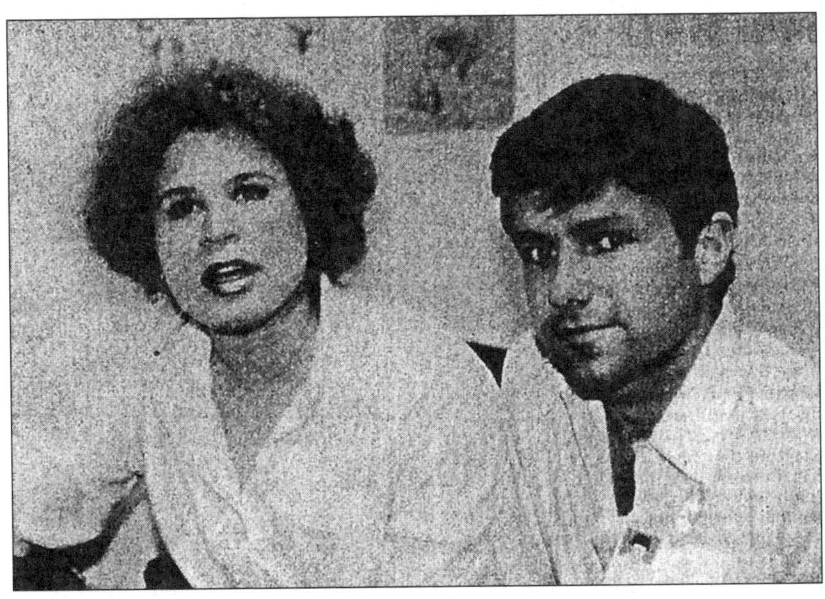

Wendy Watkins and Kevin O'Connor during their work on the Miami syphilis blitz. Source: Carol Cancila, "VDIs," American Medical News (May 4, 1984). Used with permission.

munity and increasing the flexibility of an already-burdened health system. Nighttime hours were established for clinics, and public information and radio spots disseminated information about syphilis and treatment. Wendy and Kevin would fan out into the community, visiting bars and bathhouses, brothels and street corner hangouts, and jails. In one jail, they found a twenty-six percent syphilis positivity rate among sex trade workers.[118] The work involved drawing blood for syphilis testing, conducting interviews to identify sexual contacts, bringing people in to the clinic for treatment, and field investigation to find those named as sexual contacts so that they, too, could be offered a chance for syphilis testing and treatment. As with case finding, Kevin and Wendy had to win their clients' trust. When they did, they had to be prepared to get to work wherever they were. Kevin remembers taking a blood sample from eleven people to test for syphilis in a junkyard: after one person agreed to have his blood tested, the others followed suit.[119]

"The Caskets Were Floating Down the River:" The Great Midwestern Flood of 1993

Frank Berry, PHA (ret.)

From May through September of 1993, nine states experienced significant flooding due to heavy snowfall in 1992, significant rainfall in the summer of 1993, and the failure of levees along the Mississippi and Missouri Rivers. Fifty people died, and more than fifteen billion dollars in property damages were incurred.[120] Thousands of people in North Dakota, South Dakota, Nebraska, Kansas, Missouri, Wisconsin, Iowa, and Illinois were forced to move due to the flooding. Seventy-five towns were completely submerged in floodwaters. Some of the flooding persisted for two hundred days. Prior to Hurricanes Katrina and Rita in 2005, flooding in the Midwest in 1993 was thought to be the greatest natural disaster to hit the U.S.[121]

Floodwaters were contaminated by sewage and other debris. As water continued to stand, the potential for transmission of viruses that cause St. Louis encephalitis or western equine encephalitis increased, because the water became breeding grounds for mosquitoes.[122] Drinking water from private wells was another concern, because with all the wastewater, drinking water probably was contaminated. This was a significant issue for Midwesterners, because one-third of Midwestern populations at the time obtained their drinking water from private wells.[123]

Kent Gray was supervising CDC's emergency operations during the Midwest floods. As with other natural disasters, the need for aid presented itself in a short period of time. PHAs were ready and willing to participate in the response effort. Kent remembers:

> I needed thirty or forty people. I picked up the phone, made a call, and the next day, for a period of four hours, I had people arriving from all over the country, receiving instruction, and leaving for an assignment within twelve hours.[124]

PHAs handled response logistics. They supplemented the state and local health departments' workforces. They were detailed to governors' offices to help handle media relations. They conducted surveys and damage and risk assessments. Ensuring safe drinking water was a major priority due to the Midwest's dependence on private wells. Kent Gray and his colleagues tested a sampling of wells and found them all to be contaminated:

> The private water well samples were coming back contaminated regardless of what procedures we used to clean the wells. We didn't know if this was normal. No one could provide the laboratory information since it was not a routine test. All they could say was that one third of the population is on private water supply. To get the answers we launched the largest water testing survey ever attempted. We put a ten-mile grid over nine states, and everywhere there was an intersection we sent somebody to find a well and get a sample and analyze it. And in less than six months we processed something like seven thousand wells [and] found that forty-one percent of the wells were contaminated.[125]

In 1995 the Midwest once again would see flooding, though the damage would not be as intense as in 1993. Then, during the summer of 1995, a heat wave in Chicago would target poor and elderly persons. PHAs were called to assist with the grisly follow-up.

The 1995 Chicago Heat Wave

On July 13, 1995, the temperature in Chicago hit one hundred six degrees Fahrenheit, with a heat index of one hundred nineteen.[126] The oppressive tropical temperature was exacerbated by the layer of city pollution that was trapping the heat and smog, creating what climatologists called an "urban heat island."[127] More than forty-nine thousand persons were without power due to power grids' failures. Hundreds of people were hospitalized with heat-related illnesses. More than six hundred people died as a result of that month's heat wave,[128] which was called one of the worst weather-related disasters in Illinois history.[129]

Stefan Weir is the deputy chief of the Program Services Branch in the Division of State and Local Readiness at CDC. One of his more grisly assignments occurred while working in the Chicago STD program in 1995, when he was detailed to work with the team responding to the heat wave. His work involved both operations and epidemiology. Stefan managed an interdisciplinary team of public health workers, environmental health personnel, and police. The team's role was to help discover the cause and circumstances of death so that actions could be taken to avoid future catastrophes of this kind. His skills as an investigator were easily applied, and for two months, he and his team worked tirelessly:

> [We had] to deal with coroner reports, police reports, go out to the site where the person was found, interview the people in the area, relatives, neighbors, find out what that person was doing before their death… Get all that information, find out what the situation was in the building or the apartment.[130]

The work was intense and a reminder of the harsh living conditions in this urban community at the intersection of poverty and crime. Stefan witnessed what he will not likely forget:

> We found out a lot of the people who died were elderly, who lived in high-crime areas, who could not open their windows because of the crime in their area. A lot of the windows would not open …. They had fans, but it blew hot air. Some [people] were literally found [dead] in front of their refrigerator with the door and the freezer open trying to cool off.[131]

The Risk is Part of the Job: SARS Outbreak, 2003

Severe acute respiratory syndrome, or SARS, first was identified in Asia in February 2003. That same year, a global SARS outbreak would cause illnesses and deaths that were reported in North and South America, Europe, and Asia. By the end of the outbreak, more than eight thousand people were stricken with illness. SARS is the type of illness that can be spread easily given the convenience of intercontinental travel. SARS spreads by close person-to-person contact. The SARS-associated coronavirus is spread when an infected person coughs or sneezes, or when an uninfected person touches a surface that has been contaminated and then touches his or her mouth, nose, or eyes. These infected mucous droplets can be propelled through the air at a distance of up to three feet.[132]

By March of 2003, CDC was advising air passengers traveling on direct flights from Asia to seek immediate medical care if they experienced symptoms of this respiratory illness.[133] PHAs were dispatched to major airports, such as John F. Kennedy International Airport in New York City, San Francisco International Airport, Miami International Airport, and others that received direct flights from

Asia in particular, where the SARS epidemic was unabated. There was concern not only that people would fly unknowingly with the illness, but also that others might try to enter the United States for medical treatment. Airport personnel needed to know about SARS and what to do if someone on a flight was identified with potential SARS symptoms. Passengers had to be educated so that they would recognize their own symptoms and those of others. With such an easily-traveled world, it appeared that few things could be done to protect people from SARS and to stop an epidemic from spreading into the U.S. It was important for people to learn about the severity of influenza while not becoming too afraid to have contact with others.

Frank Meyers was a PHA working for the State of Florida in the Sexually Transmitted Disease Program when he was sent on a three-month detail in the spring of 2003 to Miami International Airport and then to Orlando International Airport. His assignment involved responding to airplane arrivals where potential SARS victims were landing, and teaching airport employees and first responders about SARS and what to do in the event that someone had symptoms. Frank recalls:

> I spent three months on a TDY with SARS: two months at Miami International Airport and a month at Orlando Airport as a solo assignment there doing a lot of teaching to airport employees, explaining how the disease is and is not transmitted, that you cannot get it from being a baggage handler, and all these things to overcome their fears. At the same time we talked about what happened with the 1918 influenza outbreak, what the potentials were... I think I did some forty classes total in the three months.[134]

Frank's job also involved boarding a plane in the event a passenger was identified as potentially having SARS. He was the first person to board the plane, and this action recalled many of the PHAs' more dangerous TDY assignments in the past, where exposure to an unknown pathogen or a dangerous agent was possible despite precautions. "I was the first person to go on the airplane as soon as that door opened," he said. "I was obviously concerned because I knew I could have been exposed, but I felt well trained. It was just part of the deal."[135] He continues:

> Whether it's Ebola or anything else, it just comes with the territory. You take what precautions you can, as best you can, but you get the

> job done. I'm not afraid to die. That doesn't bother me to be put in those positions. A lot of others would walk away from that. It's more important to get the job done as effectively as possible and to preserve the public's health as best we can.[136]

Jim Beall was a PHA assigned to the State of Indiana in the Sexually Transmitted Disease and HIV program when he was detailed to meet planes at the San Francisco International Airport. He was not as cavalier as Frank Meyers, and described the moments of risk as an "out-of-body experience." But like Frank, Jim knew his calling was to get the job done. He recalled the challenges in this effort:

> I was stopping airplanes, not allowing people to deplane. I was calling hospital ambulances to meet aircraft, causing people with languages I couldn't speak to be interviewed by somebody that could speak to them before I could let them off the plane… We knew in advance which flights we were going to meet, and we also met other ones if there was a situation that wasn't routine: if somebody got off a plane and got out of there and was sick or whatever else… we were observing every person that got off the aircraft.[137]

Paul Burlack was a PHA working on the CDC Emergency Response Team when the call came on a Friday afternoon in May 2003, around two o'clock. "Can you be on a plane to Taiwan on Sunday at ten in the morning?" He spent the afternoon getting his medical and security clearances, and then called his wife, who at the time was planning a large annual party at the house. "Guess what, dear? I'm leaving for Taiwan."

> I got home about eight o'clock that night. I packed all of my stuff. Saturday morning I cleaned the deck, got ready for the party, and I was ready to go. We partied until about one in the morning. I got up at five A.M. and had someone drive me to the airport, and was soon on a twenty-six hour journey to Taiwan. I was the logistics person for a team of health professionals. Dr. Sue Maloney was in charge of the team, and I was the PHA in charge of logistics.[138]

Paul and the team would work with local Taiwanese health authorities to screen people who had been exposed to SARS and to interview quarantined SARS patients to establish household and employment contacts, "and all other daily close contacts."[139] The team needed to identify contacts in order to stop the infection's spread. Paul worked eighteen-hour days for thirty days doing this and training local personnel in logistics management related to emergency response. The environment was hectic, and the workforce had to be careful not to become infected or to spread infection themselves. Paul's team was the second to go over to Taiwan. The first team had a possible exposure to SARS:

> The reason that we went over is because they had to send back the first team because of suspicion that one of the team members was infectious. I think four of them actually had to come back because of close exposure.[140]

Phil Talboy witnessed first-hand the need for careful precautions and processes to protect the health of responders in the SARS epidemic. In the spring of 2003 he was detailed to Guam to investigate a suspected SARS case. A housecleaning staff member at a local hotel had suspicious symptoms. She was taken from the hotel by ambulance to a local hospital where emergency department staff worked hours to save her life. When she died, the medical staff suspected she might have had SARS. "The medical community and the entire island were concerned that the emergency medical personnel, the ambulance, the emergency department and the entire hospital had been contaminated,"[141] Phil said. Although SARS was ruled out in this case, Phil's work continued because Guam authorities needed logistical help to prepare for SARS. "The foremost lesson learned is that universal infection control procedures must be practiced on all patients." He continues:

> I was involved in creating a number of procedural documents, and assisted in developing procedures to investigate and manage a case of SARS, which included developing case forms and other case management tools. There were many high-level meetings that I attended with the Governor, the SARS task force, the local hospital administrators, medical associations, the World Health Organization, foreign governments, and other groups. [I would also] meet planes that had originated in known SARS countries, to either inspect arriving passengers for signs and symptoms of the illness or actually examine ill patients prior to the passengers' disembarking from the airplane on Guam. I also met ships that were coming into port in Guam to inspect the crew for signs and symptoms of illness.[142]

"Only a Really Seasoned PHA Could Survive on This Assignment:" The Rábia Balkhi Hospital Initiative

In October 2001, coalition forces removed the Taliban leadership of Afghanistan in response to their protection of the Al Qaeda terrorists who attacked the United States on September 11, 2001. Since then the United States government has been conducting simultaneously a war and reconstruction efforts in Afghanistan.[143] Critical to reconstruction efforts are humanitarian development projects, such as hospital reconstruction and the development of health and public health infrastructure. One such project, the Rábia Balkhi Hospital Project, involved PHA Steve Schindler for six months in 2003 to 2004.

Afghanistan has one of the highest infant and maternal mortality rates in the world.[144] Several decades of war have dismantled the health system, and women in particular have paltry health facilities. In 2003 then-HHS Secretary Tommy Thompson selected the Rábia Balkhi Hospital in Kabul as the focus of an initiative to improve maternal and child health outcomes.[145] The largest hospital for women in Kabul, Rábia Balkhi also is the only one to serve women after the Taliban banned women from general hospitals in 1997.[146] Today Steve Schindler is the deputy chief of the Women's Health and Fertility Branch in the CDC's Division of Reproductive Health. He was deployed to work in Kabul as part of CDC's "A" team when he served as the CDC program manager for the Rábia Balkhi project:

> Our job was to work with other agencies under HHS to implement the Secretary's Rábia Balkhi Hospital Initiative. The objective was to create an OB/GYN residency program at one of Kabul's busiest hospitals. DOD [Department of Defense] was in charge of the reconstruction of some of the hospital's infrastructure. The repairs were not fully successful or enough. Our program was often hampered by plumbing problems, cooking smoke drifting into hospital rooms, sewage back ups, equipment and supply shortages, and numerous other issues not usually faced back home. We worked with DOD to go back in and repair the hospital infrastructure, obtain fuel to burn afterbirth matter, and arrange for trucks to periodically clean out stopped-up underground sewage holding tanks.[147]

The CDC team also faced other sorts of challenges. Although training occurred for OB/GYN and other medical professionals, indicators of health problems were increasing, such as the rates of C-sections and post-operative infections. CDC and the Afghan Ministry of Health raised these and other concerns to HHS, but generally were ignored because HHS wanted to tout the project as an "unqualified success."[148] These and other challenges made Steve's job more than a coordination task. It was a diplomatic job of major proportions, requiring all of his skills: "It was a test of everything I have ever done… Only a really seasoned PHA could survive on this assignment." Steve negotiated on behalf of HHS with the U.S. Embassy, USAID, DOD, WHO, UNICEF, the Afghan Ministry of Health as well as Nangarhar Department of Public Health to fix problems created "by the incredibly difficult set of conditions caused by war, poverty, politics, cultural differences, differing expectations, competing priorities, and lack of funds."[149] Some of the problems go back to the project's selection. When Secretary Thompson chose the hospital as the HHS project, it was thought that he did so without consulting anyone in the international community already working in Afghanistan. This is unusual in global work, where countries try to coordinate with others that are working in particular areas so that true needs are known and resources are not duplicated or misdirected. Most notably, HHS also proceeded initially without consulting other U.S. departments working in Afghanistan, such as the flagship of international agencies, USAID, located in the State Department. Steve and his CDC colleagues experienced the fallout because it appeared that HHS was in competition with the State Department: "There was a little cold shoulder, but what really helped was that we were all in the same boat." Steve's experience as a PHA throughout many different placements and work situations prepared him for the challenging assignment: "I was called in to this assignment to work with the partners and to manage partners on the ground because I was used to solving problems and dealing with difficult personalities and assignments. It was tough but incredibly rewarding working on every aspect of this program."[150]

Steve was hired in 1972 to work in the New York City STD program. He spent several years working in and managing STD and AIDS programs in state and local health departments in Kansas City, Missouri, New York, New Jersey, Idaho, and California, and he worked as the Tuberculosis Control Program manager in the Central District of Los Angeles County.[151] In 1988, Steve went to CDC headquarters and served in several capacities, primarily in HIV, and including work in the Global AIDS Program.[152] All of these experiences informed Steve as he worked with Afghan, international and U.S. colleagues to improve conditions at the Rábia Balkhi Hospital.

In the midst of public health and diplomatic challenges, the risk of working in Afghanistan might be overlooked. There was and is a war in Afghanistan and every humanitarian aid worker knows that he or she is at risk of losing life and/or limb. Although he initially did not think he'd have to go to Afghanistan, Steve was honored to be part of this assignment, and to actually have the opportunity to spend time on the ground there. The work mitigated the sense of risk, even when Steve was asked be a driver of his convoy so that military personnel could use a gun to better secure it:

> When you're in the country and you know what you have to do to get the job done, you forget about your safety. You look at your task and realize that you're the person that can make a difference at that moment in time. You do what you have to do to stay safe, but you don't let that deter you from the task at hand. When the helicopters couldn't fly me to Jalalabad and land transport was being considered, I was invited by the colonel to secure the convoy. I did not even think about saying no. We [he and another civilians] drove so that the drivers could better protect the convoy. You forget about yourself and your safety, and you do what you have to do to get this job done.

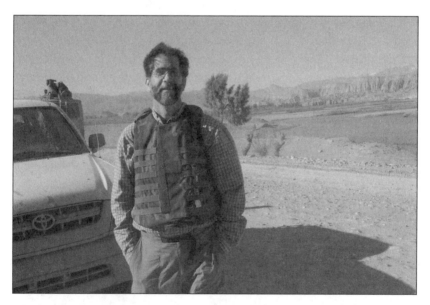

Steve Schindler in Kabul, Afghanistan, 2003.
Courtesy of Steve Schindler.

The millennium opened with terror on September 11, 2001. Kent Gray, Ron Burger, and many other PHAs were detailed to New York City, Pennsylvania, and Washington (see Chapter 1). Less than a month later, Phil Talboy, Pat McConnon, and others were detailed to Washington, D.C., and New York City in response to anthrax contamination (see Chapter 1). These events would be the harbingers of what may become a decade focused on bioterrorism preparedness and response. Such issues require highly trained and immediately deployable public health personnel. As with the many outbreak and disease events of the past, PHAs were "ready to go" at a moment's notice, and they served with distinction. Unlike past events, however, those from the late 1990s to the present required the help of the "silverbacks." Because CDC had stopped hiring entry-level PHAs in 1994, the agency does not have a sufficient number of qualified responders. So, the silverbacks—retired PHAs—are being pulled out of retirement to help.

Chapter 8

The Silverbacks

At seventy-four years of age, Dave Newberry is not spending time on a golf course. Instead, he is working in Mosul, one of the most violent cities in Iraq. Dave is on a Provincial Reconstruction Team (PRT) focused on rebuilding Iraq's health and education systems through community engagement. The team is a component of the U.S. government's surge strategy:

> The job is clearly the most challenging of my career. The PRT is a coalition of military, Department of State, and Department of Defense people... Our major assignment is to empower Iraqi professionals to reconstruct the essential services needed to restore a stable government and system of services.[1]

It is difficult to do the work and to see progress. Dave works across Iraqi sectors on a long-term capacity development effort in health and education. Some days, it is as if he takes one step forward and two steps back. Reconstructing essential services in education includes such things as figuring out how to obtain and move school supplies from place to place while avoiding improvised explosive devices (IEDs). It involves addressing challenges facing children themselves. Many children do not have enough to eat, and this clearly affects their ability to learn. Some leave school to earn money for their family. These kids are usually between the ages of twelve and seventeen years, and the insurgents target them for recruitment and pay them to plant IEDs or throw hand grenades at passing cars and trucks. Most people would find it difficult to maintain hope in such a situation. Not Dave Newberry. He sees the long-term potential for change in spite of the immediate challenges. Each challenge is an opportunity to find a solution.

Dave is an example of what some CDC employees call a "silverback"—a Public Health Advisor who continues to contribute to the health and welfare of communities after retiring from CDC. Dave says that although nothing could really prepare him for the challenges he currently faces on the ground in Iraq, his preparation as a PHA has helped him: "My assignments during the swine flu project and as senior Public Health Advisor for the Kidney Donor program provided helpful experience. We were always put on the spot for challenges and experience."[2] Dave gives credit to Dave Sencer and Bill Griggs for giving him challenging assignments at CDC that broadened his experience. He believes that the sum total of his "checkered career" as a PHA has equipped him with skills and technical knowledge that he would not otherwise possess.

Dave was hired to work as a co-op in the New York City VD program in 1964. Within eleven years, he had worked in several state and local health department VD and TB programs. In 1968, Dave was tapped to be the senior operations officer and chief of party for the Smallpox Eradication Project in Ghana, West Africa, and he served in this capacity until 1971.[3] He came to CDC headquarters with the TB Program in 1975, and in 1981 he returned to Ghana as part of an international team to interrupt the increase in yaws, a disfiguring disease caused by a spirochete not unlike syphilis, though not sexually transmitted.[4]

Dave retired in 1986 to a life of continued public health service. He began working as a consultant to several international health and aid organizations, providing technical advice, and management and operations consultation. In 1994 Dave went to work as the director of polio eradication for CARE International, one of the world's largest humanitarian organizations. In this role he provided strategic guidance to help solidify the organization's position in international health and development, with a focus on child survival programs, maternal and child health, and polio eradication. In 2003, Dave's silverback contribution intensified in its risk to life and limb; yet, for Dave, the risk was necessary because the intractable challenges needed problem solvers. That year, Dave went to Iraq on a temporary assignment for CARE Australia:

> In August 2003 I was asked to go to Iraq, representing the health component for CARE Australia, to implement rehabilitation projects involving health clinics, national laboratory restoration, and the installation of a forty-eight-inch water main to supply six million Iraqi citizens.[5]

The very next year, CARE Australia country director Margaret Hassan was murdered by insurgents. She had been working and living in Iraq for more than twenty-five years.[6] Even in the face of heightened security issues for CARE employees, Dave accepted a second assignment in Iraq in 2007. He sums up the decision as a commitment to the CDC "do-good motto" and demonstrates the PHA willingness to step up when no one else would:

> [After] Margaret Hassan was murdered, CARE Australia shut down. In August of 2007, I was asked to identify a public health person to take a one-year assignment serving as a Provincial Reconstruction Team member for health and education... Everyone I called or tried to recruit was either afraid [or] just not interested. Someone asked me, "Why don't you go?"[7]

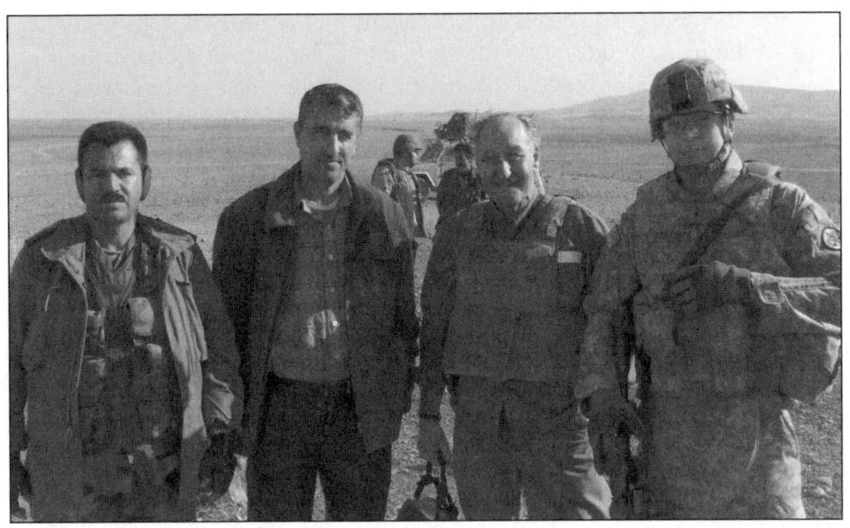

Dave Newberry (second from right) with his interpreter (second from left) and two military personnel in Mockmur, Iraq, 2008.
Courtesy of Dave Newberry.

It might be argued that the PHA tradition of service in retirement was established by Bill Watson. Although Bill is known as one of the original PHAs who rose up through the CDC ranks to serve as the agency's deputy director, he also is known for his contributions to global immunization efforts after retiring from CDC. Shortly after his retirement in 1984, Bill and former CDC director Dr. Bill Foege established the Task Force for Child Survival to raise the immunization levels of children under five years of age in developing nations. This "small non-profit" made an initial big splash, as it was able to gather the commitment of several countries for the immunization effort and achieve major strides for child survival. Bill recalls:

> The original goal was to raise the immunization levels from twenty to eighty percent in children under five, and we did it. But if you look behind that statistic, we didn't do that in every country. We didn't have to do it in Chad if we could do it in Nigeria, you see. And we didn't have to do it in Malaysia if you got Indonesia. We pulled it off, and it led to a big international meeting. We had seventy-two heads of state at that meeting. We prepared something for the people to sign off on, committing themselves to this effort in the form of a treaty with the United Nations. Practically all of them did, and it made a difference when they went back home.[8]

Bill Watson worked with the Task Force for five years. Following an invitation by former President Jimmy Carter, the Task Force became part of the Carter Presidential Center, and Watson served as the Carter Center's operations director for the next five years while Foege served as the executive director. Together, they worked on a broad array of projects in health and human rights for the Carter Center. Today Bill Watson can be found advising a project or two in his quest to live a meaningful life. As he wrote in his 1994 book, entitled First Class Privates: "In keeping with the counsel of Ecclesiastes, I have wept and laughed, mourned and danced. It's been a good show."[9]

The Bill and Melinda Gates Foundation has a strong relationship with CDC, and has hired several former CDC staff members. One such person is Kathy Cahill, a retired PHA who serves as the Foundation's deputy director for Integrated Health Solutions and Development. Kathy opted to continue to work after her career with CDC because she wanted to contribute her wealth of skills to the global health effort. Working globally now strikes Kathy as funny, because she thought she was going to get the opportunity for an international assignment when she began her career with CDC in 1983. At that time, Kathy received an offer from the Immunization Program to go to Kentucky. "I got the call, and they told me that I was going to "Frankfurt." And I said, 'My God, I'm going global?'"[10]

Kathy came to the Gates Foundation in 2005 initially to develop leadership programs for ministries of health in developing countries. Since her arrival, She

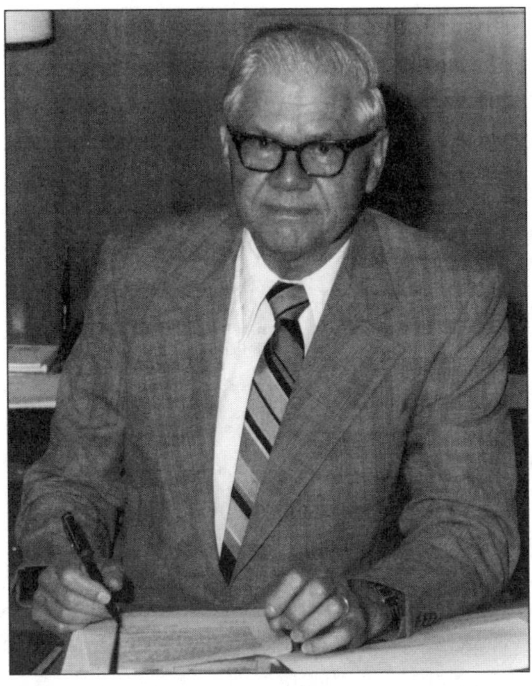

William C. Watson Jr. as deputy director of the Centers for Disease Control and Prevention, circa 1980s.
Courtesy of the Watsonian Society.

has been able to contribute much more, primarily because of accrued years of operational experience in several different programs and places during her PHA career. In 1991 as deputy director for the CDC Public Health Practice Program, Kathy developed the Public Health Leadership Institute, which provided training for state and local health department leaders in university settings.[11] Her work in Washington State, Kentucky, and California, paired with her work in immunization, public health practice, and HIV programs, prepared her for the policy and development work she would be doing at the Gates Foundation: "The whole experience of running and developing programs is valuable. With that skill set comes critical thinking, problem solving, and an action orientation. Those kinds of characteristics are important anywhere."[12] Kathy thinks that her PHA skill set contributes well to Gates Foundation efforts, particularly because the Foundation is action-oriented and is focused on solving complex issues in developing countries with innovative solutions. It is a perfect job for a PHA:

> PHAs bring the management skills and help make sure that things get done and get done in an efficient, effective way. Public Health Advisors help create programs. They help implement the programs. They are responsible for a variety of things about getting the job done: whether it's an emergency or just the day-to-day stuff. They develop the skill set to do that. I think one of the advantages of being a PHA is that you usually log enough freedom to go and do many things, and to figure out what needs to be done—so you're a problem solver of maximum value.[13]

Dave Newberry, Bill Watson, and Kathy Cahill are not unusual as retired PHAs. They are among the many who work in public health after retirement because their PHA brand of experience is needed, and because they continue to be ready to go. They are unrelenting in their commitment to public health, and particularly to CDC. "They don't do it for the money," says Joe Carter, a PHA who retired from his role as the CDC associate director of Management and Operations and now is serving as president/CEO of Carter Consulting, Inc.—a company that, among other things, specializes in placing retired PHAs with CDC and other government agencies. "Many are called out of retirement because there is a need for their particular expertise,"[14] he adds. Retired PHAs leave CDC and soon are asked to work for organizations such as the Bill and Melinda Gates Foundation, the Carter Center, the United Nations, CARE, the World Health Organization, and U.S government agencies. PHAs who have been introduced in previous chapters and are serving the health sector in their retirement include Dick Conlon, who just retired from his role as the administrator for the National Viral Hepatitis Roundtable; Pat McConnon, the executive director of the Council of State and Territorial Epidemiologists; Steve Barid, who now is fully retired but recently was the senior associate director for management at the Public Health Informatics Institute; Gary West, senior vice president for operations for the Institute for Family Health of Family Health International; Bill Parra, who is working for the CDC Foundation as the chief operating officer for the Bloomberg Global Initiative to Reduce Tobacco Use; Gary Conrad, customer relationship manager with the Science Applications International Corporation; and Dean Mason, who up until 2006 was the president and CEO of the Sabin Vaccine Institute and now is working as the assistant vice president of Global Vaccine Policy for Wyeth Pharmaceuticals.

Other PHAs retired and became permanent staff of state and local public health departments across the country. Examples from this book include Jim Beall, who retired from CDC to work in the Indiana Department of Health STD/HIV Prevention Program; Bert Malone, who retired to work in several leadership roles for the Missouri Department of Health and is now the director of the Division of Environmental Health Services with the Kansas City Health Department; Ron Burger, who retired and now is working for the State of Florida as director of the Division of Emergency Medical Operations; John Shimmens, who now is completely retired but worked for several years as the deputy director for the Division of Environmental Health and Epidemiology for the Missouri Department of Health; Ray Bly, who retired and worked for the Missouri Department of Health as the director of the STD Program; and Jack Wroten, who now is completely retired but worked for several years as the director of the STD Program for the State of Florida. All these PHAs, and many more, made a tremendous contribution of skills and experience to local public health when they became permanent staff members in local and state public health departments.

Public Health Advisors continue to serve after retirement because they are committed to public service and want to improve community health. Many contribute their time in retirement because they recognize that CDC is in tremendous need of their experience. This chapter focuses on these particular silverbacks because their contributions as retired persons working at CDC highlight an important period in PHA history, from 1994, when CDC stopped recruiting entry-level PHAs, until 2007. These silverbacks left retirement and returned to CDC as contractors in order to fill the resulting human resource gap. A confluence of issues created the setting for this historic human resource policy decision. First, throughout the United States, local and state public health capacity was becoming consistently stronger. Second, a national-level policy effort involved a review of public health roles and functions across government levels. Third, the federal government was reinventing and downsizing itself, bringing into sharp relief conflicts between FTE (full-time equivalent employee) "ceilings" designed to increase government efficiency, and exemptions from these ceilings for certain types of employees. Fourth, CDC's management of the FTE ceiling had been fairly lax in the preceding years. Finally, CDC institutional and leadership recognition of the value of field-trained PHAs had dissipated.

Since the mid-1980s, local and state public health systems were gaining strength, and appeared to have less need for the operational support the federal government provided through Public Health Advisors. PHAs certainly were not at odds with state and local health capacity building because they had spent decades helping to establish state and local health departments' public health programs, human resource systems, and positions; and they had helped many state and local health departments make the case for increasing local investment in human resource capacity.[15] As local career ladders became established and local and state governments increased investment in public health human resource capacity, some areas expressed sentiment that perhaps the management support provided by mid-level PHAs and the field activity provided by entry-level PHAs no longer was vital to state and local health functioning. In essence, the PHAs had worked themselves out of jobs, or at least it appeared this way to some of the local and state health departments that were redefining their role in public health. The emerging perspective was that states were the center of public health activity and that the federal government should "steer and not row," as articulated by a 1988 Institute of Medicine Report, *The Future of Public Health*. This seminal report called attention to the important role of states in public health coordination and leadership and identified the roles of each government level—federal, state, and local—to maximize public health benefit. The report outlined a public health leadership path and indicated that the federal government no longer should be in the business of providing operational-level help.[16] The era of Joseph Mountin's Public Health Service appeared to be over, because the federal government no longer would be called to perform routine operations for local and state public health.[17] The implication for PHAs in the field became patently clear: they no longer would be needed in their state and local-level capacities.

Parallel with these changes, CDC leadership shifted its opinion of PHAs as CDC management material. To some of the more recent CDC leaders, the PHA type of manager—one with years of management and operational experience at local, state, and regional levels in several public health programs—no longer was needed among CDC management ranks. Either this was the case, or perhaps the leadership did not realize that the type of manager who was effectively contributing as the deputy in the historic scientist-PHA duo of CDC management was a product of the PHA system of grassroots public health experience and development. The CDC leadership began to believe that while the agency was spending time and resources developing the PHA type of worker, it more urgently needed other types of public health workers. The element PHAs appeared to be missing was graduate academic training.

Although traditional PHAs came with a baccalaureate degree and years of local, state, and temporary duty experience, few came with advanced degrees in health or related fields. Many PHAs took advantage of opportunities to gain graduate degrees with agency support, and others obtained their training on their own and at their own expense. Still other PHAs did not seek a graduate degree because they felt their experience was of greater value. Efforts at CDC to help employees gain additional formal training—such as master's degrees in public health, public administration, business, and informatics—were not systemic or continuous because of the cost to the agency. In 1996, CDC established contracts with Emory University, Johns Hopkins, Tulane, and the University of Washington to provide PHAs at particular management levels with partial degrees, or certificates, in public health. The Graduate Certificate Program was designed to increase the number of PHAs who obtained some formal graduate training; however, it would not allow them to leave their assignments during the course of study so that they could obtain a full degree. Even with the challenge of working full-time and going to school, seventy-four percent of the 175 PHAs who enrolled earned a certificate in public health.

The effort was short-lived despite its success rate and was discontinued in December 2000.[18] Although cost was certainly a factor for the effort to credential the existing PHA cohort, it apparently was not the primary issue. Rather, at CDC the increasingly dominant issue was that even with credentials, the type of experience PHAs brought to CDC management did not make a valuable contribution to future CDC management, so equipping PHAs with graduate degrees was not strategically efficient for the agency. Key among leaders who held this opinion were CDC director Dr. David Satcher, deputy director Dr. Claire Broome, and Division of Sexually Transmitted Disease Prevention director Dr. Judith Wasserheit. All three had close working relationships with PHAs as deputies and senior managers. Unlike Wasserheit, who had trained as an STD and public health physician, Drs. Satcher and Broome did not arrive at CDC with any experience working with PHAs. Jack Jackson, a PHA who was working as the CDC's associate director of Management and Operations and chief financial officer at the time, remembers how difficult it was to argue for the PHA experience because these CDC leaders did not "grow up" working with PHAs:

> These leaders were very supportive of the PHAs who worked so closely with them. I worked closely with Dr. Broome and Dr.

> Satcher, as did Bill Gimson. However, these scientific leaders came up from a different system. They did not work hand-in-hand with PHAs like their predecessors. So when the time came to stop hiring PHAs, they did not realize that dismantling the system would eliminate the Jack Jacksons, the Bill Gimsons, the Jack Spencers, and others. This was especially the case for Dr. Satcher. He valued what was there but did not realize that these PHAs were the product of the system of field recruitment.[19]

The thinking was that CDC needed to expand its human resource assets to include people with formal training in business, public policy, public health, and health informatics. At the time, CDC could not expand the employee ranks to accommodate these needs. Further, there were those who expressed that if the PHA brand of experience was not necessary as part of the CDC management core, and if the local and state health departments did not appear to need PHAs any longer, why should CDC continue to train them in state and local settings? The rank and file at CDC voiced concern about this emerging leadership perspective, but CDC leadership did not hear it because the division with the greatest policy standing on any issue about PHAs was the Division of STD Prevention, and this division's leadership supported the new thinking. Dr. Judy Wasserheit felt that although the PHA program had a strong history, it recently had fallen on hard times, and the historic partnership between PHAs and scientists had eroded. Public health's dynamic needs were not reflected in what had become a more static program for PHAs, and "CDC had fallen down" in its responsibility to ensure that it had the "best and the brightest." According to Dr. Wasserheit:

> When I came to CDC it rapidly became apparent that, at least within the STD program, there were a lot of PHAs who had sort of been left behind. CDC and the STD program was the largest trainer and employer of Public Health Advisors and had really fallen down in thinking about training programs that would keep Public Health Advisors at the top of their game or at the cutting edge of where public health was going. So it seemed to me we needed to fix that.[20]

While CDC leaders were thinking about ways to develop the public health workforce of the future, they were blindsided by the wave of government efficiency efforts coming from the Clinton Administration. The federal governmental streamlining process called "reinventing government" was in full swing, and these efforts involved a thorough review of all federal agencies to improve efficiency. The elements under review included the number of FTE staff positions each agency held and whether these positions were under a maximum number, or "ceiling." The issue was not new to CDC; policy discussions about FTE ceilings had been held in the past—beginning in 1975, and especially with reference to whether the field staff assigned to a state or local government were to be counted or exempted from the ceiling because they were serving another government level on a full-time basis. CDC consistently and historically had argued that field employees such as PHAs or EIS officers were exempt from the FTE ceiling.[22]

Compounding the issue of exemption was the management of the employee ceiling itself. In the 1970s and 1980s, federal ceilings were not much of an issue for the administration. During those years CDC juggled employee vacancies to demonstrate that it had fewer FTEs than its established employee ceiling. Still, according to Jack Jackson, CDC did not watch the ceiling carefully enough, and this complicated matters for the agency. When the Clinton Administration pushed CDC to demonstrate that the agency fell short of its FTE ceiling, CDC also had to account for the number of field staff, who for the first time were deemed non-exempt. Although many CDC field personnel were affected, PHAs in the field suffered the most. In 1993 several hundred PHAs were working in the field as a result of intensified recruiting since 1988. Jack Jackson recalls:

> CDC was being hit from the ceiling standpoint and had to reduce the FTE ceiling. PHAs were not exempt… It wasn't just PHAs; it was the whole system. Nothing was exempt. The Clinton Administration looked at the total employment FTE ceiling and lumped in the field staff. Not only were we already over the ceiling, but we had not included the field staff because they had not ever been included, and now all of a sudden you're not only over but they are included in the count.[23]

CDC had no choice but to reduce the employee count. Decisions had to be made quickly. Many people opted to take retirement or early retirement. PHAs were particularly concerned because for the first time they would not be exempt. Would there be a fight to redefine their employment status, as past CDC directors had done? Would creative decisions emerge to maintain the series under these circumstances? The answer would be "no" on both counts. The division with the most PHAs, the Division of STD Prevention, stepped away from the fight—a decision that was regretted by the division's then-deputy director, Jack Spencer. He was the number-two man to Dr. Judy Wasserheit in a PHA-scientist management team. He recalls the time:

> I was very emotionally involved in that process. But there were a number of factors that all sort of came together at the same time. One was that Judy Wasserheit, whom I highly respect and who taught me the value of using the results of science to drive public health programs, came in as the director of the division. Judy was very academic in her perspective, and she wanted to see an increase in the level of academic credentials that people had before staff were hired.[24]

The decision concerned more than academics. For Judy Wasserheit, the issue was about the workforce's quality and preparedness in a changing public health environment. Support for PHAs was eroding within the Division of STD Prevention and across CDC. It was more than just a desire to have academic credentialing for PHAs; it was a need to update the program itself. Change was not emerging from the PHA program, which meant that the old system could not evolve by itself. The result was that a critical opinion of PHAs emerged among some at CDC, with the result that no one stepped forward to fight for exempt status for the PHA field staff. Judy recalled the view of PHAs outside STD and TB:

> Most of those beyond STD and TB, particularly among the non-PHA CDC staff, had a pretty negative perception about PHAs at that point... People felt that many PHAs were not well-trained and were resistant to change, or that it was very much an all-boys' club that had one way of doing things... and that the PHA series might have been helpful in the past, but that it largely had outlived its usefulness. For me, that was a manifestation of how, frankly, the STD program had failed the PHA series, because people wouldn't have felt that way if we had been doing a better job of providing career development and training and recruiting. Part of what happened was that recruitment had wound up being something that was done pretty much unilaterally by existing PHAs. At the time there was not a lot of vision among those folks about how this program could and should change.[25]

A cut in PHA field staff was necessary, as the Division of STD Prevention opted not to support the series' continuation in the face of an FTE ceiling issue.

Jack Spencer was the man who had to handle the money issues for the division. If the FTEs would not be defended, the money itself would have to be. As field PHAs left the workforce through retirement or resignation, the resources funding them were offered to the states in their grants. Why? Because just as originally designed, the PHAs who were assigned to state or local STD programs were part of the federal grant or cooperative agreement, and were given as personnel in lieu of cash. Jack found that with these changes, the STD funding was at risk. CDC had moved on to support a different kind of employee development process—the Public Health Prevention Specialist—and he believed they intended to use funding previously underwriting PHAs for the effort. He fought successfully to retain the financial resources and chalked up the problem to a CDC administration that did not understand basic principles of grant management. Jack recalls:

> It was a tough time because we had to work out issues with our state partners who for over forty years had received direct hire staff in lieu of cash. At the time there were those within the office of the director here at the agency who thought they could take the funds saved from not hiring PHAs and use it support this new cadre that eventually became what is now the Public Health Prevention Specialists [PHPS]. I believe that they thought the FTEs and the money could be used to support the PHPS who were required to have a master's degree, and who would be available to work in multiple field assignments. We were unsuccessful in keeping the FTEs as these belong to the agency, but the funding provided by Congress was categorical and could only be used for STD. The result was the development of a policy for the conversion of direct assistance [PHAs in lieu of funding] back to financial assistance [funding] so that the state STD programs could continue to provide disease intervention services. Those who made this work were the members of the Field Operations Branch at CDC, particularly Don Schwarz, Fred Martich and Gene Williams.[26]

Support for PHAs plummeted inside and outside CDC when the PHAs' major employer, the STD Division, sent the signal to the rest of CDC and to their state and local counterparts that they were changing course and no longer were going to support the hiring and placement of entry-level STD workers in state and local health departments. State and local STD programs wanted the cash resources that previously had funded their assigned PHAs' salaries, and although not all PHAs left their posts, several did, as states had the option of choosing whether they wanted the people or the money. Jack Spencer recalls that in 1994, more than five hundred PHAs were working as field assignees in the STD program, and by 2004, the number had plummeted to around 228. The people in the states who initially supported the reduction in field assignees were the first to tell CDC that there was a problem. Jack Spencer recalls:

> It was interesting that some of the people that were the most vocal opponents of PHAs were the first to come back and say, "Holy cow, we can't do this without the assistance we've had. The strength that we have in the field is primarily attributable to the presence of PHAs, who are the glue that is holding it together out here."[27]

It is difficult to appreciate how CDC could decide to discontinue entry-level hiring of PHAs at a time when PHAs themselves were serving in senior management positions throughout CDC—several in deputy director positions and several in the CDC director's office. The strongest theory is that no one among the CDC leadership understood that by eliminating the entry-level public health worker, the series itself eventually would be eliminated, and, as a consequence, the experienced manager at CDC.

The policy to stop hiring entry-level PHAs began in 1994 for the STD Division and then became agency-wide. In 1994, CDC hired fifty PHAs, half of whom were entry-level in the TB program. In 1995 there was a hiring freeze, so no PHAs were hired. In 1996 CDC was focusing on recruiting other types of employees, such as the Public Health Prevention Specialists (PHPS). Some among the remaining PHAs felt that the PHPS hires were to replace Public Health Advisors, though this cannot be clearly documented beyond recognizing that no PHAs were hired at entry level in the ensuing years. Over time, the system of hiring and assigning entry-level Public Health Advisors crumbled. The cadre of PHAs began to dwindle. In comparison to 1993 levels, there was a 62.5 percent reduction in the number of field-assigned PHAs by 2005,[28] and today the STD, TB, and Immunization Programs have a combined total of 237 field assignees, a seventy percent reduction.[29]

Local and state health departments began to feel the effects of CDC's policy decision by the late 1990s because no entry-level PHAs were available to work in the STD, HIV, and TB programs, and no mid-level managers were available for the Immunization, TB, Chronic Disease, STD, or HIV programs with sufficiently diverse field experience. By the millennium, local and state public health personnel numbers were dwindling. A 2003 study among state health departments revealed that by 2008, retirement rates among state public health personnel would be as high as forty-five percent, with vacancy rates as high as twenty percent in some states. These findings were compounded by state public health employee turnover rates of up to fourteen percent in some parts of the country. States were facing severe budget cuts, and more than half of them lacked qualified job applicants in public health.[30] At CDC, the numbers of knowledgeable and successful managers to serve as deputies—the likes of Bill Watson, Kathy Cahill, or Joe Carter—were diminished. It would only get worse. CDC was expanding its scope to include efforts abroad that compounded the need for human resources. Following the national tragedy of September 11, 2001, and the anthrax scares, CDC was expanding efforts in bioterrorism and preparedness. The new efforts needed experienced managers, but the managers who might have helped were retired or gone.

By 2005 CDC headquarters had become aware that a paucity of qualified candidates was available for management and development roles within headquarters and in several international posts—posts which were increasing in number due to CDC's expanding international activity. The need for operationally experienced public health managers at CDC and in international programs sponsored in part by CDC has been addressed by hiring retired PHAs in consulting capacities to serve in everything from project leadership in India to major CDC roles, such as employee management or program development staff for the Strategic National Stockpile (SNS). The roles these silverbacks are asked to fill are not entry-level field positions in VD contact epidemiology. Instead, they are serving in positions of responsibility which depend on a lifetime of varied public health leadership experiences. Even as CDC resumes hiring of entry-level PHAs, it will not avoid the effects of the thirteen-year hiatus. Eventually no retired PHAs will be interested or available to do the job. The silverbacks are a non-renewable resource.

Tony Scardaci did not intend to spend his retirement working for his former employer in India's polio effort. The need for experienced managers and the importance of the polio efforts in the remaining endemic countries convinced him to delay truly retiring with his family. Tony would end up making the decision to "hold off" several times. Like so many retired PHAs, he is valuable because he possesses innumerable management experiences across public health programs in various geographical locations throughout the world (see Chapter 5). He retired from CDC in April 1998, though he never really stopped working. Unlike many of his colleagues, who were contractors working for various organizations that placed retired PHAs in CDC, Tony was rehired by CDC to help provide direction with India's polio efforts. The gig seemed like a good deal because he wanted to return to India, and the assignment would only be three months long. Tony went to India and served as the senior manager working with the polio coordinator for the state of Bihar, the country's second most populous state. Initially he worked for CDC, but at CDC's request, he soon became an employee of the World Health Organization (WHO). At the end of his first three months, WHO asked Tony to remain another three months, near the end of which, Tony returned to the United States to care for his ailing mother. "That was it, I thought," and he remained retired until September 2001. Two weeks after September 11th he was asked to serve as a senior manager in CDC's efforts to create smallpox emergency response teams.

> The last thing I wanted to do was come back to work. I really did not want to come back to CDC at that point.... Another one of those discussions with my wife, and the end result was, "How do you say no under these circumstances?" So I said okay. I truly came back to work as a full-time CDC employee under an excepted appointment. I was the first person that CDC hired under the emergency authorities that they had... We put together the response teams, and at the end of seven months, in May, exactly what I was afraid was going to happen began to happen. The administration in Washington began to push on the agency to create a mass immunization program starting with hundreds of thousands of health workers. In this whole craziness I said, "This is not what I came on for. This is not what I want to be any part of. I don't believe in this. I'm leaving." And I left. That was in May of 2002. That was that. I figured that is the end.[31]

But even this experience would not end Tony's service to CDC in his retirement. By September 2003, he was working in Uttar Pradesh, India, as the senior advisor to the Polio Regional Coordinator. "Almost three years of my life now has been spent in India. It is somebody else's turn, and I really do feel that way," he says. Although he values his service to CDC, Tony recognizes the need for CDC to grow a new, more modern management workforce and not rely on retirees. The Polio Program is close to wiping out polio in India. In order to sustain the activity, "you need to hold this place together, and it is not a technical job. That's a management job." Tony continues:

> You are going to have to hold the government together. You are going to have to hold states together. You are going to have to hold your program together. These young docs that you've got out there, these SMOs [surveillance medical officers], bitch and moan and complain about round after round after round [of vaccinations] and how draining it is, and it is! And we all know what it is, but let me tell you, a year from now, do you think you are going to have a surveillance medical officer saying, "Oh, boy, I get to go out and do my third active case search in a primary healthcare center where I can't even find a doctor to talk to?" There is nobody working there. Of course you are not going to find anybody interested in doing that. It is going to be hell trying to keep this together.[32]

Standing in the CDC human resource gap are consultancies returning PHAs back to CDC to fill many important and high-level positions. Many of these consultancies are owned or managed by retired PHAs with deep contacts at CDC and tremendous knowledge and expertise regarding the CDC system and its needs. One such PHA, Jack Jackson, is the vice president and director of McKing Consulting Corporation. Jack's career with CDC is yet another example of a field-based public health worker who, through multiple transfers, varied program experiences, and management placements, came to fill an executive role at CDC. He started as a VD co-op in Pensacola, Florida, in 1965. Within two years, he was working in Mobile, Alabama, and engaged in several syphilis blitzes in response to outbreaks. He soon joined the Health Mobilization Program, focused on helping hospitals and physicians stockpile medical and pharmaceutical supplies in the event of a nuclear attack. Jack became a recognized management talent throughout his many and varied program placements, and in 1984 he was chosen as the deputy director for the National Center for Environmental Health. The last six years of his career at CDC were spent as associate director for management and chief financial officer. He retired in 1999. In every role, Jack witnessed the value of accruing experience as a PHA:

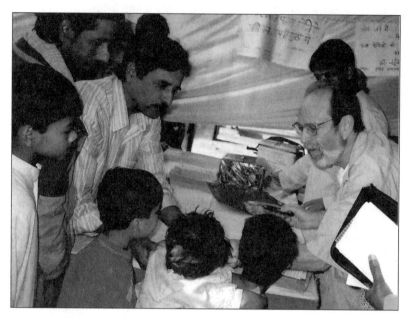

Tony Scardaci giving polio immunizations in Kanpur, Uttar Pradesh, India, 2004. Courtesy Tony Scardaci.

> The strongest thing that PHAs bring to the table is the field experience. They really had to work with a variety of different people to get the job done. It was just basic get-the-job-done, figuring out how to do it in different environments. I think the state and local experience was critical. You just can't quickly replicate this kind of experience.[33]

By the time Jack retired from CDC, it was clear that the agency needed the help of recently-retired PHAs to work in several key CDC programs and initiatives. This need for topic experts or experienced and senior officials is not unique to CDC. Many organizations hire recently-retired personnel on a short-term basis to provide assistance in one area or another. CDC's need for retired PHAs, however, went far beyond this customary scenario. The range of work tasks was vast—from lower-level work, such as grant application reviews or project area site visits, to mid-level management tasks, such as program and policy development or evaluation. There was also a need for senior-level management and leadership. By the early years of the twenty-first century, McKing Consulting Corporation and other consultancies like it (COMFORCE Corporation, Northrop Grumman Corporation, Science Applications International Corporation, and Carter Consulting, Inc.) had provided retired PHAs to CDC.

Former PHA Russ Havlak is a contractor working at CDC in a major capacity. In 1999 he was retired for less than a year when Steve Bice convinced Russ that he needed to come and help him develop the Strategic National Stockpile Program at CDC. One of many terrorism countermeasures, the Strategic National Stockpile attempts to store sufficient vaccine and key pharmaceuticals for use in the event of a terrorist attack or some other major catastrophe. Russ retired from CDC at the tail end of the "perfect storm," when downsizing the federal government converged with concerns about the FTE ceiling and PHAs. He did not necessarily want to stop working, but did not think he would want to return to work in the negative climate that was developing at CDC. Russ said that he was "seduced" into working with the Strategic National Stockpile by Steve Bice, a PHA who knew just how to use other PHAs' expertise to further the program:

> Steve had very few FTEs and was looking for a few old hands who could help pull a complicated program together. [He wanted someone who] knew the ropes and was versatile enough to handle most any crappy job tossed his way. It turned out that I was his only old hand and so was handed just about every crappy job that came along. I wrote position descriptions, work plans, strategic plans, Congressional testimony and budgets, proposals on SNS ethics, education, training, field operations, and just about any topic you can imagine. Along the way I recruited several other retired PHAs. As I absorbed the logistics, materiel management, and pharmaceutical aspects of the SNS, I also participated in analyzing and deliberating on just about every issue pertaining to these topics that came down the line. It was Steve's management style to solicit the judgment of his people—FTE or contractor, it made no difference to him. It was all about what you could deliver.[34]

Russ, like many PHAs, is known for his "cut to the chase" work style and his ability to make things happen. This professional persona developed over many years and placements as a PHA. The VD program hired him in 1963 and placed him in his hometown of Pittsburgh. Russ soon was transferred to Sharon,

Pennsylvania, where he served as the district rep. This was at the height of the U.S. effort to eradicate syphilis in the 1960s, and the tools available were not always as efficient as one might like. This was not a time of rapid diagnostics, so PHAs often had to jostle local or state public health laboratories to get blood samples examined in short time periods. Although any public health lab would recognize that time was of the essence in syphilis epidemiology, for efficiency's sake, local laboratories often required VD investigators to wait until the lab could batch their samples—gather sufficient numbers. "At the time I was covering six large rural counties," Russ said. "If I drew a blood on a syphilis contact, suspect or potential patient, my only option was to mail it off to the state lab in Harrisburg and wait a week to ten days for the result to be mailed back. That hardly supported rapid syphilis epidemiology."

During the course of routine laboratory visits, Russ found a man named Pete Mancino, who ran a lab in his garage: "My information said that Pete ran a lab approved by the state for premarital and prenatal testing, which meant he passed their periodic quality control testing and knew what he was doing." Pete not only knew what he was doing, but he agreed to run the samples whenever Russ needed them. Although this might raise eyebrows, the lab was legitimate, and it was a good solution for what otherwise would be a seven-day wait. When Russ called in the results from this lab, it sounded as if he were calling from a junkyard with a bunch of barking dogs:

> Pete was an elderly microbiologist who ran his own lab out of a detached garage behind his house in New Castle, Pennsylvania, a very nice residential area. I see the address of his lab and pull into his driveway and around the back of this big house. Suddenly I'm attacked by four dogs that, I was to learn, had total freedom to roam in and out of Pete's lab. The place was an absolute mess, but he sure did know his business. He ran syphilis serologic tests there along with most of the other basic tests you'd expect from a clinical lab.[34]

Once Russ got to know Pete and explained the problem with the turnaround time for laboratory samples, Pete told Russ to bring him bloods any time. "So I snapped up his offer, and things really began to move," Russ said. "Whenever I'd have anything, I'd investigate, draw a blood, and run it to Pete. Even if I got there at ten or eleven at night, he'd put everything on hold and run a VDRL (test for syphilis) for me." The cost of doing business together was high for Pete because the State of Pennsylvania had no mechanism to reimburse him for his laboratory services. Although Russ offered to pay him "out of my own shallow pockets," Pete refused to discuss payment. Pete Mancino's contribution to syphilis epidemiology enabled Russ to turn around contacts in a matter of hours—something unheard of in the state STD program. Russ used Pete's lab services so often that the state STD program recognized Russ' call even before he spoke: "It got so they knew at once it was me and where I was by the background chorus of four barking dogs."[36]

In contrast to other types of managers and executives, the more senior and experienced PHAs become, the more they continue to miss the field and the development experience. Like Tony Scardaci, Russ had a stellar career of management and operations activity, and reveled in the chance to build a program from scratch with the Strategic National Stockpile. Such creativity and the flexibility to problem-solve became a hallmark of the SNS program. Russ thinks that Steve Bice's leadership as a PHA made the difference, and helped the program respond as planned on September 11, 2001. According to Russ, Steve Bice and fellow PHA Steve Adams had anticipated that aircraft would be grounded in the event of a terrorist attack. Six months before September 11, 2001, they approached the Federal Aviation Administration to request and receive priority flight status for the Strategic National Stockpile (see Chapter 1). "Throughout the two weeks of domestic aircraft grounding, our priority flight status was accepted without question," Russ said. During that period, CDC was the only means of supplying respirators, boots, gloves, and other protective materiel needed by the volunteers at Ground Zero. Russ continues:

> I would venture to say that under non-PHA leadership we would not have been nearly as prepared to respond as we did on 9/11 and during the ensuing anthrax crisis. I can think back on several PHA-like creative twists and turns we took that made it possible for the SNS to perform as it did, and save Tommy Thompson's butt the Sunday after 9/11, when he had to face questioning from Mike Wallace on *60 Minutes* about what HHS did to help NYC in the crisis. Tommy got this smile across his face and said, "We delivered fifty tons of medical materiel there within seven hours of the request by New York City, and we also flew in medical supplies and CDC epidemiologists despite the grounding of all domestic aircraft."[37]

Russ's value for the Strategic National Stockpile increases geometrically when combined with that of other retired PHAs working for this program: Dave Adcock, Orlando Blancato, Dave Brownell, and Jack Stubbs. With new efforts, it will take time to develop the kind of public health human resources PHAs offered. By the time these resources are fully developed and deployable throughout the CDC system, the Russ Havlaks, Tony Scardacis, and hundreds of other retired PHAs who now work in the public health system will be long gone.

But hope is on the horizon. Following a 2005 McKing report that focused on the Public Health Advisor series,[38] CDC began to formally recognize the impact of the human resource bubble that had been created by hiring policies in the 1990s. The agency's recognition was reflected in a 2006 policy statement reinforcing the strategic value of field assignments. The policy stated that Public Health Advisors had a direct impact on national health goals "through their assignments in the broader public health system," and that these assignments would ensure practical and local experience for CDC headquarters succession planning and expedite deployment in times of public health crisis or need, since a cadre of PHAs would be in the field at any given time.[39] Jack Jackson believes this change is positive, but he knows that the human resource gap will not be resolved easily because the PHA field placement system was dismantled more than a decade ago: "If tomorrow you decide to assign people to the states and you don't have the infrastructure in place, you can't just send people out there." He continues:

> I think CDC recognizes there's a need, and I think they realize that it is field experience that they need to get. So I see a bright future. The challenge is going to be how do you get—after you in essence have not had the structure in place and you have so many gaps—how do you get from where they were to where you need to be?[34]

Chapter 9

The New Experiment

It all began with an experiment on Maryland's Eastern Shore in 1948. A cadre of men trained to become VD investigators for the federal government. They immediately were joined by others and would contribute significantly to the development of sexually transmitted disease programs throughout the U.S. Since the 1960s, PHAs had been called on to help eliminate smallpox, polio, measles, syphilis, and tuberculosis, and they had responded to countless health and humanitarian disasters. By the end of the 1970s, Public Health Advisors had gained experience in many types of public health programs throughout the world. By this time, these unique workers had become a central part of CDC's management backbone and were credited with contributions to numerous public health efforts. With the wisdom and flexibility gained through years of field experience, PHAs earned a reputation as problem solvers, as "can-do" and "go-to" people at CDC. Yet despite their significant contributions, CDC stopped hiring entry-level Public Health Advisors in 1994—just four years short of the PHA series' fiftieth anniversary. It soon looked as if CDC were going to allow the Public Health Advisor to fade away.

Within five years, CDC began to recognize the impact of the decision not to hire entry-level PHAs. Several major tasks at the agency were being handled by retired PHAs because the current agency workforce had no experience. When Dr. Julie Gerberding was appointed CDC director in 2002, CDC already had managed ably through response efforts following September 11th, 2001, with critical help provided by retired PHAs. Dr. Gerberding and her deputy Bill Gimson knew the value of the Public Health Advisors they had at CDC. They also recognized that it was in the agency's strategic interest to rekindle the PHA series. Mike Sage, a PHA and director of CDC's Portfolio Management Project (PMP), recalls how the CDC's thinking about PHAs began to change when he and others developed the PMP effort:

> In 2005, Dr. Gerberding asked us to revisit the field staff at CDC, to look at it anew and start to think about how we would develop

> a future for field placements of PHAs with CDC and its programs. There had not been much hiring or concerted strategy around a plan for PHAs and field staff at CDC for quite some time, so as we started to look into this whole issue, it became apparent that the entry-level PHA was something that we really needed to explore.[1]

Bill Gimson directed Mike and the PMP to reinvigorate the PHA career track. Mike recruited PHA Glen Koops away from the Office of Preparedness to help identify a modernized version of the PHA series. Glen was valuable to this effort because he had spent the past two years exploring the potential for an employee development program as director of field services in the Office of Preparedness. Glen recalls that his effort revealed a truth about CDC: "there just wasn't a field based pipeline for CDC management any longer."[2] When Glen joined the Portfolio Management Project, he began to see the field staff "as both an investment in the states in terms of technical assistance, and also as an investment in future CDC leaders and managers."[3] The PMP was a new initiative geared toward the management of agency resources by establishing executive-level relationships with state and local public health partners across programs. The program was an effort to create agency-wide coordination that would move beyond the "silos" that often formed as a result of disease-specific funding. This was a perfect program home for a reinvigorated PHA series.

As Glen began his work with the PMP, he consulted with his PHA colleague Kristin Brusuelas, who previously had worked with him in the Office of Preparedness and in the National Immunization Program. She recalled the challenge facing the Immunization Program: "We always had requests for people at the program level, but we could not fill the need. It was very different than when I was hired as a PHA."[4] When CDC hired Kristin in 1990, the agency was engaged in an intensive recruitment effort which by 1993 would yield an historic high of eight hundred field PHAs.[5] Like other PHAs hired in the early 1990s, Kristin had a multitude of valuable work experiences that contributed to her knowledge as a CDC leader. She began in South-Central Los Angeles in syphilis elimination and HIV notification. Within one year, she had transferred to Dallas with the STD and HIV Program, followed by transfers to Chicago, New Mexico, and back to Los Angeles with the Immunization Program. Kristin was also detailed to Mombasa, Kenya, and nearby coastal communities to work in a CDC effort to stop polio and measles. She came to CDC headquarters in 2000 as the co-team leader (with Tom Hicks) of the immunization field staff within the Immunization Division, but soon was drawn into working with Glen Koops to expand the CDC field staff's involvement in bioterrorism and preparedness and later with the Portfolio Management Program. It was possible to involve current field staff in assisting with preparedness, but finding new field staff to meet the current challenges was daunting because there was no extant mechanism to recruit and train them. By 2005, the PHA field system had been effectively dismantled. PHAs were still in the field, though in fewer numbers (see Chapter 8). Public health workforce development was further complicated by emerging needs. Public health workers at local, state, and federal levels were aging out of the system,[6] and although entry-level local public health workers were badly needed, local systems, whose training assets were varied and in some cases nonexistent, no longer were poised to support a federal recruitment effort. Kristin recognized then that if CDC decided to reinvigorate the PHA series and initiate some type of entry-level hiring, the agency would need some assurance of solid entry-level experience and training.

When Kristin became the senior management official (SMO) for Florida's Portfolio Management Project, she hoped there would be an opportunity to continue working toward reinvigorating the PHA series. As the SMO, Kristin served as the CDC executive team contact in a strengthened relationship between CDC, the state health officer, and other public health leaders in the state.[7] Public health workforce issues were critical to Florida, because the state believed itself to be disproportionately impacted by the workforce trends. Florida is a destination for retirement, and this means that many public health workers choose Florida as a job destination toward the end of their careers. This observation was confirmed by Florida staffing projections. Kristin recalls that Florida found that a "large number of management, business management, and people who were running county health departments and programs were projected to retire soon."[8]

As Kristin delved into Florida's state and local workforce challenges, Glen Koops continued his work inside CDC to identify ways to reinvigorate the PHA series, though he was soon at an impasse. Although PHAs were generalists and accrued a wealth of experience across public health programs, they were primarily the products of siloed programs—historically, STD Prevention. The effort to revive entry-level PHA hiring was received well by several CDC programs, though they could not envision how it would be possible given current priorities:

"Many programs supported the concept of new PHA development in categorical programs, but no one had money for it."[9] Glen knew that the primary issue would be money, but he did not anticipate that it would also be vision. Glen believes that when programs considered a revived PHA model, they tended to think of a supply-side model: "We train up a good-sized cohort of PHA Associates, ask states 'how many do you want?', then we'd push them out there." The old model was not getting any traction inside CDC. Mike Sage recalls that the momentum changed when they started to think about this as a state-initiated project or experiment:

> Why don't we start with a state and see what happens? It would be a little experiment within an experiment. We thought of Florida. Glen, Kristin, and Bonnie Sorenson, who was then the deputy director of the Florida Health Department, gathered a group to put the meat to the bones.[10]

A group of Florida public health leaders assembled to talk about the shared problem, and it soon became clear that to revive a system of placement, training, and mentoring for entry-level Public Health Advisor types, federal and state governments would have to have a more active partnership. The effort could not be centered in a particular program at CDC, nor could it be solely a CDC effort. Florida's director of health at the time, Dr. Rony Francois, had workforce development expertise and provided the needed leadership to develop a program that would meet both CDC's and Florida's future workforce needs. The outcome was a new take on what an entry-level PHA program might be. The new model would begin with state need. According to Kristin Brusuelas, it also incorporated features from the previous PHA model and CDC fellowship programs. Florida had very specific needs and experiences:

> Florida needed people to be worker bees in their counties and on the front lines of public health. Some of the discussions recognized and valued the public health fellowships that CDC offered in the past, such as with EIS, PHPS and others; however, Florida said that they needed the front line workers. Plus, Florida would never be able to compete for the salaries once fellows entered the market after receiving training with the state. So when people finished their training in the new system, Florida wanted to compete in terms of hiring.[11]

Historically, state and local health departments have been training areas for PHAs and for fellows such as Epidemic Intelligence Service Officers, Public Health Prevention Specialists, and Presidential Management Interns. With the exception of state and local experience with PHAs, Florida witnessed CDC fellows who completed training and then left the state to work in more lucrative environments. The better-paying jobs were at CDC headquarters, in universities, and in states with higher wages. According to Kristin, the emerging solution was to develop a PHA entry-level training program that would offer comparable remuneration to the host state's public health pay scale at placement time in order to remove the financial incentive to leave after completing a training period: "We sat down with the state and tried to establish a program where we would pay at a level equivalent to their salary levels." Florida and CDC wanted to improve on the previous PHA model in another respect: cross-training. Instead of immersing trainees in one program for a few years, the new model would attempt to place new PHAs in a few programs during the initial training period. Kristin called this approach "taking the best of the former system and incorporating the modern needs."[12]

The Florida workgroup produced the vision for a reinvigorated PHA system. However, vision alone was not enough to get something off the ground. They needed money. Mike Sage and Glen Koops took the proposal to Bill Gimson, who gave the go-ahead for the pilot project: "We went to Bill with the Florida proposal, saying that we want to start with ten people, and this is the cost. He was instrumental in ensuring that we got the resources to get it started."[13] In light of history, Bill Gimson's contribution could be compared with that of the Madam who paved the way for the Doctor to initiate his experiment in 1948. The comparisons continue, because just as the VD Division moved decisively toward a policy of federal operational support prior to initiating the original experiment (see Chapters 2 and 3), the present-day CDC shifted its policy position on the value of field assignments; paving the way for the new experiment. In 2006, CDC issued a policy statement reinforcing the strategic benefit of field assignments in public health. The policy affirmed the value of field PHAs and their direct contribution to national health goals through their assignments in the broader public health system. Field assignments would ensure practical and local experience for CDC headquarters succession planning, and they would expedite deployment in times of public health crisis or need, since a complement of PHAs would be in the field at any given time.[14] In this new CDC environment, Glen and his colleagues procured the initial resources for the experiment.

The actual startup money came from the Office of Workforce and Career Development through the efforts of Candice Nowicki-Lehnherr, the senior management official for the State of Georgia. At the time, Candice was with the Office of Workforce and Career Development as the senior advisor to the director and the associate director of Program Development. She was able to gain agency support for this workforce project by demonstrating "how this project was a link for the local and state health departments. We want to develop the workforce that would carry out specific activities."[15] One could not think of a better person to help sell the idea of the new PHA experiment throughout CDC. Candice, a PHA, had spent years working in several different public health programs across CDC and in many state and local areas. She was also an understudy to Jack Spencer in the Division of STD Prevention at the time when the hiring of entry-level PHAs was discontinued. Candice saw this new program as the continuation of the PHA series, and she understood how to communicate the value to a variety of partners within the agency:

> The role and the delivery of program services, the outreach, and the relationships among the levels of the public health system—these are roles of the PHA. PHAs function at the local level interpreting federal program or policies, or they are working at the federal level using their vast experience gained through years in the field.[16]

CDC was able to initiate a pilot of Florida's project with a one-time influx of resources through the efforts of several PHAs: Glen Koops, Kristin Brusuelas, Candice Nowicki-Lehnherr, Bill Gimson, and Mike Sage. The pilot experiment, called the Public Health Apprenticeship Program, was established in 2007. Like its predecessor, the program hires public health personnel on a temporary basis to gain skills and experiences at the entry level of public health programs. Unlike the original PHA system, this new model is driven by the needs of state and local health departments, and program assignments are not limited to STD, HIV, and TB. As with the co-ops of long ago, the apprentices are understood to be in an excepted hiring position. They are on a three-year training cycle, or apprenticeship. Upon completing their apprenticeship, they will be able to compete for local, state, and federal jobs.[17]

Cooperatively designing a system for entry-level PHAs with a state was a departure from the previous PHA model. The outcome would allow more flexibility based on state need, which theoretically would increase state long-term investment in the program. In the original PHA model, CDC partnered with states through cooperative agreements to place PHAs in program-specific roles. The PHA was part of a grant resource from the federal government to state or local governments. State or local health departments could request PHAs, and they might get them, if PHAs were available and if the assignment was appropriate as a training ground. This model, however, was far from a partnership. The new experiment called for a different type of relationship between CDC and a state health department, with program components negotiated based on individual and evolving state needs. According to Glen Koops:

> A strong collaborative approach is one of the characteristics that make the Apprentice Program different from the old co-op system. We are engaging states one at a time, and asking them whether they are interested in the program. If they are, we begin with a discussion of their workforce needs in the area of program operations. From there we build the process of identifying specific apprentice assignments that suit the needs of the state and local public health entities as well as the needs of CDC. Those states that are interested see it as an opportunity to improve their own workforce. They want to compete with CDC to hire these individuals. The PHAP experiment is essentially a needs-driven approach to staff development.[18]

The career path set out for apprentices includes several skill and experience areas: knowledge of the components, roles, and functions of the public health system; entry-level experience in public health practice across multiple programs; skills in public health program implementation; and experience in public health preparedness and response activities.[19] Recognizing the paucity of federal mentors due to the dissolution of the previous PHA placement structure, new apprentices are assigned mentors with broad public health experience at several levels of government (local, state, and federal).

The new experiment began in Florida on July 23, 2007—almost sixty years after the original experiment began in July of 1948 on the Eastern Shore of Maryland. Ten of ninety-nine apprentice applicants were selected and placed in various local health department programs across Florida. During their first two years they will rotate among two of the following efforts: HIV, STD, tuberculosis,

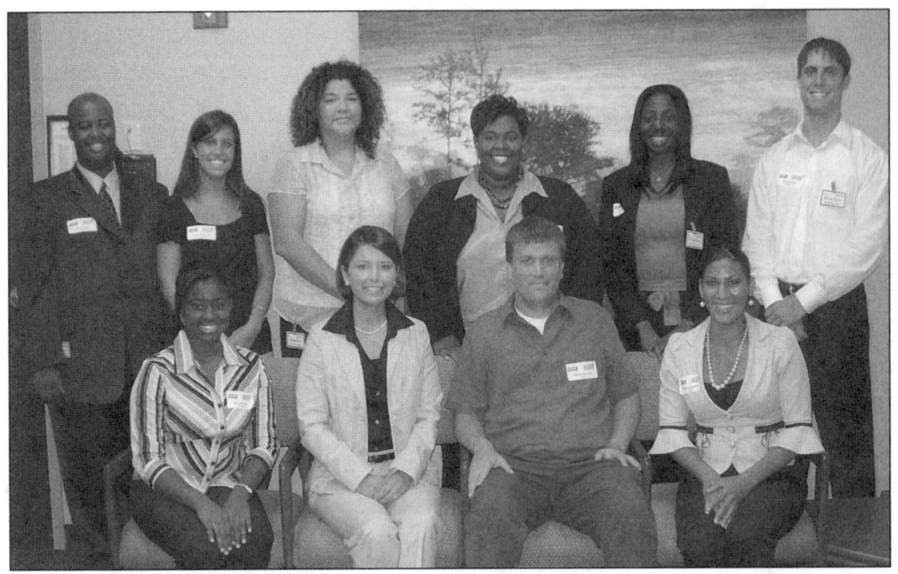

The inaugural class of CDC Public Health Apprentices. Back row (left to right): Jabari Paul, Adrienne Huneke, Cecilia Galvan, Kara Johnson, Toyin Ademokun, Clayton Weiss. Front row (left to right): Donyelle Russ, Bobbie Strickland, Martin Honisch, Camille Gonzalez.
Courtesy of Glen Koops.

quarantine, general epidemiology and surveillance, refugee health, public health emergency preparedness, environmental health, and health education programs. In the third year, they will work in cross-cutting areas, including women's health coordination, public health planning, grants development, and program development.[20] The first year of training introduces the apprentices to epidemiology, disease, and health hazard investigation, as well as public health promotion and social marketing. Within three years, apprentices will receive progressively more varied and complex assignments in at least two public health programs. As the Florida pilot is proving successful, additional states have been selected as hosts for an apprenticeship pilot program based on how rapidly and efficiently they can establish one. These new pilot locations include Georgia, North Carolina, Texas, and Arkansas. According to Glen Koops, the vision is to evaluate the program after five years:

> Ideally, we hope to have sixty to ninety apprentices participate in a five-year pilot in five or six states. This number will help us to

> honestly evaluate the effectiveness of this strategy and its use in helping us meet the staffing gaps at the local, state, and federal levels for years to come.[21]

The Public Health Apprentice Program exists in response to a need for a "consistent pipeline" of public health workers with accrued field and varied public health program experience, who have an understanding of state and local public health realities. CDC has much to gain by reinitiating the entry-level hiring of such public health workers. Glen Koops recognizes that CDC shares the personnel challenge facing local and state public health departments: "[A] significant percentage of career PHAs are nearing retirement age, and CDC has not systematically recruited and trained new PHAs since the mid-1990s."[22] The need within CDC for an experienced and operationally-skilled workforce with strong local and state relationships, paired with the expressed need by state and local health departments for entry-level workers, was sufficiently acute to justify CDC's policy turnaround regarding the hiring of entry-level PHAs.[23] As CDC clearly views the Public Health Apprentice Program as an effort to "revitalize the Public Health Advisor pipeline,"[24] lessons from history should be observed.

The success of the revitalized cadre and its ability to meet the future needs of not only local and state public health but also CDC management and public health efforts worldwide depends upon the replication of several elements from the original model. First, opportunities for CDC field positions at intermediate supervisory levels (GS-9 and GS-11) must be available, so that the newly trained apprentices can continue to accumulate valuable management and operational experiences in the field. The dismantled system of PHA placement and transfer should be reassembled at the management and supervisory levels for the Apprentice Program to be of any lasting value as a CDC supply chain of highly-trained and experienced logisticians and operations management personnel. History tells us that after an initial period of years in the field, successful co-ops were given the opportunity to fully join the series, and then they were transferred to yet another set of field experiences. Although state and local health departments will position themselves to compete for the newly trained Apprentices, CDC also should be ready—not with desk jobs at headquarters, but with field management opportunities. Otherwise, an important experiential disconnect will occur, and the scarcity of management and operational acumen at

CDC will continue to burden the agency and impact its effectiveness. Essentially, this means that if the new experiment is to be a lasting contribution to CDC, the agency will need to intentionally create career trajectories for Public Health Advisors/Apprentices. Combining the old and new models on this point would be highly innovative. The Portfolio Management Program is a tremendous centralizing home for planning and directing such career laddering.

Second, the developing PHA culture should be nurtured to engender international collegiality, and to instill the workforce qualities that are unique to Public Health Advisors and highly sought today. The enculturation process will necessarily engage all PHAs past and present, and will require steadfast CDC support. "Once a PHA, always a PHA" is the kind of thinking that CDC should instill in all new Apprentices. Establishing esprit de corps appears easy in theory. It will be enormously challenging in a decentralized system that probably will lose a percentage of the group to turnover prior to pilot completion and another percentage after the fellowship's completion. What, then, is the remnant that comprises the culture? Although PHAs historically wore 'two hats,' they still recognized themselves to be part of the federal cohort. With the shift in focus from the CDC (old model) to states (new model), how will Apprentices become part of the culture that transcends the state?

Finally, although pressures from federal ceilings, government restructuring, and struggles over organizational core management credentialing combined to dismantle the PHA system, an ongoing issue should not be overlooked: academic credentialing of Public Health Advisors. The Apprentice Program rightly takes the lesson from PHA history that the PHAs' singular contributions came not from formal education but from community-based education accumulated through years of front-line and mid-program-level experiences across public health programs in various geographic locations. This accumulated experience, paired with additional formal educational opportunities later in the PHA career, makes tremendous sense. Whether CDC invests in a Graduate Certificate Program or develops a personnel strategy to provide a targeted number of PHAs at certain levels the opportunity to earn advanced degrees full-time, as they did with several of the PHAs mentioned in this book, is a question that CDC must answer.[25] Avoiding the issue, however, abandons the important responsibility so well articulated by Dr. Judy Wasserheit (see Chapter 8). CDC must attend to the development of all public health workers that serve the agency and its mission. It must not fall down in its obligation to provide a prepared and appropriately-credentialed public health workforce. PHA history teaches that the field and credentialing aspects of a full career are falsely in conflict. Characteristics and varied experiences, placements and culture will create this inimitable public health worker, and for maximum value, these experiences must occur early in a PHA's career and at the public health entry level. Concomitantly, there must be a plan to equip emerging leaders with additional credentials when doing so furthers public health strategic interests.

The good news is that these challenges are not insurmountable because "can-do" people and problem solvers are still within CDC's reach. They are among the men and women working for CDC today as employees and contractors, they are retired PHAs working in sibling organizations, they are PHAs who now are employees of state and local health departments, and they are among those who are retired but accessible through the vast network of Public Health Advisors. There must be an intentional effort to integrate—structurally, culturally, and historically—the old and new experiments for the long-term benefit of health programs globally and for CDC as an agency.

In 1948, the first experiment began. Dr. Johannes Stuart had a vision for the nascent endeavor, and Lida J. Usilton opened doors to make it happen and ensure its success. One wonders what this pair would think about the contributions made thus far by U.S. Public Health Advisors at home and abroad. In 2007, a new experiment began. If this modern version of the earlier system provides a similar wealth of experienced, flexible, capable public health workers and leaders, the new cadre of men and women soon will be *ready to go* and contribute to health and human service efforts worldwide, today and tomorrow.

Notes

Chapter 1

1. E. Kent Gray, interview by PHA History Project, February 4, 2004.

2. Kenneth Archer, as quoted in Kathy Nellis, "Remembering 9/11," *CDC Connects* [internal CDC newsletter] (September 9, 2004). Retrieved from CDC intranet.

3. The Strategic National Stockpile originally was named the National Pharmaceutical Stockpile. Following September 11, 2001 it was renamed as the Strategic National Stockpile (SNS). The SNS is a countermeasure to major events which may threaten health security. The stockpile contains large quantities of medicines, vaccines, and medical supplies which can be deployed at a moment's notice should local supplies be exhausted or contaminated. Source: e-mail from Russell Havlak to author Beth Meyerson on April 17, 2008. Information about the SNS obtained online from the Centers for Disease Control and Prevention on April 25, 2008. http://www.bt.cdc.gov/stockpile. Information about the name change obtained online from Military Medical Technology online edition on May 27, 2008. Kenya McCullum, "National Stockpiling," *Military Medical Technology* 10, no. 7 (November 8, 2006) http://www.military-medical-technology.com/article.cfm?DocID=1771 (accessed May 27, 2008).

4. E-mail from Russell Havlak to author Beth Meyerson, April 23, 2008.

5. Steven Adams, as quoted in Nellis, "Remembering 9/11,"

6. E-mail from Kenneth Archer to author Beth Meyerson, May 15, 2008.

7. Valerie Kokor, interview by PHA History Project, October 29, 2004; Kent Gray, interview by PHA History Project, February 4, 2004; Phillip Finley, interview by PHA History Project, January 30, 2004. See also Nellis, "Remembering 9/11"; e-mail from Russell Havlak to author Beth Meyerson, April 17, 2008.

8. E. Kent Gray, interview by PHA History Project, February 4, 2004.

9. Kenneth Archer, as quoted in Nellis, "Remembering 9/11."

10. E-mail from Ronald Burger to author Beth Meyerson, May 28, 2008. See also: e-mail from E. Kent Gray to author Beth Meyerson, May 26, 2008.

11. E. Kent Gray, interview by PHA History Project, February 4, 2004.

12. Steven Adams, as quoted in Nellis, "Remembering 9/11." See also E-mail from Ronald Burger to author Beth Meyerson, May 28, 2008.

13. E-mail from Kenneth Archer to author Beth Meyerson, May 15, 2008.

14. E-mail from Kenneth Archer to author Beth Meyerson, May 15, 2008. See also E-mail from Ronald Burger to author Beth Meyerson, May 28, 2008.

15. E. Kent Gray, interview by PHA History Project, February 4, 2004.

16. Steven Adams, as quoted in Nellis, "Remembering 9/11."

17. Paraphrase of Ronald Burger's comment from Nellis, "Remembering 9/11"; E-mail from Ronald Burger to author Beth Meyerson, May 28, 2008; Kent Gray, interview by PHA History Project, February 4, 2004.

18. Based on Steven Adams comments in Nellis, "Remembering 9/11." See also E-mail from Ronald Burger to author Beth Meyerson, May 28, 2008.

19. E-mail from Ronald Burger to author Beth Meyerson, May 28, 2008.

20. Ronald Burger comments in Nellis, "Remembering 9/11."

21. William Parra, interview by PHA History Project, June 18, 2004, edited via e-mail on October 20, 2007.

22. Historically and until 1983, CDC referred to work in diseases that were sexually transmitted as VD or venereal disease work. Hence, programs were referred to as VD programs, and disease investigators were known as VDIs or venereal disease investigators. In 1983, Dr. Willard "Ward" Cates, in his role as the director of the Division of STD Prevention, changed the term VD to STD, or sexually transmitted diseases. He recalls the change in 1983: "At that time, the Division was called DVDC, Division of VD Control… I chose [PHA] Bill Parra to be the DVDC deputy director and together, Bill and I realized the 'VD' field had evolved greatly beyond syphilis and gonorrhea, to include an extra fifteen or so new infections spread sexually. Different public health approaches were necessary to address this expanded list of organisms. We wanted to change the name to indicate this evolution, symbolically if for no other reason. Also, the terminology 'VD' was somewhat stigmatizing, and we wanted the more descriptive term 'STD' to open up wider channels of communication about sex and sexuality." E-mail from Willard Cates to author Beth Meyerson, April 26, 2008. For the purpose of this book, we will use the terms "VD" and "STD" as appropriate to the era referenced. Therefore, persons who were hired or working before 1983 will be referred to as VD investigators working in VD programs. When

talking about STD programs theoretically or referencing them from the period of 1983 to the present, the term STD or sexually transmitted disease(s) will be used.

23. It is important to state that some Public Health Advisors did not begin their careers at the entry level of public health, or in the field with patients. PHAs without such experience are relatively new phenomena, or they were women who were working at CDC headquarters at the time that women began to join the ranks of PHAs in the early 1970s (see Chapter 5). For the purposes of this chapter, we will reference the traditional and primary PHA model—the one that involves placement throughout the public health system over a period of several years before a PHA reaches senior management level.

24. William Gimson, interview by PHA History Project, April 1, 2004.

25. Edward Powers, interview by PHA History Project, August 13, 2004.

26. Bernard Malone, interview by PHA History Project, May 28, 2004.

27. Bernard Malone, interview by PHA History, May 28, 2004.

28. Edward Powers, interview by PHA History Project, August 13, 2004.

29. Kevin O'Conner, interview by PHA History Project, March 19, 2004.

30. Richard Conlon, interview by PHA History Project, May 17, 2004.

31. James Chin, ed., *Control of Communicable Diseases*, 17th ed. (Washington, D.C.: American Public Health Association, 2000).

32. Phillip Talboy, interview by PHA History Project, April 21, 2004.

33. Phillip Talboy, interview by PHA History Project, April 21, 2004.

34. E-mail from Dennis McDowell to author Beth Meyerson on October 26, 2007.

35. Dennis McDowell, interview by PHA History Project, June 21, 2007.

36. Kathryn Koski, interview by PHA History Project, August 27, 2004.

37. James Beall, interview by PHA History Project, March 10, 2004.

38. Wendy Wolf, interview by PHA History Project, March 10, 2004.

39. Wendy Wolf, interview by PHA History Project, March 10, 2004.

40. Allan M. Brandt, *No Magic Bullet: A Social History of Venereal Disease in the United States Since 1880* (New York: Oxford University Press, 1987).

41. Charles Joseph Webb, interview by PHA History Project, February 9-10, 2004.

42. William Parra, interview by PHA History Project, June 18, 2004.

43. Philip Talboy, interview by PHA History Project, April 21, 2004.

44. Philip Talboy, interview by PHA History Project, April 21, 2004.

45. Steven Bice, interview by PHA History Project, April 2, 2004.

46. The Compact of Free Association was negotiated between the U.S. government and the Pacific Island nations of the Republic of the Marshall Islands and the

Federal States of Micronesia. For more information, see *U.S. Code 48* (1986), § 1931.

47. Steven Bice, interview by PHA History Project, April 2, 2004.

48. Steven Bice, interview by PHA History Project, April 2, 2004

49. Steven Bice, interview by PHA History Project, April 2, 2004.

50. Anne-Renee Heningburg, interview by PHA History Project, March 29, 2004.

51. Anne-Renee Heningburg, interview by PHA History Project, March 29, 2004.

52. Alan Hinman, interview by PHA History Project, July 29, 2004.

53. E-mail from David Sencer to author Beth Meyerson, May 12, 2008. According to Sencer, the title Executive Officer no longer exists. Today the position would be Deputy or Assistant Director of Management.

54. E-mail from David Sencer to author Beth Meyerson, May 12, 2008.

55. Lawrence Posey, interview by PHA History Project, March 31, 2004; David Sencer, interview by PHA History Project, March 31, 2004; Billy Griggs, interview by PHA History Project, April 2, 2004.

56. David Sencer, interview by PHA History Project, March 31, 2004.

57. David Sencer, interview by PHA History Project, March 31, 2004.

58. William Foege, interview by PHA History Project, September 23, 2004.

59. William Roper, interview by PHA History Project, September 29, 2004.

60. E-mail from Kathleen Irwin to author Beth Meyerson, May 7, 2008.

61. Kathleen Irwin, interview by PHA History Project, May 20, 2004.

62. Kathleen Irwin, interview by PHA History Project, May 20, 2004.

63. Patrick McConnon, interview by PHA History Project, March 31, 2004.

64. Patrick McConnon, interview by PHA History Project, March 31, 2004.

65. Steven Bice, interview by PHA History Project, April 2, 2004.

66. Steven Bice, interview by PHA History Project, April 2, 2004.

67. Steven Bice, interview by PHA History Project, April 2, 2004.

68. Richard Conlon, interview by PHA History Project, May 17, 2004.

69. Anne-Renee Heningburg, interview by PHA History Project, March 29, 2004.

70. Anne-Renee Heningburg, interview by PHA History Project, March 29, 2004.

71. William Foege, interview by PHA History Project, September 23, 2004.

72. William Foege, interview by PHA History Project, September 23, 2004.

73. Jerry Lama, interview by PHA History Project, June 8, 2004.

74. Julie Gerberding, interview by PHA History Project, August 5, 2005.

Chapter 2

1. Allan M. Brandt, *No Magic Bullet: A Social History of Venereal Disease in the United States Since 1880* (New York: Oxford University Press, 1987). See also Raymond A. Vonderlehr and Lida J. Usilton, *"The Extent of the Syphilis Problem at the Beginning of World War II."* New York State Journal of Medicine 43 (October, 1943): 1825. Also found in *American Journal of Syphilis, Gonorrhea and Venereal Diseases*, 27 (November 1943): 686.

2. Brandt, *No Magic Bullet*. See also James H. Jones, *Bad Blood: The Tuskegee Syphilis Experiment* (New York: The Free Press, 1981). See also Fitzhugh Mullan, *Plagues and Politics: The Story of the United States Public Health Service* (New York: Basic Books, 1989), 74

3. Jones, *Bad Blood*, 49.

4. See Brandt, *No Magic Bullet*; also Jones, *Bad Blood*, 50.

5. John Pendleton, interview by PHA History Project, August 14, 2007.

6. See Mullan, *Plagues and Politics*, 86; Thomas Parran, "Why Don't We Stamp Out Syphilis?" *Reader's Digest* (July 1936): 65-74. See also Centers for Disease Control and Prevention "Venereal Disease Administrative Communication from Venereal Disease Branch" [sic.][c. 1968]: 8-9. Source: Kenneth Latimer archives. See also "Venereal Disease Campaign," *Time*, January 11, 1937: 38-39.

7. Thomas Parran (1937), *Shadow on the Land: Syphilis* (Baltimore, MD: Waverly Press, 1937); Parran, "Why Don't We Stamp Out Syphilis?" 65-74; Thomas Parran, "Syphilis: A Public Health Problem," in *Syphilis*, ed. Forest Ray Moulton, (Lancaster, PA: The Science Press, 1938), 187-193.

8. Parran, *Shadow*, 54, 62. See also Raymond A. Vonderlehr, Herman N. Bundesen, Lida J. Usilton, et al., "Recommendations for a Venereal Disease Control Program in State and Local Health Departments." Report of the Advisory Committee to the U.S. Public Health Service. *Venereal Disease Information* 17, no. 1, reprint No. 54. Also found in Journal of the American Medical Association 106 (January 1936): 115-117. Washington, January 1936; Video of an interview with Richard "Dick" Bowman, 2002. Interview conducted by Robert Emerson. Source: Robert Emerson archive.

9. Parran, *Shadow*, 60-61. See also Parran, "Syphilis: A Public Health Problem," 87-193; Lida J. Usilton, "Mortality Trends for Syphilis," *Journal of Venereal Disease Information*, 27 (February, 1946): 47-52.

10. Dick Bowman, former financial officer of the VD Division in the 1940s.

Source: Video of an interview with Richard "Dick" Bowman, 2002. Interview conducted by Robert Emerson. Source: Robert Emerson archive.

11. Mullan, *Plagues and Politics*, 107; Brandt, *No Magic Bullet,* 143.

12. Jones, *Bad Blood*. See also Evan W. Thomas, *Syphilis: Its Course and Management* (New York: Macmillan 1949).

13. John Pendleton, interview by PHA History Project, August 14, 2007.

14. Mullan, *Plagues and Politics*, 90, 122. By World War II, the Commissioned Corps expanded to include nurses, scientists, dieticians, physical therapists, and sanitarians. These professionals were precursors to the Public Health Advisors. Like the PHAs, these men and women were assigned to local areas and expected to be deployable to other areas if need be. Sanitarians were the first non-medical professionals commissioned by the PHS through the Parker Act of 1930. See also Jones, *Bad Blood*; John Pendleton, interview by PHA History Project, August 14, 2007; and William Watson, interview by PHA History Project, November 17, 2003.

15. Mullan, *Plagues and Politics*, 107; Jones, *Bad Blood*; Thomas, *Syphilis*; See also John Pendleton, interview by PHA History Project, August 14, 2007; William Watson, interview by PHA History Project, November 17, 2003; Walter Hughes, interview by PHA History Project, May 9, 2007.

16. Brandt, *No Magic Bullet*, 143; Video of an interview with Richard "Dick" Bowman, 2002. Interview conducted by Robert Emerson. Source: Robert Emerson archive. See also Jones, *Bad Blood*; John C. Cutler and R. C. Arnold, "Venereal Disease Control by Health Departments in the Past: Lessons for the Present" *American Journal of Public Health* 78, no. 4 (1988): 372-376.

17. William Parra, interview by PHA History Project, June 28, 2007. See also Thomas R. Eng and William T. Butler, eds. *The Hidden Epidemic: Confronting Sexually Transmitted Diseases* (Washington, DC: National Academy Press, 1997).

18. Video of an interview with Richard "Dick" Bowman, 2002. Interview conducted by Robert Emerson. Source: Robert Emerson archive.

19. U.S. Public Health Service Reorganization Order No. 1, December 30, 1943, implementing Public Health Service Act (57 Stat. 587), November 11, 1943. See 90.8.

20. William Watson, interview by PHA History Project, April 13, 2007.

21. William Watson, interview by PHA History Project, November 17, 2003.

22. Lida J. Usilton curriculum vitae, Source: John Pendleton archives. See also Lida J. Usilton, "A Mechanical System for Record Keeping of Morbidity, Treatment Progress, and Control of Venereal Disease Information," *American Journal of Public Health* 30 (August 1940): 928.

23. Video of an interview with Richard "Dick" Bowman, 2002. Interview conducted by Robert Emerson. Source: Robert Emerson archive; telephone conversation with William Watson, April 24, 2008.

24. John Pendleton, interview by PHA History Project, August 14, 2007.

25. Walter Hughes, interview by PHA History Project, May 9, 2007.

26. Lida J. Usilton curriculum vitae. Source: John Pendleton archives. American Social Hygiene William Snow Award Brochure, 1954. Source: John Pendleton archives.

27. Elizabeth W. Etheridge, *Sentinel for Health: A History of the Centers for Disease Control* (Berkeley: University of California Press,1992), 20.

28. John Pendleton, interview by PHA History Project, August 14, 2007.

29. John Pendleton, interview by PHA History Project, August 14, 2007.

30. "Woman, Pioneer in VD Control, Wins Hygiene Association Award," *New York Times*, April 27, 1954.

31. Lida J. Usilton (1954) acceptance speech for Snow Award presented by the American Social Hygiene Association in April 1954. Source: John Pendleton archives.

32. William Hamlin, interview by PHA History Project, November 18, 2003.

33. John Pendleton, interview by PHA History Project, August 14, 2007.

34. Video of an interview with Richard "Dick" Bowman, 2002. Interview conducted by Robert Emerson. Source: Robert Emerson archive.

35. Kenneth Latimer. Excerpts from unpublished and untitled story written by Kenneth Latimer and submitted to author Beth Meyerson in 2004.

36. Kenneth Latimer, interview by PHA History Project, September 3, 2004.

37. *The Early Years of the Public Health Advisor,* VHS, (Atlanta, GA: Centers for Disease Control and Prevention, 1994). Joseph Giordano quoted. Source: Watsonian Society Archives.

38. John Pendleton, interview by PHA History Project, August 14, 2007.

39. William Watson, interview by PHA History Project, July 12, 2007.

40. E-mail communication from Frederick "Stu" Kingma, nephew of Johannes Stuart. E-mail to author Fred Martich dated June 26, 2007.

41. E-mail communication from Frederick "Stu" Kingma, nephew of Johannes Stuart. E-mail to author Fred Martich dated June 26, 2007. Video of an interview with Richard "Dick" Bowman, 2002. Interview conducted by Robert Emerson. Source: Robert Emerson archive. See also David Sencer, interview by PHA History Project, September 14, 2007; William Watson, interview by PHA History Project, July 12, 2007.

42. William Watson, interview by PHA History Project, July 12, 2007.

43. William Watson, interview by PHA History Project, July 12, 2007 and July 13, 2007. David Sencer, interview by PHA History Project, March 31, 2004 and September 14, 2007.

44. William Watson, interview by PHA History Project, July 12, 2007.

45. William Watson, interview by PHA History Project July 12, 2007.

46. David Sencer, interview by PHA History Project, March 31, 2004

47. William Watson, interview by PHA History Project, July 12, 2007 and July 13, 2007. David Sencer, interview by PHA History Project, July 12, 2007.

48. David Sencer, interview by PHA History Project, September 14, 2007.

49. Dick Bowman, interview by PHA History Project, July 22, 2007; David Sencer, interview by PHA History Project, September 14, 2007 and E-mail communication between David Sencer and author Beth Meyerson September 2007.

50. David Sencer, interview by PHA History Project interview, September 14, 2007.

51. Harold Mauldin conversation with author Fred Martich 2007; William Watson, interview by PHA History Project, July 12 and 13, 2007. Kenneth Latimer, interview by PHA History Project, September 3, 2004.

52. Charles Joseph Webb, interview by PHA History Project, February 9-10, 2004. E-mail communication from William Watson to authors Meyerson, Martich, and Naehr, April 13, 2007.

53. William Watson E-mail to author Beth Meyerson, April 13, 2007. See also Mullan, *Plagues and Politics*, for discussion of non-physician commission corpsmen and women.

54. William Watson, interview by PHA History Project, July 12 and 13, 2007.

55. Telephone conversation between Kenneth Latimer and author Fred Martich, April 26, 2007.

56. Charles Joseph Webb, interview by PHA History Project, February 9-10, 2004.

57. Harold Mauldin, interview by PHA History Project, May 19, 2004.

58. Harold Mauldin, interview by PHA History Project, May 19, 2004; Kenneth Latimer, interview by PHA History Project, September 3, 2004; E-mail communication from Kenneth Latimer to authors Fred Martich and Beth Meyerson in 2007.

59. Harold Mauldin conversation with author Fred Martich, August 15, 2007.

60. William Watson, interview by PHA History Project, July 12, 2007.

61. Jones, *Bad Blood*; Brandt, *No Magic Bullet*; Video of an interview with Richard "Dick" Bowman, 2002. Interview conducted by Robert Emerson.

Source: Robert Emerson archive.

62. Video of an interview with Richard "Dick" Bowman, 2002. Interview conducted by Robert Emerson. Source: Robert Emerson archive. See also Parran, Shadow; Norman R. Ingraham, "Syphilis Epidemiology Applied: Fifteen Years' Experience with Contact-Tracing and Case-Holding in New Jersey," *Journal of Venereal Disease Information* 19 (March, 1938). Reprint no. 83.

63. Video of an interview with Richard "Dick" Bowman, 2002. Interview conducted by Robert Emerson. Source: Robert Emerson archive. See also U. J. Wile, "Syphilis Control: General Considerations," in Forest Ray Moulton, ed. *Syphilis*. (Lancaster, PA: The Science Press, 1938), 184-186.

64. Parran, "Syphilis: A Public Health Problem," 187-193.

65. See Brandt, *No Magic Bullet*, and also Mullan, *Plagues and Politics*.

66. Brandt, *No Magic Bullet*,124, 132.

67. Video of an interview with Richard "Dick" Bowman, 2002. Interview conducted by Robert Emerson. Source: Robert Emerson archive. See also S. J. Axelrod, "The Five-Day Treatment for Syphilis," *American Journal of Nursing* 41 (Sept., 1941): 1039-1044.

68. Donna Pearce, "Rapid Treatment Centers for Venereal Disease Control," *American Journal of Nursing* 43, no. 7(1943): 658-660. See also Title II of the Lanham Act of 1941 (55 Stat. 361; U.S. Code 42 (1941) § 1523). Quote from the United States Government Manual of 1945, 1st ed. (Washington: Federal Works Agency, 1945), 468. http://www.ibiblio.org/hyperwar/ATO/USGM/A.html (accessed March 27, 2008); William Watson, interview by PHA History Project, July 12, 2007.

69. Donna Pearce, "Rapid Treatment Centers," 658-660. Pearce quotes Surgeon General Thomas Parran regarding the hope that Rapid Treatment Centers would demonstrate treatment efficacy to the medical community. The source of the quote was not cited in this article.

70. Donna Pearce, "Rapid Treatment Centers," 658. See also Thomas, *Syphilis*, 1949:290.

71. Harold Mauldin, interview by PHA History Project, May 19, 2004.

72. Donna Pearce, "Rapid Treatment Centers," in *Syphilis Symptoms and Treatment Facilities* (Arkansas State Board of Health, circa 1940s). Source: Monte Meador archive, and "Ground Zero 1941: A Jacksonville Experiment," *Jacksonville Medicine: 1853 to 2003:* Sesquicentennial Issue, 24-25. http://www.dcmsonline.org/jax-medicine/2004journals/historical/150-24-25-1946syphillis.pdf. (accessed September 8, 2007); Kenneth Latimer,. Excerpts from unpublished and untitled story written by

Kenneth Latimer and submitted to author Beth Meyerson in 2004.

73. Centers for Disease Control and Prevention, *The Early Years*.

74. "Ground Zero 1941: A Jacksonville Experiment," 24-25.

75. William Watson, interview by PHA History Project, July 13, 2007.

76. Thomas, *Syphilis*, 292ff. See also *VD Case-Finding Manual: For Use in Training Programs* (Raleigh, NC: VD Education Institute, May, 1945), Trial Edition, sec. 4, p. 5. Thomas Parran, *Shadow*, 258; Brandt, *No Magic Bullet*,150; See also C.C. Pierce, "Syphilis and Gonorrhea Control: Principles of Case-Finding and Case-Holding," *Journal of Venereal Disease Information* (February 1941): 43-52.

77. Mullan, *Plagues and Politics*, 72.

78. Brandt, *No Magic Bullet*,138.

79. Brandt, *No Magic Bullet*,151; Thomas, *Syphilis*.

80. The physicians' role in VD control and the need for their support of case finding and reporting of cases often was discussed in the literature of the 1940s. See Parran, *Shadow*; Thomas, *Syphilis*; Brandt, *No Magic Bullet*,. See also William G. Hollister, "Self Interview Forms in Private Physician Contact Reporting—a New Technic [sic.] in Case Finding: A Preliminary Report," *Journal of Venereal Disease Information* 27 (October 1946). Reprint 272.

81. R. F. Sondag and A. J. Sweeney, "Syphilis Morbidity Reporting by Private Physicians in the State of Florida," *Journal of Venereal Disease Information* (December 1947): 276; Brandt, No Magic Bullet.

82. Anne Sweeney, "Studies in the Epidemiology of Syphilis: Methods of Contact Investigation," *Journal of Venereal Disease Information* 23 (April 1942): 137-143. Reprint 177.

83. Ingraham, "Syphilis Epidemiology." See also William G. Hollister, "Self Interview Forms."

84. Parran, "Why Don't We Stamp Out Syphilis?," 65-73. Also Ingraham, "Syphilis Epidemiology."

85. Howard P. Steiger and Barbara Jane Taylor, "Venereal Disease Interviewing," *Journal of Venereal Disease Information* 28 no. 4 (April 1947): 55-60. Reprint 279.

86. A. J. Casselman and Anabel Cadwallader, "Venereal Disease Contact-Tracing in Camden, New Jersey," *Journal of Venereal Disease Information* (July 1939). See also Brandt, *No Magic Bullet*, and Thomas, *Syphilis*.

87. Ingraham, "Syphilis Epidemiology"; Casselman and Cadwallader, "Venereal Disease Contact Tracing"; Henry Packer, "A Comparison of Case-Finding Methods in a Syphilis Control Program," *Journal of Venereal Disease Information* (December

1942). Bundesen, et al., "Recommendations"; Steiger and Taylor, "Venereal Disease Interviewing." See also Brandt, *No Magic Bullet*, 15, and "Persuasive Methods in the Control of Syphilis," *Science*, Supplement 84 (December 18, 1936).

88. Ingraham, "Syphilis Epidemiology"; Casselman and Cadwallader, "Venereal Disease Contact Tracing."

89. Bundesen, et al., "Recommendations."

90. Theodore Rosenthal and George Kerchner, "Experiences with Registered Letter Follow-Up in the New York City Health Department," *Journal of VD Information* 27 (October 1946). Reprint 272.

91. Packer, "A Comparison."

92. Casselman and Cadwallader, "Venereal Disease Contact Tracing."

93. Casselman and Cadwallader, "Venereal Disease Contact Tracing."; Sweeney, "Studies in the Epidemiology of Syphilis." See also William Hamlin, interview by PHA History Project, November 18, 2003; Jack Wroten, interview by PHA History Project, September 23, 2004; Larry Posey, interview by PHA History Project, March 31, 2004; Edith M. Baker, "Scope of Activities of the Follow-Up Worker," *Journal of Venereal Disease Information* (June 1938).

94. Emerson L. Crowley and C. B. Tucker, "The Cost of Venereal Disease Contact Investigation in Tennessee," *Journal of Venereal Disease Information* (May 1947): 81-82.

95. Crowley and Tucker, "The Cost of Venereal Disease."

96. Lena R.Waters and Louise Brown Ingraham. "The Organization and Function of Follow-Up Service in Venereal Disease Clinics." *Journal of Venereal Disease Information* (July 1938): 220-226.

97. Edgar J. Easley, George E. Parkhurst, Robert R. Swank, "The 100-Day Experiment in Contact Investigation in Arkansas," *Journal of Venereal Disease Information* 29, no. 1 (January 1948):13-19. Reprint 303.

98. William Watson, interview by PHA History Project, November 17, 2003.

99. William Watson, interview by PHA History Project, November 17, 2003. William Hamlin, interview by PHA History Project, November 18, 2003.

100. Walter Hughes, interview by PHA History Project, May 9, 2007.

101. Video of an interview with Richard "Dick" Bowman, 2002. Interview conducted by Robert Emerson. Source: Robert Emerson archive.

102. S. Ross Taggart, Stanley B. Russel, Eleanor V. Price, "Report of Syphilis Follow-Up Program Among Veterans After World War II," *Journal of Chronic Disease* 4, no. 6 (December 1956): 579-587.

103. Video of an interview with Richard "Dick" Bowman, 2002. Interview conducted by Robert Emerson. Source: Robert Emerson archive.

104. Rosenthal and Kerchner, "Experiences with Registered Letter Follow-Up"; Richard A. Koch, Marian Thornton, "Use of Telegrams in Venereal Disease Case Holding," *Journal of Venereal Disease Information* 27 (October 1946). Herman J. Bundesen, Theodore J. Bauer, Amelia H. Baker, "Evaluative Study of Three Types of Epidemiology Activity on 360 Syphilis Contacts." *Journal of Venereal Disease Information* 27 (October 1946).

Chapter 3

1. *Public Health Advisor: Four Decades and the Future*, (VHS), (Atlanta, Georgia: Centers for Disease Control and Prevention, 1994). From the Watsonian Society Archives. William Watson quoted.

2. See M. J. White, "Steps in the Field of Venereal Disease Control from the Standpoint of the United States Public Health Service," *Journal of Venereal Disease Information* 7, no. 6 (June, 1926):171–177.

3. See Thomas Parran, "Syphilis: A Public Health Problem," in *Syphilis*, ed. Forest Ray Moulton (Lancaster, PA: The Science Press, 1938),187–193. See the notation about a 1936 PHS special advisory committee of local and state health officials and syphilologists that recommended (among other things) that each state and city should have a trained public health staff to deal with syphilis. See also Edgar J. Easley, George E. Parkhurst, Robert R. Swank, "The 100-Day Experiment in Contact Investigation in Arkansas." *Journal of Venereal Disease Information* 29, no. 1 (January 1948):13–19. Reprint 303.

4. Elizabeth W. Etheridge, *Sentinel For Health: A History of the Centers for Disease Control* (Berkeley: University of California Press,1992), 90, quoting Mountin from a Thomas Parran article, "A Career in Public Health," *Public Health Reports* 67 (October 1952):937.

5. John Pendleton, interview by PHA History Project, August 14, 2007.

6. William Hamlin, interview by PHA History Project, November 18, 2003. John Pendleton, interview by PHA History Project, August 14, 2007. Walter Hughes, interview by PHA History Project, May 9, 2007. William Watson, interview by PHA History Project, November 17, 2003.

7. William Watson, interview by PHA History Project, July 13, 2007.

8. William Watson, interview by PHA History Project, November 17, 2003 and

April 13, 2007. See also "Celebrating 50 Years: Public Health Advisor," *History of the Public Health Advisor* (Atlanta, GA: Centers for Disease Control and Prevention, 1998), 1. See also Etheridge, Sentinel.

9. William Watson, interview by PHA History Project, November 17, 2003.

10. William Watson, interview by PHA History Project, April 13, 2007.

11. The practice of excepted appointments was not created with the Public Health Advisor. Such appointments were just becoming part of federal practice by the late 1940s. Excepted appointment means literally that the position is excepted from regular General Schedule salaries and from standard federal competitive procedures (such as the federal entrance exam). See Federal Personnel Manual, Schedule A.6.114(b)(4); Classification ACT of 1949, as amended – Sec. 202 (14). See also Perry, James E. "Federal Recruiting Under Specialized Excepted Authority." Paper submitted to the Centers for Disease Control and Prevention, March 1970. Obtained by author Fred Martich.

12. Emerson L Crowley and C. B. Tucker, "The Cost of Venereal Disease Contact Investigation in Tennessee," *Journal of Venereal Disease Information* (May 1947):81–82.

13. Don Lederman, interview by PHA History Project, December 20, 2007.

14. William Watson, interview by PHA History Project, April 13, 2007.

15. *The Early Years of the Public Health Advisor* (VHS), (Atlanta, GA: Centers for Disease Control and Prevention, 1994). From the *Watsonian Society Archives*; Video of an interview with Richard "Dick" Bowman, 2002. Interview conducted by Robert Emerson. Source: Robert Emerson archive.

16. William Watson, interview by PHA History Project, November 17, 2003.

17. William Watson, interview by PHA History Project, November 17, 2003.

18. The original list of PHAs was compiled from interviews with members of this group as well as one CDC publication: William Watson, interview by PHA History Project, July 12, 2007; William Hamlin, interview by PHA History Project, November 18, 2003; Don Lederman, interview by PHA History Project, December 20, 2007; e-mail from Patricia Keitchen, daughter of William Hamlin, to author Fred Martich, January 14, 2008; "Notice," Watsonian Society Advisor (Winter 1995), 4. The authors recommend continued research regarding those hired in this initial period. There are no extant PHS personnel records, and CDC records are incomplete because the early co-ops were hired in the VD Division, which, at the time, resided in the Public Health Service (see Chapter 5 regarding the VD Division's move to CDC in 1957). A question remains as to whether the members of the original group on Maryland's Eastern

Shore were in fact the only co-ops working for the VD Division at the time. Others may have been hired by Johannes Stuart or Lida Usilton at the same time and trained elsewhere.

19. William Watson, interview by PHA History Project, November 17, 2003 and July 12, 2007.

20. Ibid.

21. William Hamlin, interview by PHA History Project, November 18, 2003.

22. "Notice," 4.

23. William Watson, interview by PHA History Project, April 13, 2007. See also William Hamlin, interview by PHA History Project, November 18, 2003; E-mail from Patricia Keitchen, daughter of William Hamlin to author Fred Martich reporting Bill's recollection of the original PHAs. E-mail dated January 14, 2008; William Watson, interview by PHA History Project, January 24, 2008.

24. William Hamlin, interview by PHA History; November 18, 2003.

25. Ibid. See also William Watson, interview by PHA History Project, November 17, 2003 and conversation with author Beth Meyerson on September 21, 2007. See Chapter 2 for a discussion of the 100-Day Experiment.

26. For a memorial article on Robert Swank, see CDC, "In Memoriam," *Contact* (February 21, 1966), 1. Contact was a CDC internal newsletter. See also Robert R. Swank, Venereal Disease Contact Interviewing (manual). February 5, 1951. Archives of Ken Latimer.

27. "In Memoriam," 1.

28. William Hamlin, interview by PHA History Project, November 18, 2003.

29. See Brandt, *No Magic Bullet*; Fitzhugh Mullan, *Plagues and Politics: The Early Years of the PHA* (New York: Basic Books, 1989).

30vWilliam Watson, interview by PHA History Project, November 17, 2003.

31. Ibid.

32. William Hamlin, interview by PHA History Project, November 18, 2003.

33. William Watson, interview by PHA History Project, November 17, 2003.

34. Ibid.; see also William Hamlin, interview by PHA History Project, November 18, 2003.

35. A. P. Iskrant, Q. R. Remein, J. F. Donohue, "Evaluation of Antisyphilitic Therapy with Intensive Follow-Up. III. Statistical Method of Analysis and its Critical Evaluation," *Journal of Venereal Disease Information* 32, no. 12, (December, 1951):371–375; T. J. Bauer, "Evaluation of Antisyphilitic Therapy with Intensive Follow-Up. I: The Plan," *Journal of Venereal Disease Informationn* 32, no. 12 (Decem-

ber, 1951):355–359. See also J. Q. Blackwood, V. Scott, E. G. Clark, "Treatment of Early Syphilis with Sodium Penicillin: A Preliminary Report with a Comparison of Results with 4,800,000 Units Administered in 7 ½ days with Smaller Dosages," *Archives of Dermatology and Syphilology* 57, no. 6 (June 1948):1028–1041. T. J. Bauer, E. V. Price. "Results of Therapy by Race, Sex and Stage of Syphilis," *Journal of Venereal Disease Information*, 30, no. 1. (January 1949):1–7; F. G. Pegg, "Penicillin in the Treatment of Syphilis," *North Carolina Medical Journal* 10, no. 2 (February 1949):82–84; Thomas, *Syphilis*.

36. William Watson, interview by PHA History Project, September 21, 2007.

37. William Hamlin, interview by PHA History Project, November 18, 2003; Don Lederman, interview by PHA History Project, December 20, 2007; William Watson, interview by PHA History Project, November 17, 2003.

38. A. P. Iskrant and H. A. Kahn, "Statistical Indices Used in the Evaluation of Syphilis Contact Investigation," *Journal of Venereal Disease Information* 29, no. 1 (1948):1–6. See also J.S. Stuart, "Venereal Disease Contact Investigation," *Journal of Venereal Disease Information* (September 1951):242–246.

39. Don Lederman, interview by PHA History Project, December 20, 2007; *The Early Years of the PHA*. Watsonian Society Archives. William Watson quoted. William Watson, interview by PHA History Project, November 17, 2003 and interviews on April 13, July 12, and July 13, 2007.

40. *The Early Years of the PHA*. William Watson quoted. William Watson, interview by PHA History Project, July 12, 2007.

41. Stuart, JS (1951). Venereal Disease Contact Investigation. *Journal of Venereal Disease Information* (September):242–246.

42. *The Early Years of the PHA*. William Watson quoted. See also Don Lederman, interview by PHA History Project, December 20, 2007.

43. William Hamlin, interview by PHA History Project, November 18, 2003.

44. William Watson, interview by PHA History Project, November 17, 2003, and September 21, 2007.

45. William C. Watson, *First Class Privates*. (Atlanta, GA: William Watson, 1994). See also William Watson, interview by PHA History Project, November 17, 2003.

46. William Watson, interview by PHA History Project, November 17, 2003. See also Watson, First Class Privates.

47. William Hamlin, interview by PHA History Project, November 18, 2003.

48. Walter Hughes, interview by PHA History Project, May 9, 2007.

49. Delwin Hammons, interview by PHA History Project, October 6, 2004.

50. Delwin Hammons, interview by PHA History Project, October 6, 2004.

51. Early personnel records dating back to the days of the Public Health Service VD Program are not available. See: CDC document "Celebrating 50 Years: Public Health Advisor" (1998). Extant information in the CDC document was updated using interviews among the initial PHAs: Watson, Lederman, Hamlin, Hughes, and Pendleton. See: CDC document "Celebrating 50 Years: Public Health Advisor" (1998).

52. William Watson, interview by PHA History Project, April 13, 2007. See also *Public Health Advisor: Four Decades and the Future*.

53. Video of an interview with Richard "Dick" Bowman, 2002. Interview conducted by Robert Emerson. Source: Robert Emerson archive.

54. *The Early Years of the PHA*. Jack Benson quoted.

55. Etheridge, *Sentinel*, 58–59. See also Mullan, *Plagues and Politics*.

56. *Public Health Advisor: Four Decades and the Future*. Joseph Giordano quoted.

57. Video of an interview with Richard "Dick" Bowman, 2002. Interview conducted by Robert Emerson. Source: Robert Emerson archive. According to Dick Bowman, the early classification was specifically Public Health Advisor. Extant PHS documents date back to 1963 and cite a previous iteration (probably the original) of the classification. The 1963 source document is: United States Civil Service, United States Civil Service Commission, Bureau of Programs and Standards, Standards Division (October 1963). Position Classification Standard for the GS-685 Series. The cover of the document explains that "[a]s a result of an occupational study, the Public Health Administration Series, GS-685-0 has been redefined, with modified coverage, and retitled as Public Health Program Specialist Series, GS-685-0, and a new standard issued." This document was sent from the Office of Personnel Management of the Strategic Human Resources Policy, Center for Talent and Capacity Policy in Washington, DC, to author Beth Meyerson on January 10, 2008. The original series and classification standard was issued under the authority of Title IV of the Classification Act of 1949. The 1963 classification document is the earliest extant document related to the GS-685 series. See also Etheridge, *Sentinel*, for a brief discussion of the series development.

58. Video of an interview with Richard "Dick" Bowman, 2002. Interview conducted by Robert Emerson. Source: Robert Emerson archive.

59. The Department of Health Education and Welfare was the sponsor for the classification, and this ultimately indicates that the earliest date for the series creation is 1953 (when HEW was formed). The latest date would be 1956, based on interviews

with Public Health Advisors and extant video files. Richard "Dick" Bowman is the only living person who was involved in this process, but he does not recall the precise year of creation. He does indicate that it was early in the experiment. Video of an interview with Richard "Dick" Bowman, 2002. Interview conducted by Robert Emerson. Source: Robert Emerson archive; Richard "Dick" Bowman, interview by PHA History Project, July 22, 2007; *Public Health Advisor: Four Decades and the Future*. Joseph Giordano quoted. Kenneth Latimer, interview by PHA History Project, September 3, 2004.

60. CDC, "Change in Retirement Credit for Cooperative Employees," *Contact* (January 17, 1964), 4. See also Perry, "Recruiting Under Specialized Excepted Authority;" Federal Civil Service Retirement System – See Subchapter III, Chapter 83, Title 5, United States Code.

61. Video of an interview with Richard "Dick" Bowman, 2002. Interview conducted by Robert Emerson. Source: Robert Emerson archive.

62. Raymond Bly, interview by PHA History Project, May 28 and August 17, 2004.

Chapter 4

1. J. S. Stuart, "Venereal Disease Contact Investigation," *Journal of Venereal Disease Information* (September, 1951):242–246. See also Raymond Bly, interview by PHA History Project, May 28, 2004; A. L. Gray, T. J. Bauer, L. J. Usilton, R. O. Carlson (1951), "Case Finding Through an Understanding of Known Syphilitic Patients," *Journal of Venereal Disease Information* 32, no. 6 (1951):144–149; W. L. Warner, M. C. Hill, C. D. Bowdoin, J. W. Rion, B. McCall (1951), "Syphilis Prevalence and Community Structure," *Journal of Venereal Disease Information* 32, no. 6 (1951):157–166.

2. Jack Wroten, interview by PHA History Project, September 23, 2004.

3. Ken Latimer, interview by PHA History Project, September 30, 2004. See also e-mail correspondence from Jack Wroten to author Beth Meyerson on January 17, 2008.

4. See also Chapter 5 for a discussion of the racial, ethnic and gender diversification of the PHA cohort. Personnel records from the Public Health Service are not available (or perhaps lost), and CDC personnel files do not predate the VD Division move to Atlanta in 1957. The data are from interviews among PHAs at the time: Bill Doyle, interview by PHA History Project, April 27, 2007; William Watson, interview

by PHA History Project, July 12, 2007; Franklin Miller, interview by PHA History Project, December 17, 2003; E-mail from Kenneth Latimer to author Fred Martich on April 26, 2007. See also telephone conversation between author Fred Martich and John Gallagher August 12, 2007; telephone conversation between author Fred Martich and Harold Mauldin August 13, 2007; Personal conversation between Bill Doyle and author Fred Martich, April 26, 2007.

5. E-mail from Robert Baldwin to Fred Martich, June 4, 2007. According to this e-mail, Bob hired Penny prior to 1971, but she could not begin federal service until the federal hiring freeze was lifted in 1971. It is important to note that a Sally Roy was identified by several interview participants as an early PHA. Sally was in fact a statistician who was transferred to the GS-685 series and served as the city representative (city rep) for the New Orleans VD program in the early 1950s. Like the "New Dealers" who served in the VD program, Sally was not a co-op, and did not hire in at field level. Bill Watson also recalled a 1955 experiment of Johannes Stuart to hire six women as co-ops in Chicago. According to Bill, these women did not last a year in the program. See William Watson, interview by PHA History Project, July 13, 2007. Unfortunately, this could not be corroborated by others who were working in and around Chicago at the time. Given the lack of PHS hiring data from the 1950s, we cannot verify these and other early hires.

6. See Jack Wroten, interview by PHA History Project, September 23, 2004, Harold Mauldin, interview by PHA History Project, April 14, 2007. Don Lederman, interview by PHA History Project, December 20, 2007. See also H. Shortal, "The Nurse as a Case Finder in Venereal Disease," *Journal of Venereal Disease Information* (November 1946):270–272.

7. Emerson, Robert (circa 2003). Untitled written submission to the PHA History Project received 11, 24, 2003.

8. Raymond Bly, interview by PHA History Project, May 28, 2004. See also Windell Bradford, interview by PHA History Project, October 27, 2004; John Miles, interview by PHA History Project, January 15, 2004; Jack Wroten, interview by PHA History Project, September 23, 2004.

9. Jim Fowler, interview by PHA History Project, July 16, 2007.

10. John Shimmens, interview by PHA History Project, August 17, 2004.

11. See Jack Benson, interview by PHA History Project, November 18, 2003; Jack Wroten, interview by PHA History Project, September 23, 2004.

12. Elizabeth W. Etheridge, *Sentinel for Health: A History of the Centers for Disease Control*, (Berkeley: University of California Press, 1992), 91. See also William

Watson, interview by PHA History Project, November 17, 2003, William Hamlin, interview by PHA History Project, November 18, 2003, Donald Lederman, interview by PHA History Project, December 20, 2007, Delwin Hammons, interview by PHA History Project,, October 6, 2004, and Walter Hughes, interview by PHA History, May 9, 2007.

13. Jack Benson, interview by PHA History Project, November 18, 2003.

14. *The Early Years of the Public Health Advisor* (VHS). (Atlanta, GA: Centers for Disease Control and Prevention, 1994). Pete Campassi quoted.

15. J. R. Heller, L. J. Usilton, A. B. Clark, "A Plan for Revitalizing National Venereal Disease Control," *Journal of Venereal Disease Information* (February 1946):29–33; T. J. Bauer, A. P. Iskrant, "Epidemiology of Syphilis," *American Journal of Medicine* 6, no. 3 (1949):341–344; T. J. Bauer, "Venereal Disease Program in Transition," *Public Health Reports* 67, no. 1 (1952):17–20; T. J. Bauer. "The VD Hunt is Still On," *Journal of Social Hygiene* 38, no. 7 (1952):290–296; T. J. Bauer, "Public Health Problems in Syphilis Control," *Journal of the American Medical Association* 152, no. 4 (1953):300–303; J. K. Shafer, "The Scope of Public Health in Venereal Disease Control," *Medicine Illustrated* 8, no. 10 (1954):670–673; J. F. Donohue, G. A. Gleeson, K. H. Jenkins, E. V. Price, "Venereal Disease among Teen-Agers: Its Relationship to Juvenile Delinquency," *Public Health Reports* 70, no. 5 (1955):453–461.

16. G. Goodwin, "Mass Disease Hunt to Start in Atlanta," *Atlanta Journal*, May 11, 1950 Latimer archive. See also Dick Bowman video.

17. *The Early Years of the Public Health Advisor*, William Watson quoted.

18. J. Stuart, W. T. Davis, J. J. Jolly, "Location of Testing Stations in a Mass Survey," *American Journal of Syphilis, Gonorrhea and Venereal Diseases*, St. Louis 36, no. 6 (1952):571–578.

19. William Hamlin, interview by PHA History Project, November 18, 2003.

20. Kenneth Latimer to author Beth Meyerson dated February 2, 2008.

21. Kenneth Latimer (1994). Excerpts from unpublished and untitled story written by Kenneth Latimer and submitted to author Beth Meyerson in 2004. See also PHA History Project interview with Kenneth Latimer, September 30, 2004.

22. Kenneth Latimer, interview by PHA History Project, September 30, 2004.

23. Kenneth Latimer, interview by PHA History Project, September 30, 2004; Kenneth Latimer (1994). Excerpts from unpublished and untitled story written by Kenneth Latimer and submitted to author Beth Meyerson in 2004. See also Harold Mauldin, interview by PHA History Project, May 19, 2004; J. S. Moorhead, G. S. Usher, J. F. O'Brien, D. G. O'Brien, H. N. Bossak, K. H. Jenkins, "Blood Testing for

Syphilis in an Island Population," *American Journal of Syphilis, Gonorrhea, and Venereal Diseases* 37, no. 1 (1953):46–59; E. Quintero, "Variations in Syphilis Prevalence as Indicated in the Puerto Rico Case Finding Activities," *Boletin de la Associacion Medica de Puerto Rico* 45, no. 6 (1953):198–205; E. Quintero, "The Door to Door Blood Testing Project in Puerto Rico," *Boletin de la Associacion Medica de Puerto Rico* 47, no. 4 (1955):162–165.

24. Correspondence from Harold Mauldin to author Beth Meyerson, May 24, 2008.

25. Kenneth Latimer, interview by PHA History Project, September 30, 2004. See also Kenneth Latimer (1994). Excerpts from unpublished and untitled story written by Kenneth Latimer and submitted to author Beth Meyerson in 2004.

26. Harold Mauldin, interview by PHA History Project, May 19, 2004.

27. Kenneth Latimer (1994). Excerpts from unpublished and untitled story written by Kenneth Latimer and submitted to author Beth Meyerson in 2004; Kenneth Latimer, interview by PHA History Project, September 30, 2004.

28. Kenneth Latimer, interview by PHA History Project, September 30, 2004.

29. A. P. Iskrant, Q. R. Remein, J. F. Donohue, "Evaluation of Antisyphilitic Therapy with Intensive Follow-Up.–III. Statistical Method of Analysis and its Critical Evaluation," *Journal of Venereal Disease Information* 32, no. 12 (December 1951):371–375; T. J. Bauer,. "Evaluation of Antisyphilitic Therapy with Intensive Follow-Up.–I: The Plan," *Journal of Venereal Disease Information* 32, no. 12 (1951):355–359. See also J. Q. Blackwood, V. Scott, E. G. Clark,. "Treatment of Early Syphilis with Sodium Penicillin: A Preliminary Report with a Comparison of Results with 4,800,000 Units Administered in 7 ½ Days with Smaller Dosages," *Archives of Dermatology and Syphilology* 57, no. 6 (June 1948):1028–1041. T. J. Bauer, E. V. Price, "Results of Therapy by Race, Sex and Stage of Syphilis," *Journal of Venereal Disease Information* 30, no. 1 (January, 1949):1–7; F. G. Pegg), "Penicillin in the Treatment of Syphilis," *North Carolina Medical Journal* 10, no. 2 (February 1949):82–84; Evan W. Thomas, *Syphilis: Its Course and Management*, (New York: Macmillan, 1949).

30. T. J. Bauer, "Evaluation of antisyphilitic therapy with intensive follow-up, I. The Plan" *Journal of Venereal Disease Information* 32 (1951):355–59. T. J. Bauer, J. F. Donohue, V. Larsen, A. P. Iskrant, Q. R. Remein, "Do Persons Lost to Long Term Observation Have the Same Experience as Persons Observed?: Evaluation of Antisyphilitic Therapy," *Journal of the American Statistical Association* 49, no. 265 (1954):36–50. See also Richard "Dick" Bowman, interview by PHA History Project,

July 22, 2007; Centers for Disease Control and Prevention, *The Early Years of the Public Health Advisor*. William Watson quoted.

31. T. J. Bauer, J.F. Donohue, V. Larsen, A. P. Iskrant, Q. R. Remein.

32. Jack Benson, interview by PHA History Project, November 18, 2003.

33. John Pendleton, interview by PHA History Project, August 14, 2007.

34. S. R. Taggart, S. B. Russell, E. V. Price,. "Report of Syphilis Follow-up Program among Veterans after World War II," *Journal of Chronic Diseases* 4, no. 6 (1956):579–588.

35. Kenneth Latimer to author Beth Meyerson dated May 24, 2007.

36. Jack Benson, interview by PHA History Project, November 18, 2003.

37. Kenneth Latimer, interview by PHA History Project, September 30, 2004; see also e-mail from Harold Mauldin dated April 14, 2007.

38. Bill Doyle, interview by PHA History Project, January 8, 2004.

39. Delwin Hammons, interview by PHA History Project, October 6, 2004.

40. H. H. Handsfield, D. Hoel, "Sex, Science, and Society: A Look at Sexually Transmitted Diseases," *Postgraduate Medicine* 101, no. 5 (May 1997):268–73, 277–78. See also Allan M. Brandt, *No Magic Bullet: A Social History of Venereal Disease in the United States Since 1880* (New York: Oxford University Press, 1987); See also. *Public Health Advisor: Four Decades and the Future* (VHS) (Atlanta, GA: Centers for Disease Control and Prevention, 1994).

41. *The Early Years of the Public Health Advisor*. William Watson quoted.

42. Billy Griggs, interview by PHA History Project, April 2, 2004. Bill credits this to Bill Schwartz, but mentioned that it was known as Bill Brown's Law. See also William Watson, interview by PHA History Project, November 17, 2003.

43. William Watson, interview by PHA History Project, July 13, 2007.

44. Jack Benson, interview by PHA History Project, November 18, 2003.

45. Kenneth Latimer, interview by PHA History Project, September 30, 2004.

46. The Early Years of the Public Health Advisor, William Watson quoted.

47. William Watson, interview by PHA History Project, July 13, 2007.

48. *The Early Years of the Public Health Advisor*; Kenneth Latimer, interview by PHA History Project, September 30, 2004

49. *The Early Years of the Public Health Advisor*. Jack Benson quoted.

50. Raymond Bly, interview by PHA History Project, May 28, 2004.

51. Ibid.

52. See Etheridge, *Sentinel*, 160ff., 235ff. for discussion of CDC's challenge with VD and gonorrhea historically.

53. E-mail from Jack Benson to author Beth Meyerson on January 21, 2008, and e-mail from Jack Benson to author Fred Martich on January 22, 2008. See also Billy Griggs, interview by PHA History Project, April 2, 2004.

54. E-mail from Jack Benson to author Fred Martich, January 22, 2008. Jack wrote: "You have to remember that back in the old days some of us were isolated. At the time I wrote about, there were only three or four PHAs on the entire West Coast. I was in San Francisco, one was in Portland, and Bob Lugar was in Los Angeles."

55. E-mail from Jack Benson to author Beth Meyerson on January 21, 2008.

56. Jack Wroten, interview by PHA History Project, September 23, 2004.

57. Billy Griggs, interview by PHA History Project, April 2, 2004; E-mail from Jack Benson to author Beth Meyerson on January 21, 2008.

58. Kenneth Latimer archive of the Houston 1957 outbreak chart; Billy Griggs, interview by PHA History Project, April 2, 2004. Centers for Disease Control and Prevention, "Shreveport Epidemic Continues…," Contact (CDC internal newsletter) (1961): 1.

59. United States under Public Law 45 of 1942. House joint resolution 96); Public Broadcasting Service (PBS). *The Border*, http://www.pbs.org/kpbs/theborder/history/timeline/17.html (accessed January 11, 2008). See also Ronald J. Mize, "Mexican Contract Workers and the U.S. Capitalist Agricultural Labor Process: The Formative Era, 1942-1964," *Rural Sociology* 71, no. 2 (2006):85–108.

60. Mize, "Mexican Contract Workers," 85-108. Several states received Bracero workers: Colorado, Idaho, Illinois, Indiana, Iowa, Kansas, Michigan, Minnesota, Montana, Nebraska, Nevada, New Mexico, North Carolina, North Dakota, Oregon, South Dakota, Utah, Washington, Wisconsin, Wyoming, Arkansas, Georgia, Mississippi, Texas, Ohio, Missouri, Tennessee, and Louisiana (from Mize); Sin Fronteras Organizing Project, http://www.farmworkers.org/bracerop.html (accessed January 11, 2008).

61. National Museum of American History. "Opportunity or Exploitation: The Bracero Program." *America on the Move* (exhibit). http://americanhistory.si.edu/ONTHEMOVE/themes/story_51_5.html (accessed January 11, 2008): See also "527 Braceros Cross to U.S.," The El Paso Times, May 30, 1963: "With the crossing of [527] braceros through the Santa Fe Street Bridge Tuesday night, current contracting of Mexican laborers for work in U.S. farms ended, [an] official of the National Railways of Mexico reported Wednesday. The railroad in charge of transporting the braceros to Juárez from all parts of the state disclosed the total number of workers contracted amounted to 12,127. Of this number, only a few were sent back after fail-

ing to pass their physical examination at the Bracero Center." Online at: http://www.farmworkers.org/bracerop.html (accessed January 11, 2008).

62. Billy Griggs, interview by PHA History Project, April 2, 2004.

63. William Watson, interview by PHA History Project, July 13, 2007.

64. Billy Griggs, interview by PHA History Project, April 2, 2004.

65. Ibid.

66. Ibid.

67. Jack Benson, interview by PHA History Project, November 18, 2003.

68. Ibid.

69. Raymond Bly, interview by PHA History Project, May 28, 2004.

70. Ibid.

71. Thomas Parran, *Shadow on the Land: Syphilis* (Baltimore, MD; Waverly Press, 1937); See also Chapter 2 of this work.

72. Kenneth Latimer, interview by PHA History Project, September 30, 2004.

73. *The Early Years of the Public Health Advisor*, Joe Giordano quoted.

74. Jack Benson, interview by PHA History Project, November 18, 2003. See also Chapter 6 for a continued discussion of darkfield microscopy.

75. Jack Wroten, interview by PHA History Project, September 23, 2004.

76. E-mail from Jack Wroten to author Beth Meyerson on January 17, 2008.

77. Ibid.

78. Robert Kingon, interview by PHA History Project, February 19, 2004.

79. U.S. Department of Health, Education, and Welfare Public Health Service Public Health Service, *Syphilis: Modern Diagnosis and Management*, [Publication No. 743; revised July 1961], (Washington D.C.: U.S. Government Printing Office, 1961).

80. Frank Berry, interview by PHA History Project, June 15, 2004

81. U.S. Department of Health, Education, and Welfare Public Health Service, Bureau of Disease Prevention and Environmental Control, National Communicable Disease Center Venereal Disease Program, *Syphilis: A Synopsis*, [Public Health Service Publication No. 1660], (Washington, D.C.: U.S. Government Printing Office, 1967)

82. Lawrence Posey, interview by PHA History Project, March 31, 2004.

Chapter 5

1. Elizabeth W. Etheridge, *Sentinel for Heath: A History of the Centers for Disease Control*, (Berkeley, University of California Press, 1992), 87 ff. See also tran-

script from a telephone conversation between Kenneth Latimer and author Beth Meyerson on January 21, 2008.

2. During the course of research, we came upon a few stories regarding Lida Usilton's exit from the VD Division. Primary among them was her ouster by the VD Division leadership after the tenure of Surgeon General Thomas Parran. Parran and Lida were close colleagues, collaborating on several projects including the writing of *Shadow on the Land*. Following Parran's departure in 1948, Lida remained with the VD Division until around 1954(?), or perhaps until the VD Division moved to Atlanta. A few of the earliest PHAs suggest that Lida was forced out of her role in the VD Division. According to Don Lederman, "I always admired Lida Usilton and worked closely with her. I was disappointed when she was forced out of the program. They ganged up on her… Dr. Bill Brown transferred from Arkansas to take over the VD Division… She survived a year and then was given the shaft." Source: Don Lederman, interview by PHA History Project, December 20, 2007. Bill Watson recalled that Lida lost her support after Parran left PHS: "Doctors in the PHS were an elite group and did not take kindly to Lida J. Usilton having this much power. She lost her power base when Parran left." William Watson, interview by the PHA History Project, April 24, 2008. Lida's nephew Jack Pendleton recalled that she transferred to the TB Program, though this would have been before David Sencer arrived there (circa 1955), as he does not recall Lida being part of the TB Program. There is some evidence that Lida may have had a short stint with the Indian Health Service. See John Pendleton, interview by PHA History Project, August 14, 2007; David Sencer, interview by PHA History Project, September 14, 2007. Dr. Sencer suggested that Lida left the VD Division when it made the move to Atlanta.

3. Elvin Hilyer, interview by PHA History Project, July 30, 2007 and David Sencer, interviews by PHA History Project, March 31, 2004, and September 14, 2007.

4. Etheridge, *Sentinel*, 87 ff., 119 discussing a 1962 story from PHAs William Darrow and William Watson regarding an African American PHA who had been refused service in a restaurant.

5. William Watson, CDC oral history dated September 25, 1985, as quoted in Etheridge, *Sentinel*, 88.

6. Etheridge, *Sentinel*, 88. See also William Watson, interview by PHA History Project, November 17, 2003.

7. William Watson, CDC oral history dated September 25, 1985, as quoted in Etheridge, *Sentinel*, 88.

8. Etheridge, *Sentinel*, 130. See also Centers for Disease Control and Prevention,

"TB Program Joins CDC: Blomquist Assistant Chief," memorandum (November 1960): 1–2.

9. John Seggerson, interview by PHA History Project, April 15, 2004. John was hired as a TB rep in December 1965.

10. Centers for Disease Control and Prevention, *Contact* newsletters: February 1, 1961, September 7, 1961, and December 1, 1961. Transfers were noted from the VD Division to the Division of Chronic Diseases for field assignments in San Francisco, Denver, Washington, DC, Chicago, and New Jersey; and for the Division of Dental Public Health and Resources in Detroit and New Jersey.

11. Centers for Disease Control and Prevention (1968). VD Administration Communication. February 25, 1968. Archives of Frank Piecuch.

12. E-mail from Jack Benson to author Beth Meyerson, December 11, 2003. See also McKing Consulting Corporation, *Review of the GS-685 Public Health Advisor Series*. Final report, Task 2. CDC Task Order 027. Contract 200-2003-01396 (June 30, 2005). Atlanta, GA.

13. Etheridge, *Sentinel*, 140–141.

14. William Watson, interview by PHA History Project, April 16, 2008. Watson is quoted. See also Jack Benson, interview by PHA History Project, November 18, 2003.

15. William Watson, interview by PHA History Project, November 17, 2003.

16. Jack Benson, interview by PHA History Project, November 18, 2003.

17. Ibid.

18. James Fowler, interview by PHA History Project, July 16, 2007.

19. William Watson, interview by PHA History Project, April 16, 2008.

20. William Watson, interview by PHA History Project, November 17, 2003.

21. Ibid. See also Venereal Disease Branch, CDC, "Watson Leaves VD. Centers for Disease Control and Prevention" *Contact* [CDC newsletter] (February 1, 1961): 1.

22. E-mail from David Sencer to author Beth Meyerson, May 12, 2008.

23. David Sencer, interview by PHA History Project, March 31, 2004. See also William Watson, interview by PHA History, November 17, 2003. See also Etheridge, *Sentinel*, 144.

24. Centers for Disease Control and Prevention, "TB Program Joins CDC: Blomquist Assistant Chief," memorandum (November 1960): 1–2. See also David Sencer, interview by PHA History Project, March 31, 2004.

25. Etheridge, *Sentinel*, 130–131.

26. William Watson, interview by PHA History Project, November 17, 2003.

27. Etheridge, *Sentinel*, 154.

28. See Etheridge, *Sentinel*, for a sense of the organizational cultures of the VD division and the then-Communicable Disease Center. See also William Watson, interview by PHA History Project, November 17, 2003.

29. David Sencer, interview by PHA History Project, March 31, 2004.

30. Gerald Naehr, *CDC Public Health Advisor Field Staff: History, Functions and Current Deployment* (March 11, 1987). Archives of the Watsonian Society.

31. John Shimmens, interview by PHA History Project, August 17, 2004.

32. John Seggerson, interview by PHA History Project, April 15, 2004.

33. R. Reves, D. Blakey, D. E. Snider, L. S. Farer, "Transmission of multiple drug-resistant tuberculosis: report of a school and community outbreak," *American Journal of Epidemiology* 113, no. 4 (1981):423–435. See also John Seggerson, interview by PHA History Project, April 15, 2004, and E-mail from John Seggerson to author Beth Meyerson, May 14, 2008.

34. E-mail from John Seggerson to author Beth Meyerson, May 14, 2008.

35. Ibid.

36. Edward Thompson, interview by PHA History Project, September 16, 2004.

37. Naehr, *CDC Public Health Advisor Field Staff* (March 11, 1987). Archives of the Watsonian Society.

38. Etheridge, Sentinel, 144, 175; Harold Mauldin, interview by PHA History Project, May 19, 2004. See also Jack Benson, interview by PHA History Project, November 18, 2003; letter from Harold Mauldin to author Beth Meyerson received May 28, 2008.

39. Harold Mauldin, interview by PHA History Project, May 19, 2004.

40. Etheridge, *Sentinel*, 144.

41. Etheridge, *Sentinel*, 149.

42. Etheridge, *Sentinel*, 169.

43. Naehr, *CDC Public Health Advisor Field Staff* (March 11, 1987).

44. John Shimmens, interview by PHA History Project, August 17, 2004.

45. Etheridge, *Sentinel*, 176. See also Harold Mauldin, interview by PHA History Project, May 19, 2004.

46. Etheridge, *Sentinel*, 172–174ff.

47. Steven Barid, interview by PHA History Project, March 29, 2004.

48. William Foege, interview by PHA History Project, September 23, 2004.

49. Etheridge, *Sentinel*, 293ff.

50. Tony Scardaci, interview by PHA History Project, June 14, 2004. See also Etheridge, *Sentinel*, 156ff.

51. Tony Scardaci, interview by PHA History Project, June 14, 2004.

52. Naehr, CDC Public Health Advisor Field Staff See also: Archives of the Watsonian Society (document circa 1979), *"TAB A" Staffing Level Trends by Division*.

53. Naehr, *CDC Public Health Advisor Field Staff*

54. Centers for Disease Control and Prevention, Center for Prevention Service, *Field Assignees by Program 1974-June 1984*, (CDC: Atlanta, GA, 1984). Archives of the Watsonian Society.

55. Telephone conversation between author Fred Martich and Barbara Park, Chief of the Program Development Branch, and Pat Mitchell, Deputy Chief of the Program Development Branch, March 25, 2008. According to Barb and Pat, there are three PHAs in the field with Diabetes Control Programs today. Two are in Albuquerque and one is with the Nevada Health Department. All other PHAs were called in from the field in the mid- to late-1990s.

56. Naehr, *CDC Public Health Advisor Field Staff.*

57. Archives of the Watsonian Society *"TAB A" Staffing Level Trends by Division* (c. 1979).

58. William Foege, interview by PHA History Project, September 23, 2004.

59. Windell Bradford, interview by PHA History Project, October 27, 2004.

60. James Curran, interview by PHA History Project, March 30, 2004.

61. Ibid.

62. E-mail from Russell Havlak to author Beth Meyerson, May 6, 2008.

63. Robert Kingon, interview by PHA History, February 19, 2004.

64. Windell Bradford, interview by PHA History Project, October 27, 2004.

65. James Curran, interview by PHA History Project, March 30, 2004.

66. E-mail from Russell Havlak to author Beth Meyerson, April 17, 2008.

67. E-mail from Russell Havlak to author Beth Meyerson, May 6, 2008.

68 Phillip Finley, interview by PHA History Project, January 30, 2004; see also E-mail from Phillip Finley to author Beth Meyerson, May 14, 2008.

69. Robert Kohmescher, interview by PHA History Project, March 4, 2004.

70. E-mail from Fred Martich to author Beth Meyerson on May 6, 2008.

71. James Curran, interview by PHA History Project, March 30, 2004.

72. Telephone conversation between author Fred Martich and Harold Mauldin August 13, 2007; E-mail from Ken Latimer to author Fred Martich on April 26, 2007.

73. Franklin Miller, interview by PHA History Project, December 17, 2003.

74. Personal conversation between Bill Doyle and author Fred Martich, April 26, 2007.

75. Telephone conversation between author Fred Martich and Jack Wroten, August 13, 2007.

76. William Watson, interview by PHA History Project, July 12, 2007. See also E-mail from Kenneth Latimer to author Fred Martich on April 26, 2007; Telephone conversation between author Fred Martich and John Gallagher, August 12, 2007; Telephone conversation between author Fred Martich and Harold Mauldin, August 13, 2007. For information about the Appalachian Regional Program, see http://www.federalgrantswire.com/appalachian-area-development.html (accessed April 3, 2008).

77. Franklin Miller, interview by PHA History Project, December 17, 2003.

78. Ibid.

79. William Watson, interview by PHA History Project, July 12, 2007.

80. E-mail from John Narkunas to Fred Martich June 4, 2007.

81. John Heath, interview by PHA History Project, March 10, 2004.

82. Franklin Miller, interview by PHA History Project, December 17, 2003.

83. Charles Watkins, interview by PHA History Project, March 31, 2004.

84. Ibid.

85. Ibid.

86. William Watson, interview by PHA History Project, July 13, 2007.

87. Ibid.

88. E-mail from John Narkunas to author Fred Martich on June 4, 2007.

89. E-mail from Orlando Blancato to author Fred Martich on June 4, 2007; E-mail from John Narkunas to author Fred Martich, June 4, 2007; E-mail from Roger Bernier to author Fred Martich, June 3, 2007.

90. E-mail from John Narkunas to author Fred Martich on June 4, 2007.

91. E-mail from Norman Scherzer to authors Beth Meyerson, Jerry Naehr and Fred Martich on June 10, 2007.

92. E-mail from Robert J. Baldwin to author Fred Martich, June 3, 2007.

93. Ibid.

94. E-mail from John Heath to author Jerry Naehr on February 27, 2008: "The year was in 1971, there were 13 females in the program."

95. E-mail from Norman Scherzer to the authors on June 10, 2007.

96. Virginia Bales Harris, interview by PHA History Project, July 20, 2007.

97. Ibid.

98. Pam Chin, interview by PHA History Project, May 21, 2004.

99. Centers for Disease Control and Prevention, National Center for Prevention Services, *Review of Recruitment and Placement*. Internal agency document. (1992).

Watsonian Society Archives.

100. Anne-Renee Heningburg, interview by PHA History Project, March 29, 2004.

101. Anne-Renee Heningburg, interview by PHA History Project, March 29, 2004.

102. David Sencer to John Droke, May 2, 1975, re: CDC Comments on the Draft Report on the Review of the CDC Assignment of Personnel to State and Local Governments and the Draft Recommendation Concerning the Future of the Program, 4. Dr. Sencer cites a 1974 "informal but fairly intensive survey" focused on the placement of former assignees. Archives of the Watsonian Society.

Chapter 6

1. Gary West, interview by PHA History Project, June 15, 2004.

2. Centers for Disease Control and Prevention, Division of Sexually Transmitted Diseases. Hiring data provided to author Fred Martich from the Division of Sexually Transmitted Diseases, 2001.

3. National Center for Prevention Services, *Review of Recruitment and Placement*. [Internal agency document.] (Atlanta, GA: Centers for Disease Control and Prevention, National Center for Prevention Services, 1992), Watsonian Archives.

4. Steven Barid, interview by PHA History Project, March 29, 2004.

5. Victor Tomlinson, interview by PHA History Project, August 24, 2004.

6. Tracy Ford, interview by PHA History Project, March 11, 2004.

7. Michael Cassell, interview by PHA History Project, March 10, 2004.

8. See Gerald Naehr, CDC Public Health Advisor Field Staff: History, Functions and Current Deployment, (March 11, 1987). Archives of the Watsonian Society. The report cites several past field staff reviews: a 1969 review by Health Services and Mental Health Administration (HSMHS) in connection with the review of Federal health staffing issues; a 1975 review by the Department of Health, Education and Welfare responding to an Office of Management and Budget directive in the markup of FY1976 budget; a 1984 review conducted internally at CDC by the Assistant Director for Management to examine the rationale for field staff. See also Coopers and Lybrand, "Final Report of a Management Study of Public Health Advisor Field Staff" (1987); V. S. Bales and W. R. Bradford, Developing Public Health Program Specialists, (Atlanta, GA: Centers for Disease Control and Prevention, July 1996); DB Consulting Group, Inc,. Consultation and Assessment of Potential Placement of CDC Public Health Professionals Off-Site, (2004); McKing Consulting Corporation, Review of the GS-685 Public Health Advisor Series. Final Report. Task 2. CDC Task

Order 027. Contract 200-2003-1396. (June 30, 2005); Watsonian Society, History of the CDC/ASTDR Public Health Advisor Series. [1993?]; Unpublished document shared with author. Watsonian Archives (undated, but probably around 1980) Tab D: Previous Reviews of Field Staff, part of another document which was not part of the archive. According to this final document, the 1969 Health Services and Mental Health Administration review was contracted with a private consulting firm which reviewed the assignees program in Pennsylvania and Maryland. The conclusion was that the assignees were "filling a valuable liaison role between the states and (CDC)" and that they were performing useful and valuable public health service. The document described a 1975 review by the Public Health Service of the assignee program in ten state and local health departments which recommended that PHS continue to strengthen the assignee program with greater emphasis on state capacity-building. The document also cites a planned review in 1980 conducted by the CDC as part of an overall evaluation plan for FY1981.

9. Katherine Cahill, interview by PHA History Project, August 25, 2004.

10. E-mail from Russell Havlak to author Beth Meyerson, April 17, 2008.

11. CDC, "In Memoriam," *Contact* (February 21, 1966):1.

12. Ibid.

13. Robert R. Swank, "Role of the Interviewer in Syphilis Control," in *Proceedings of the World Forum on Syphilis and Other Treponematoses*. (Washington, DC, September 4–8, 1962). U.S. Department of Health, Education and Welfare.

14. Jack Wroten, interview by PHA History Project, September 23, 2004.

15. E-mail from Russell Havlak to author Beth Meyerson, April 17, 2008.

16. David Sencer, interview by PHA History Project, March 31, 2004.

17. Willard Cates, interview by PHA History Project, June 16, 2004.

18. Robert R. Swank, "The Old Pro Takes a Look Inside the Contact Index," *Contact* (December 21, 1962).

19. Robert R. Swank, "The Old Pro Says..." [column] *Contact* (May 15, 1963): 4–5.

20. E-mail from Louis Salinas to author Beth Meyerson, May 15, 2008.

21. Louis Salinas, interview by PHA History Project, August 27, 2004.

22. Swank, "Role of the Interviewer."

23. Ken Latimer, handwritten note to author Beth Meyerson when sharing Kinsey photo on May 18, 2004.

24. Paul Burlack, interview by PHA History Project, February 26, 2004.

25. E-mail from William Doyle to author Beth Meyerson, April 24, 2008.

26. E-mail from Russell Havlak to author Beth Meyerson, April 17, 2008.

27. Ibid.

28. Elizabeth W. Etheridge, *Sentinel For Health: A History of the Centers for Disease Control* (Berkeley: University of California Press, 1992), 119–121; See also *U.S. Public Health Service, The Eradication of Syphilis: A Task Force Report to the Surgeon General of the Public Health Service on Syphilis Control in the United States*, (Washington, DC: U.S. Public Health Service, 1962). See also F. S. Kingma, "From the Desk Of," *Contact* (May 15, 1963):3. See also Etheridge, *Sentinel*, 119–121, 160.

29. William J. Brown, "A Word from the Chief," *Contact* (August 21, 1962).

30. William J. Brown (1962). Statement at a 1962 (precise date unknown) meeting of the branch at Hotel Moraine in Highland Park. Source: Centers for Disease Control and Prevention, *Contact* (3/20/62):1. See also Etheridge, *Sentinel*, 121.

31. Centers for Disease Control and Prevention, *Contact* (March 1, 1963):2.

32. Kingma, "From the Desk Of," 3.

33. The interviewing school in New York City was mentioned in a 1963 *Contact* (8/16/63):4.

34. Centers for Disease Control and Prevention, *Contact* (August 16, 1963):1. This newsletter includes a reference to the regional VD seminars as an opportunity for information exchange at regional level, targeted to field personnel. See also *Contact* (April 10, 1964):3; *Contact* (July 31, 1964):3. According to this latter newsletter issue, nationwide coverage in seminars occurred over a cycle of five seminars located in Minneapolis, Detroit, Miami, Denver, and Portland from September 1964 to February 1965. Topics included the epidemiology of syphilis, working with physicians in syphilis eradication, medical aspects of syphilis and gonorrhea, working with the laboratory and follow-up of reactive tests for syphilis, behavioral science as a factor in syphilis eradication, and education for eradication. Regional seminars were noted as being held as early as 1960 (per CDC info memo dated October-November 1959).

35. Centers for Disease Control and Prevention, "Epidemiologic Consultation and Training Unit: Background and Function," *Venereal Disease Administrative Communication* (undated). See also Kenneth Latimer, handwritten note to author Beth Meyerson, January 24, 2008, accompanying several photographs.

36. Centers for Disease Control and Prevention, *Contact* (January 22, 1965): 2.; Telephone conversation between Kenneth Latimer and author Beth Meyerson, February 11, 2008.

37. Kenneth Latimer, handwritten note to author Beth Meyerson, June 29, 2007.

38. Centers for Disease Control and Prevention, "Epidemiologic Consultation and Training Unit"; Ken Latimer, handwritten note to author Beth Meyerson dated

January 24, 2008.

39. Windell Bradford, interview by PHA History Project, October 27, 2004.

40. E-mail from Windell Bradford to author Beth Meyerson, April 20, 2008.

41. E-mail from Russell Havlak to author Beth Meyerson, February 14, 2008.

42. Ibid.

43. Swank, "Role of the Interviewer."

44. Swank, "The Old Pro Takes a Look," 6–7.

45. William Parra, interview by PHA History Project, June 18, 2004.

46. William Parra, interview by PHA History Project, June 28, 2007.

47. E-mail from Russell Havlak to author Beth Meyerson, May 5, 2008.

48. Ibid.

49. E-mail from Russell Havlak to author Beth Meyerson, April 17, 2008.

50. Ibid.

51. James Curran, interview by PHA History Project, March 30, 2004.

52. E-mail from Russell Havlak to author Beth Meyerson, May 5, 2008.

53. William Parra, interview by PHA History Project, June 28, 2007.

54. E-mail from Russell Havlak to author Beth Meyerson, April 17, 2008.

55. William Parra, interview by PHA History Project, June 28, 2007.

56. Ibid.

57. E-mail from Russell Havlak to author Beth Meyerson, May 5, 2008.

58. William Parra, interview by PHA History Project, June 28, 2007.

59. E-mail from Russell Havlak to author Beth Meyerson, April 17, 2008.

60. Kathryn Kosky, interview by PHA History Project, August 27, 2004.

61. Bassam Jarrar, interview by PHA History Project, October 21, 2004.

62. Laura Shelby, interview by PHA History Project, March 10, 2004.

63. Louise Galaska, interview by PHA History Project, April 22, 2004.

64. John Miles, interview by PHA History Project, January 15, 2004.

65. Jack Spencer, interview by PHA History Project, May 4, 2004.

66. Ibid.

67. Dean Mason, interview by PHA History Project, March 29, 2004.

68. Centers for Disease Control and Prevention, "Case Management Chalk-Talk meetings Standardized—New Jersey," *CDC Venereal Disease Administrative Communication* (February 1, 1967): 8.

69. Gary Conrad, interview by PHA History Project, January 21, 2004.

70. Tracy Ford, interview by PHA History Project, March 11, 2004.

71. Ibid.

72. Lisa Speissegger, interview by PHA History Project, March 8, 2004; e-mail from Lisa Speissegger to author Beth Meyerson, April 24, 2008.

73. Gary Conrad, interview by PHA History Project, January 21, 2004.

74. Robert Keegan, interview by PHA History Project, February 26, 2004.

75. Gary Conrad, interview by PHA History Project, January 21, 2004.

76. Phillip Talboy, interview by PHA History Project, April 21, 2004.

77. Louise Galaska, interview by PHA History Project, April 22, 2004.

78. Raymond Bly, interview by PHA History Project, May 28, 2004.

79. Robert Kohmescher, interview by PHA History Project, March 4, 2004.

80. Signor, Roger, "Computer Used in Fight Against Syphilis," *St. Louis Post Dispatch*. (n.d., 1981). Raymond Bly archives.

81. Russell Havlak letter to author Beth Meyerson, April 14, 2004.

82. Robert Kohmescher, interview by PHA History Project, March 4, 2004.

83. Patrick McConnon, interview by PHA History Project, March 31, 2004.

84. To maintain the client's privacy, the cross streets were removed from the story.

85. Richard Conlon, interview by PHA History Project, May 17, 2004.

Chapter 7

1. United States Nuclear Regulatory Commission, "Fact Sheet on the Three Mile Island Accident," http://www.nrc.gov/reading-rm/doc-collections/fact-sheets/3mile-isle.html (accessed December 1, 2007).

2. Paul Forman and Roger Sherman, "Three Mile Island: The Inside Story," Smithsonian Institution, http://americanhistory.si.edu/tmi/tmi04.htm, (accessed December 17, 2007). See also Joseph Carter, interview by PHA History Project, April 1, 2004.

3. Joseph Carter, interview by PHA History Project, April 1, 2004.

4. Fitzhugh Mullan, Plagues and Politics: *The Story of the United States Public Health Service,* (New York: Basic Books, 1989), 22ff.

5. In April 1947, CDC engaged in disaster response when multiple explosions in Texas City, Texas killed hundreds of people. CDC assisted local and state-level health agencies in their response to local emergency. CDC initiated help directly and in doing so, went outside the process established by the Public Health Service, primarily because the PHS regional communication system hampered efficient follow-up. See Elizabeth Etheridge, *Sentinel for Health: A History of the Centers For Disease Control,* (Los Angeles: University of California Press, 1992).

6. Etheridge, *Sentinel*, 94, 141.

7. See also the American Academy of Family Physicians, "Parvovirus B19 Infections," http://www.aafp.org/afp/991001ap/1455.html (accessed December 17, 2007).

8. Joseph Betros, interview by PHA History Project, March 9, 2004, and E-mail from Joseph Betros to author Beth Meyerson, May17, 2008.

9. Alison Young, "CDC Loses Key Official to Iraq Job," *Atlanta Journal-Constitution*, November 1, 2007.

10. William Gimson, interview by PHA History Project, April 1, 2004.

11. Billy Griggs, interview by PHA History Project, April 2, 2004.

12. Ibid.

13. Windell Bradford, interview by PHA History Project, October 27, 2004.

14. Phil Talboy, interview by PHA History Project, April 21, 2004.

15. Gerald Naehr, "PHA Response to International and Domestic Crises" (Attachment IV). Attachment to unspecified recruitment document. E-mail communication with author Beth Meyerson dated December 6, 2007; Centers for Disease Control and Prevention, "Bureau of State Services Field Assignee Participation in Special Details 1965–1979" (July 11, 1979). (Partial Data). Found as "Tab B" to a document that was not present in the Watsonian Society Archives and could not be located.; Centers for Disease Control and Prevention, "Field Assignee Participation in Special Details Partial List Center for Prevention Services 1965–1984" (July, 1984). Found as "Appendix D" to a document that was not present in the Watsonian Society Archives and could not be located; Centers for Disease Control and Prevention, "Examples of Short-and-Medium-Term PHA Responses" (July, 1984). Found with a document marked "Table 9" of a document that was not present in the Watsonian Society Archives and could not be located.

16. Centers for Disease Control and Prevention, "Field Assignee Participation."

17. James Fowler, interview by PHA History Project, July 16, 2007.

18. Preston P. Reynolds, "Hospitals and Civil Rights, 1945–1963: The Case of Simkins v. Moses H. Cone Memorial Hospital," *Annals of Internal Medicine* 126, no. 11 (June 1, 1997):898–906. See also Windell Bradford, "Investigation of Complaints: Integration of Hospitals and Other Health Facilities, 1965" (2004). Unpublished paper shared with the Public Health Advisor History Project. See also Jill Quadagno, "Promoting Civil Rights through the Welfare State: How Medicare Integrated Southern Hospitals," *Social Problems* 47, no. 1 (February, 2000):68–89.

19. Reynolds, "Hospitals and Civil Rights." See also Windell Bradford, interview by PHA History Project, October 27, 2004; Bradford, "Investigation of Complaints."

20. E-mail correspondence from David Sencer to author Beth Meyerson on December 11, 2007.

21. Robert Kingon, interview by PHA History Project, February 19, 2004; Robert Kingon, interview by PHA History Project, June 21, 2007.

22. Bradford, "Investigation of Complaints."

23. Ibid.

24. James Fowler, interview by PHA History Project, July 16, 2007.

25. Robert Longenecker, "Recollection of Robert Longenecker" (2003). Unpublished document submitted to the PHA History Project on November 25, 2003.

26. *Public Health Advisor: Four Decades and the Future*, VHS, (Atlanta, Georgia: Centers for Disease Control and Prevention, 1994). From the Watsonian Society Archives. William Watson quoted.

27. Longenecker, "Recollection"; Bradford, "Investigation of Complaints."

28. James Fowler, interview by PHA History Project, July 16, 2007.

29. Bradford, "Investigation of Complaints."

30. Longenecker, "Recollection."

31. Bradford, "Investigation of Complaints."

32. Mary Stanton, *From Selma to Sorrow: the Life and Death of Viola Liuzzo* (Athens, GA: University of Georgia Press, 1998).

33. James Fowler, interview by PHA History Project, July 16, 2007.

34. William Griggs, interview by PHA History Project, April 2, 2004.

35. J. P. Luby, G. Miller, P. Gardner et al, "The Epidemiology of St. Louis Encephalitis in Houston, Texas, 1964," *American Journal of Epidemiology* 86 (1967):584–97; Cooperative Study Group, "Epidemic St. Louis Encephalitis in Houston, 1964," *Journal of the American Medical Association* 193 (1965):139–46.

36. Centers for Disease Control and Prevention, "Epidemiologic Notes and Reports: St. Louis Encephalitis—Baytown and Houston, Texas," *Morbidity and Mortality Weekly Report* 35, no. 44 (November 07, 1986):693–5. See also Luby, Miller, Gardner et al., "The Epidemiology of St. Louis Encephalitis"; L. J. Chandler, R. Parsons, Y. Randle, "Multiple Genotypes of St. Louis Encephalitis Virus (Flaviviridae Flavivirus) Circulate in Harris County, Texas," *American Journal of Tropical Medicine and Hygiene* 64, nos. 1, 2 (2001):12–19.

37. Chandler, et al., "Multiple Genotypes of St. Louis Encephalitis Virus."

38. Donald Eddins, interview by PHA History Project, January 9, 2004.

39. Luby, et al., "The Epidemiology of St. Louis Encephalitis."

40. Donald Eddins, interview by PHA History Project, January 9, 2004.

41. Radford Davis and Danelle Bickett-Weddle, Danelle, "Viral Encephalitis." PowerPoint presentation. Center for Food Security, Iowa State University, "http://www.cfsph.iastate.edu/DiseaseInfo/ppt/ViralEncephalitis.ppt" www.cfsph.iastate.edu/DiseaseInfo/ppt/ViralEncephalitis.ppt (accessed 2004).

42. Charles Watkins, interview by PHA History Project, March 31, 2004.

43. Charles Watkins, interview by PHA History Project, March 31, 2004.

44. David J. Sencer, "CDC's 60th Anniversary: Director's Perspective," *Morbidity and Mortality Weekly Report* 55, no. 27 (July 14, 2006):745–749. See also Mike Lane, interview by PHA History Project, July 30, 2007.

45. Centers for Disease Control and Prevention, "Smallpox Eradication: Memories and Milestones," *CDC Connects* (October 26, 2007).

46. Mullan, *Plagues and Politics*, 165. See also Billy Griggs, interview by PHA History Project, April 2, 2004; and William Foege, interview by PHA History Project, September 23, 2004.

47. William Griggs, interview by PHA History Project, April 2, 2004; and William Foege, interview by PHA History Project, September 23, 2004. See also Sencer, "CDC's 60th Anniversary," 745–749.

48. Centers for Disease Control and Prevention, "Smallpox Eradication: Memories and Milestones."

49. David Sencer, interview by PHA History Project, March 31, 2004; Larry Posey, interview by PHA History Project, March 31, 2004.

50. Centers for Disease Control and Prevention, "Global Effort Pays Off… Smallpox Target at 'Zero.'" *Dateline* CDC 11, no. 10 (October, 1979):4.

51. Naehr, Gerald. "PHA Response to International and Domestic Crises" (Attachment IV). Attachment to unspecified recruitment document as sent by e-mail communication with author Beth Meyerson dated December 6, 2007.

52. Michael Lane, interview by PHA History Project, July 30, 2007.

53. Centers for Disease Control and Prevention, "Smallpox Eradication: Memories and Milestones."

54. Michael Lane, interview by PHA History Project, July 30, 2007.

55. Centers for Disease Control and Prevention, "Smallpox Eradication: Memories and Milestones."

56. Michael Lane, interview by PHA History Project, July 30, 2007.

57. Ibid.

58. Centers for Disease Control and Prevention, "Global Effort Pays Off."

59. Centers for Disease Control and Prevention, "Smallpox Eradication:

Memories and Milestones."

60. Ibid.

61. Michael Lane, interview by PHA History Project, July 30, 2007.

62. Ibid.

63. Michael Lane, interview by PHA History Project, July 30, 2007.

64. Centers for Disease Control and Prevention, "Smallpox Eradication: Memories and Milestones." See also Patrick McConnon, interview by PHA History Project, March 31, 2004.

65. Patrick McConnon, interview by PHA History Project, March 31, 2004.

66. Gary Conrad, interview by PHA History Project, January 21, 2004.

67. Gary Conrad, interview by PHA History Project, January 21, 2004.

68. William Foege, interview by PHA History Project, September 23, 2004.

69. Peter Buxtun, interview by PHA History Project, July 11, 2007. See also James H Jones, *Bad Blood: The Tuskegee Syphilis Experiment* (New York: The Free Press, 1981).

70. Peter Buxtun, interview by PHA History Project, July 11, 2007.

71. Ibid.; Etheridge, *Sentinel*, 237; Jones, *Bad Blood*.

72. Etheridge, *Sentinel*. See also Windell Bradford, interview by PHA History Project, October 27, 2004.

73. Bill Watson, interview by PHA History Project, April 16, 2008.

74. Peter Buxtun, interview by PHA History Project, July 11, 2007.

75. U.S. Public Health Service Syphilis Study at Tuskegee, "Tuskegee Timeline," http://www.cdc.gov/tuskegee/timeline.htm (accessed November 25, 2007).

76. Tuskegee Syphilis Study Ad Hoc Advisory Panel, "Initial Recommendation of the Tuskegee Syphilis Study Ad Hoc Advisory Panel," (October 25, 1972) http://www.research.usf.edu/cs/library/docs/finalreport-tuskegeestudyadvisorypanel.pdf (accessed November 25, 2007).

77. Franklin Miller, interview by PHA History Project, December 17, 2003.

78. Ibid.

79. Richard Conlon, interview by PHA History Project, May 17, 2004.

80. Ibid.

81. Ibid. See also Patrick McConnon, interview by PHA History Project, March 31, 2004, and Franklin Miller, interview by PHA History Project, December 17, 2003. See also telephone and e-mail communications by author Fred Martich with Richard Conlon, Lawrence Burt, Robert Kingon, Frank Miller, Jack Jackson, Casey Riley, Dan Vander Meer, and Willie Green, January 2008. Russell Havlak indicated that

Pete Campassi and John Supinski were among the original group, in an e-mail to author Beth Meyerson dated April 28, 2008.

82. Patrick McConnon, interview by PHA History Project, March 31, 2004.

83. Richard Conlon, interview by PHA History Project, May 17, 2004.

84. E-mail from Russell Havlak to author Beth Meyerson, April 28, 2008.

85. James Fowler, interview by PHA History Project, July 16, 2007.

86. Dennis McDowell, interview by PHA History Project, June 21, 2007.

87. Mullan, *Plagues and Politics*, 191ff.

88. James Coan, interview by PHA History Project, August 11, 2004; See also Etheridge, Sentinel, 245ff.

89. Robert Keegan, interview by PHA History Project, February 26, 2004.

90. James Coan, interview by PHA History Project, August 11, 2004.

91. Dennis McDowell, interview by PHA History Project, June 21, 2007.

92. Ibid.

93. Ibid.

94. Ibid.

95. Alex Stepick, "Haitian Boat People: A Study in the Conflicting Forces Shaping U.S. Immigration Policy," *Law and Contemporary Problems* 45, no. 2 (Spring, 1982):163–196.

96. Alex Larzelere, *The 1980 Cuban Boatlift*, (Washington DC: National Defense University Press, 1988).

97. Trinity College Haiti Program, "The Evolution of the Haitian Diaspora in the USA," http://www.haiti-usa.org/modern/evolution.php (accessed November 30, 2007).

98. Mullan, *Plagues and Politics*, 191ff.

99. Laurie Garrett, *The Coming Plague: Newly Emerging Diseases in a World Out of Balance* (New York: Farrar, Straus and Giroux, 1994), 154ff.

100. John M. Barry, *The Great Influenza: The Epic Story of the Greatest Plague in History* (New York: Viking, 2004).

101. Sencer, "CDC's 60th Anniversary."

102. Lawrence K. Altman, "With Every Epidemic, Tough Choices," *The New York Times*, March 28, 2006.

103. John Shimmens, interview by PHA History Project, August 17, 2004. see also Steven Barid, interview by PHA History Project, March 29, 2004.

104. Robert Delaney, interview by PHA History Project, October 12, 2004; Sencer, "CDC's 60th Anniversary."

105. Robert Delaney, interview by PHA History Project, October 12, 2004.

106. Etheridge, *Sentinel*,121.

107. James Chin, *Control of Communicable Diseases Manual*, 17th ed. (Washington, DC: American Public Health Association, 2000).

108. "Gonorrhea—United States, 1983," *Morbidity and Mortality Weekly Report* 33, no. 25 (June 29, 1984):361–3.

109. Carol Cancila, "VDIs," *American Medical News* (May 4, 1984):21–25.

110. Jack Wroten, interview by PHA History Project, September 23, 2004.

111. Cancila, "VDIs."

112. E-mail from Russell Havlak to author Beth Meyerson, April 23, 2008.

113. E-mail from Mark Schrader to author Beth Meyerson, May 14, 2008.

114. Mark Schrader, interview by PHA History Project, January 21, 2004. and E-mail from Mark Schrader to author Beth Meyerson, May 14, 2008.

115. Cancila, "VDIs."

116. Ibid.

117. Ibid. See also Kevin O'Connor, interview by PHA History Project, March 19, 2004.

118. Cancila, "VDIs."

119. Ibid.

120. U.S. Federal Emergency Management Agency, "The 1993 Great Midwest Flood: Voices Ten Years Later." Document published by the U.S. Department of Homeland Security May 2003.
http://www.fema.gov/library/file;jsessionid=397E1DF4C6E3D5D69D030E0AAA625B5E.WorkerLibrary?type=publishedFile&file=voices_anthology.pdf&fileid=2b366f70-2d46-11db-ad64-000bdba87d5b (accessed May 21, 2008).

121. Lee W. Larson, "The Great USA Flood of 1993." (Paper presented at the IAHS conference entitled "Destructive Water: Water-Caused Natural Disasters—Their Abatement and Control," Anaheim, California, June 24–28, 1996).
http://www.nwrfc.noaa.gov/floods/papers/oh_2/great.htm (accessed December 17, 2007), See also Mason Booth, "Looking Back: The Great Midwest Floods of 1993," *Red Cross News* (August 5, 2003).
http://www.redcross.org/article/0,1072,0_312_62,00.html (accessed December 17, 2007).

122. Centers for Disease Control and Prevention, "Rapid Assessment of Vector-borne Diseases During the Midwest Flood—United States 1993," *Morbidity and Mortality Weekly Report* 43, no. 26 (July 08, 1994):481–3.

123. Kent Gray, interview by PHA History Project, February 4, 2004.

124. Ibid.

125. Ibid.

126. Centers for Disease Control and Prevention, "Heat Related Mortality—Chicago, July 1995," *Morbidity and Mortality Weekly Report* 44, no. 31 (August 11, 1995):577–579.

127. Jim Angel (Illinois State Climatologist Office), "The 1995 Heat Wave in Chicago, Illinois," http://www.sws.uiuc.edu/atmos/statecli/General/1995Chicago.htm (accessed 12/17/07).

128. Eric Klinnenberg, *Heat Wave: A Social Autopsy of Disaster in Chicago* (Chicago: University of Chicago Press, 2002). See also Centers for Disease Control and Prevention, "Heat Related Mortality—Chicago, July 1995"; Jan C. Semenza, Carol H. Rubin, Kenneth H. Falter et al. "Heat-Related Deaths during the July 1995 Heat Wave in Chicago," *New England Journal of Medicine* 335, no. 2 (July 11, 1996):84–90.

129. Angel, "The 1995 Heat Wave."

130. Stefan Weir, interview by PHA History Project, February 20, 2004.

131. Ibid.

132. Centers for Disease Control and Prevention, "Basic Information about SARS" (May 3, 2005). http://www.cdc.gov/ncidod/sars/factsheet.htm (accessed 12/20/07).

133. Centers for Disease Control and Prevention, "Outbreak of Severe Acute Respiratory Syndrome." *Morbidity and Mortality Weekly Report* 52, no. 11 (March 21, 2003):226–228.

134. Frank Meyers, interview by PHA History Project, March 11, 2004.

135. Ibid.

136. Ibid.

137. James Beall, interview by PHA History Project, March 10, 2004.

138. Paul Burlack, interview by PHA History Project, February 26, 2004.

139. E-mail from Paul Burlack to author Beth Meyerson, May 23, 2008.

140. Paul Burlack, interview by PHA History Project, February 26, 2004.

141. E-mail from Phillip Talboy to author Beth Meyerson, May19, 2008.

142. E-mail from Phillip Talboy to author Beth Meyerson, May19, 2008.

143. U.S. General Accounting Office, "Afghanistan Reconstruction: Despite Some Progress, Deteriorating Security and Other Obstacles Continue to Threaten Achievement of U.S. Goals," *Report to Congressional Committees*, July 2005. http://www.gao.gov/new.items/d05742.pdf (accessed April 6, 2008).

144. J. Williams, B. McCarthy, "Observations from a Maternal and Infant Hospital

in Kabul, Afghanistan—2003," *Journal of Midwifery and Women's Health* 50, no. 4 (July/August 2005):e31–e35.

145. U.S. Department of Defense, "Defense's Wolfowitz Visits Women's Hospital in Kabul: Says Work in Afghanistan Entering New Phase," transcript of January 15, 2003 visit. http://usinfo.state.gov/sa/Archive/2004/Jan/29-793437.html (accessed April 6, 2008).

146. Allison Young, "Big Success or Sad Story?" *Atlanta Journal-Constitution*, November 18, 2007. http://www.ajc.com/news/content/news/stories/2007/11/16/CD-CAfghan_1118.html (accessed May 5, 2008).

147. E-mail from Steve Schindler to author Beth Meyerson, April 9, 2008.

148. Young, "Big Success or Sad Story?"

149. E-mail from Steve Schindler to author Beth Meyerson, May 28, 2008.

150. Steve Schindler, interview by PHA History Project, April 15, 2008.

151. E-mail from Steve Schindler to author Beth Meyerson, April 4, 2008.

152. Steve Schindler, undated bio/curriculum vitae sent to author Beth Meyerson, March 27, 2008; e-mail from Steve Schindler to author Beth Meyerson, April 4, 2008.

153. Steve Schindler, interview by PHA History Project, April 15, 2008.

Chapter 8

1. E-mail from David Newberry to author Beth Meyerson, March 18, 2008.

2. E-mail from David Newberry to author Beth Meyerson, March 18, 2008.

3. E-mail from author Jerry Naehr to author Beth Meyerson using data from the Watsonian Archives, March 17, 2004. E-mail from David Newberry containing curriculum vitae to author Beth Meyerson, February 2, 2008.

4. E-mail from David Newberry to author Beth Meyerson, March 18, 2008. See also Centers for Disease Control and Prevention, "International Notes Yaws and Yellow Fever Project—Ghana," *Morbidity and Mortality Weekly Report* 31, no. 12 (April 2, 1982): 149–50.

5. David Newberry to Watsonian Society and the National Active and Retired Federal Employees Association (NARFE), January 20, 2008. Shared with author Fred Martich, January 20, 2008.

6. BBC News, "Profile: Margaret Hassan" (October 20, 2004). http://news.bbc.co.uk/1/hi/uk/3756552.stm (accessed March 25, 2008). See also Guardian News and Media Limited, "Margaret Hassan: Relief Worker Who Dedicated Her Life to Helping the Iraqi People: (November 17, 2004).

http://www.guardian.co.uk/society/2004/nov/17/internationalaidanddevelopment.guardianobituaries (accessed March 25, 2008).

7. David Newberry to Watsonian Society, January 20, 2008.

8. William Watson, interview by PHA History Project, November 17, 2003.

9. William C. Watson, *First Class Privates*, (William Watson: Atlanta, GA, 1994), 235ff. See also Tom Griffen "The Man Who Helped Banish Smallpox from the Earth is the 1994 Alumnus of the Year," Columns: *The University of Washington Alumni Magazine* (June, 1994). http://www.washington.edu/alumni/columns/top10/calling_the_shots.html (accessed March 18, 2008).

10. Katherine Cahill, interview by PHA History Project, August 25, 2004.

11. Katherine Cahill, interview by PHA History Project, March 25, 2008.

12. Ibid.

13. Katherine Cahill, interview by PHA History Project, August 25, 2004.

14. Joseph Carter, interview by PHA History Project, March 21, 2008.

15. Several state and local public health STD career ladder systems were developed by Public Health Advisors. E-mail from Russell Havlak to author Beth Meyerson, April 17, 2008. Russ stated that PHA D. L. Gunter "pushed through in California an impressive career ladder." Bob Wenger also established the career ladder for New York State, and Norm Scherzer created a career ladder for New York City. "By any definition, I believe this has to be one of the enduring legacies of PHAs, since the people who now populate the career ladders in these and other areas represent almost the total current infrastructure of STD, TB and Immunization programs there."

16. Institute of Medicine, *The Future of Public Health* (Washington, DC: National Academy of Sciences, 1998).

17. See Chapter 2 and also Elizabeth W. Etheridge, *Sentinel for Health: A History of the Centers for Disease Control and Prevention* (Berkeley: University of California Press, 1992), 90, quoting Mountin from a Thomas Parran article, "A Career in Public Health," *Public Health Reports* 67 (October, 1952):937.

18. McKing Consulting Corporation, *Review of the GS-685 Public Health Advisors Series Final Report*, Task 2 CDC Task Order 027, Contract 200-2003-01396 (June 30, 2005). See also letter from David Satcher, CDC director, to all CDC and ATSDR Employees re: "The Future Role of CDC Field Assignees," dated May 25, 1993. Watsonian Society archives. The McKing report indicates that there were eight hundred field assignees in 1993, while the Satcher letter indicates that there were six hundred fifty field assignees.

19. Telephone conversation between Jack Jackson and author Beth Meyerson, March 21, 2008; Telephone conversation between Jack Jackson and author Beth Meyerson, May 2, 2008.

20. Judith Wasserheit, interview by PHA History Project, February 2, 2005.

21. R.P. Hillman, *Reinventing Government: Fast Bullets and Culture Changes,* (Austin, TX: University of Texas, 2001). See also: Vice President Gore's National Partnership for Reinventing Government. http://govinfo.library.unt.edu/npr/index.htm (accessed March 24, 2008).
For PHA staff levels in 1994, see McKing Consulting Corporation, *Review of the GS-685 Public Health Advisors Series.*

22. Letter from James D. Bloom, CDC executive officer, to deputy assistant secretary for Health Operations, dated October 9, 1979, re: "Exploration of Different Ways of Accomplishing a Reduction in the VD Field Staff." Watsonian Archives. This letter indicates that federal policies on FTE ceilings exerted pressure on CDC to reduce field staff. An option was offered to redefine employment reporting requirements to allow field staff to be exempt from federal employee counts. CDC cites a 1965 General Counsel opinion that provision of personnel in lieu of cash grants to states is part of the grant to states and should be treated as such for accounting purposes. The opinion apparently was reaffirmed in 1969, according to this letter. See also letter from Charles M. Gozonsky, Office of the General Counsel of CDC, to James Bloom, CDC executive officer, dated September 28, 1979, re: "CDC—Employment ceiling—VD assignees—Necessity for inclusion in count—Obligation of funds—Retention of benefits as Federal employees—section 311 of Civil Service Reform Act—Leach amendment." Watsonian Archives. See also Office of Personnel Management Federal Personnel Manual System FPM Letter 298-7 Subject: "Revision of the Monthly Report of Federal Civilian Employment (SF 113-A) As a Result of the CSRA (Civil Service Reform Act) and Other Changes," August 13, 1979. Watsonian Society Archives. According to the memo, the Civil Service Reform Act, signed October 13, 1978, states that the number of civilian employees in the Executive Branch on September 30, 1979, September 30, 1989, and September 30, 1981, should not exceed the number of employees on September 30, 1977.

23. Jack Jackson, interview by PHA History Project, November 17, 2003.

24. Jack Spencer, interview by PHA History Project, May 4, 2004.

25. Judith Wasserheit, interview by PHA History, February 5, 2005.

26. Jack Spencer, interview by PHA History Project, May 4, 2004.

27. Ibid.

28. McKing Consulting Corporation, *Review of the GS-685 Public Health Advisors Series.*

29. E-mail from Joe Scavatto to author Beth Meyerson, April 25, 2008; E-mail from Norman Fikes to author Beth Meyerson, April 24, 2008; E-mail from Robert Cicatallo to author Beth Meyerson, April 23, 2008.

30. Association of State and Territorial Health Officials, *State Public Health Employee Worker Shortage Report: A Civil Service Recruitment and Retention Crisis* (Washington, DC: ASTHO, 2004). See also Health Resources and Services Administration, *Public Health Workforce Study* (Washington, DC: Department of Health and Human Services, 2004).

31. Anthony Scardaci, interview by PHA History, June 14, 2004.

32. Ibid.

33. Jack Jackson, interview by PHA History Project, November 17, 2003.

34. E-mail from Russell Havlak to author Beth Meyerson on March 17, 2008.

35. Russell Havlak, interview by PHA History Project, March 31, 2004; and e-mail from Russell Havlak to author Beth Meyerson, April 17, 2008.

36. E-mail from Russell Havlak to author Beth Meyerson, April 17, 2008.

37. E-mail from Russell Havlak to author Beth Meyerson, March 17, 2008; edited via e-mail to author Beth Meyerson, April 17, 2008.

38. McKing Consulting Corporation, *Review of the GS-685 Public Health Advisors Series.*

39. CDC policy entitled "Coordination and Management of Field Staff Assignments," CDC-GA-2006-05, issued September 20, 2006.

40. Jack Jackson, interview by PHA History Project, November 17, 2003.

Chapter 9

1. Michael Sage, interview by PHA History Project, April 15, 2008.

2. Glen Koops, interview by PHA History Project, March 21, 2008.

3. E-mail from Glen Koops to author Beth Meyerson, May 16, 2008.

4. Kristen Brusuelas, interview by PHA History Project, March 24, 2008.

5. McKing Consulting Corporation, *Review of the GS-685 Public Health Advisors Series Final Report*, Task 2 CDC Task Order 027, Contract 200-2003-01396 (June 30, 2005).

6. Ibid.; Association of State and Territorial Health Officials, *State Public Health Employee Worker Shortage Report: A Civil Service Recruitment and Retention Crisis*

(Washington, DC: ASTHO, 2004). See also Health Resources and Services Administration, *Public Health Workforce Study* (Washington, DC: Department of Health and Human Services, 2004).

7. Centers for Disease Control and Prevention, *CDC Portfolio Assessment Prospectus Reports* (October, 2006).

8. Kristin Brusuelas, interview by PHA History Project, March 24, 2008.

9. E-mail from Glen Koops to author Beth Meyerson, May 16, 2008.

10. Michael Sage, interview by PHA History Project, April 15, 2008.

11. Kristin Brusuelas, interview by PHA History Project, March 24, 2008.

12. Ibid.

13. Michael Sage, interview by PHA History Project, April 15, 2008.

14. CDC policy entitled, "Coordination and Management of Field Staff Assignments," CDC-GA-2006-05, issued September 20, 2006.

15. Candice Nowicki-Lehnherr, interview by PHA History Project, March 24, 2008.

16. Ibid.

17. Centers for Disease Control and Prevention, "Apprenticeships in Public Health, Executive Overview" (March, 2008).

18 Glen Koops, interview by PHA History Project, March 21, 2008.

19. Centers for Disease Control and Prevention, "Program Overview: The Public Health Apprenticeship Program" (February 5, 2008).

20. Centers for Disease Control and Prevention, "Public Health Apprenticeships: A Collaborative Project to Revitalize the Public Health Advisor Pipeline." Update dated January 28, 2008. See also Centers for Disease Control and Prevention, "PHAP Successes" (2008). Unpublished document provided by program director Glen Koops to author Beth Meyerson.

21. Centers for Disease Control and Prevention, "CDC Helps Pilot PH Apprentices," *CDC Connects* (October 17, 2007).

22. Glen Koops, in Centers for Disease Control and Prevention, "CDC Helps Pilot PH Apprentices."

23. Centers for Disease Control and Prevention, "Public Health Apprenticeships: A Collaborative Project."

24. Ibid.

25. Examples of Public Health Advisors mentioned in this book who over the years have been sent by CDC to earn academic degrees on a full-time basis without being burdened by their CDC jobs (called "long-term training") include Bill Watson

(Harvard), Anne-Renee Heningburg (Harvard), Gary West (Berkeley and Cal State), Kathy Cahill (University of North Carolina), Windell Bradford (Syracuse-Maxwell), Louise Galaska (University of North Carolina), and Dick Conlon (Lyndon B. Johnson School of Public Affairs, University of Texas). Others obtained degrees on their own (Louis Salinas, Larry Posey, and Bill Parra, for example).

Index

A

Adams, Steve, 7–9, *8*

Adcock, Dave, 7–9, 228

Agle, Andy, 31, 32

Anthrax scare (2001), 21–22, 29

Apodaca, Janella, 69, 120

Appalachian Regional Program, 113, 268

Archer, Ken, 7–9, *8*

Army Appropriation Act of 1918, 35

arsenotherapy, 46

B

Babies and Breadwinners campaign, 94–96, *95*, 164

Baldwin, Robert, 118, 120, 122

Bales Harris, Virginia, 121–122

Barid, Steve, 103–104, 127–128, 212

Bass, Susan, 69, 120

Bauer, Theodore, 66, 81

Baumgartner, Leona, 138

Beall, James, 18, 200, 213

Benson, Jack

Blue Star Research Program, 77

  career diversity, 85

  hiring of, 65–66

  in Immunization Program, 95, *95*, 103–104

  patient contact facilitation by, 82

  Syphilis Follow-up Program, 78–80

  syphilis testing by, 87–88

Bernier, Roger, 118
Berry, Frank, 90
Betros, Joseph, 165–166
Biafran War, 173
Bice, Steve
  career, 22–23
  Hurricane Andrew (1992), 29
  on PHA work, 23–25, 28
  September 11, 2001 attacks, 7–9
  in SNS development, 225
Bill and Melinda Gates Foundation, 210–212
Billingslea, Albert, 69, 112–114, *113*
Black Creek Canal Virus, 16
Blancato, Orlando, 118, 228
blitz (syphilis), 193–194
blood testing/screening (*See also* Phlebotomy)
  Bracero Program, 83–85, 262–263
  confidentiality issues, 78, 89
  early efforts, 72–75, *74*
  HIV/AIDS, 110–111
  human resources for, 56
  issues in, 70, 83–86
  military, 54, *76*
  PHAs on, 73, 157
  in Puerto Rico, 75–77, *76*
  in RTCs, 48–49
  safety, 85-86, 155-157
  Sheppard tubes, *87*, 157
  staff, *107*
  training in, 14, 60, 61, 72, 155–157
Blue Star Research Study, 77–79
Bly, Ray, 70, 81, 85–86, 159, 213
Boudreaux, Stathan "S.A.", 58, 59, 64
Bowman, Richard
  on co-op benefits, 65
  described, *42*
  on Johannes Stuart, 45

on Lida Usilton, 41
on PHA creation, 256–257
as PHA interviewer, 67
on VD control funding, 37, 38
Bracero Program, 83–85, 262–263
Bradford, Windell
on the case management system, 139–140
HIV work by, 108
on hospital integration, 169–171
temporary duty assignments, 167
and the Tuskegee experiments, 184
Brennan, Larry, 46
Broome, Claire, 215
Brown, William, 138
Brownell, David, 228
Brusuelas, Kristin, 230–234
Burger, Ron, 7–9, 205, 213
Burlack, Paul, 137, 200–201
Burney, Leroy, 93
Burt, Larry, 184
Buxtun, Peter, 181–182, 185

C

Cahill, Kathy, 131, 210–212
Califano, Joseph, 104
Callan, Art, 46
Campassi, Pete, 72, 184
Carter, Joseph, 116–117, 163, 167, 184, 212
case finding. *See also* Contact epidemiology
blitzing, 193–194
competitions, 71
described, 49–50
history of development, 39–40
outcomes, improving, 52
patient interviewing in, 131–147
as PHA role, 10, 14, 69, 92, 130, 167
requirements of, 85

syphilis, 49–50, 85
system, limitations of, 140–141
trust and, 195
case management system, 139–141
Cassell, Michael, 129
Cates, Willard "Ward," 133–134, 242
CDC. *See* Centers for Disease Control and Prevention (CDC)
culture, 97
consultancies, 208, 223
diversification of
gender, 117–122, *118, 119*, 258
racial, 69, 113–116
closed offers, 114–115
field staff reductions by, 221, 283
history, 13, 242
hospital integration, 168–171
in disaster response, 273–274
on field assignments in public health, 233–234
management philosophy, 26, 215–217
management requirements, 121–122, 214
PHA funding by, 217–220, 234
PHA recruitment by, 213–217, 228, 229–234
PHA roles in, 104–106, 163–166
Portfolio Management Project, 229–231, 238
Regional Office system closure, 116
retired PHA roles in, 221–225
Saigon, fall of, 165, 166, 185–190, *187*
smallpox eradication, 84–85, 166–167, 173–180
Tuskegee experiment, 137, 181–185
VD Division's move to, 92–98
Chicago Heat Wave, (1995), 197–198
children. *See also* Immunization Program
blood testing of, 73
congenital syphilis births, 37, 73
immunization of, 104, 209–210
STD screening of, 155, 165
thalidomide in, 171–172

tuberculosis screening of, 98–99
Chin, Pam, 122–123
cholera, 22, 186–187
Chronic Disease Program, 105
Civil Rights Act of 1964, 168
Coan, James, 186–187, *187*
Commissioned Corps, 2, 10, 45, 65, 246
Compact of Free Association, 23, 243–244
Conlon, Richard
on Frank Miller, 160
on PHAs as problem solvers, 29
post-retirement work, 212
qualifications/training, 15
and the Tuskegee experiments, 183, 184
Connor, Marvin "Paul," 61
Conrad, Gary, 152, 155–157, 179–180, 212
consultancies, 208, 223
contact epidemiology. *See also* Case finding
benefits of, 62–63, 89
cholera, 186–187
described, 50, 193–194
diphtheria, 37, 48–50
human resources for, 56
issues in, 50–54, 86, 88–90
legal basis, 51
patient interviewing in, 131–147
smallpox eradication, 176–178
success, measurement of, 62
in syphilis control, 37, 48–54
in TB Program, 97
training in, 14, 60
vs. counseling, 146
worker qualifications, 51–52
worker recruitment for, 55–57
contact Investigation. *See* Contact epidemiology
Contact tracing. *See* Contact epidemiology
co-ops. *See also* Public Health Advisors (PHAs); specific individuals

benefits of, 69
competitions, 160–161
culture, 69–72
early history, 38, 42, 56, 58–67
gender diversification in, 117–122, *118, 119*
issues faced by, 69
qualifications/training, 69 (*See also* Training of PHAs)
racial diversification in, 113–116
roles of, 10, 16, 20–22, 26–29, 48, 79
crack cocaine, 14, 83, 154, 192
Crankshaw, Richard, 118
Curran, James, 108, 109, 112, 144

D

darkfield microscopy, 87–90, 88
Davis, Tom, 46
Delaney, Robert, 191–192
Diabetes Control Programs, 105–106, *107*, 267
diphtheria, 37, 48–50, 102
Do, Kim, 157
Donahue, James, *42*
Doyle, William, 137
Dutta, Mahendra, *106*

E

Eddins, Don, 172
Emerson, Robert, 147
Epidemic Intelligence Service (EIS), 10, 22, 164
Epidemiologic Consultation and Training Unit, 138–140, *139*
Equal Rights Amendment, 119
Erlich, Cy, 58, 62
excepted service appointments, 57, 65, 66, 253

F

Fall of Saigon, 165, 166, 185–190, *187*
fieldwork. *See also* Training of PHAs
as CDC management requirement, 121–122, 214

challenges, 147–149, 171, 177, 204
confidentiality issues, 152–155
described, 14–18, 128, 148
importance of, 122, 158–159, 220, 224, 228
motivation issues, 150–152
performance requirements, 149–150
PHA training in, 147–162
problem-solving skills, 152
rapport building, 17–20, 51, 89, 152–155
Finley, Phillip, 111
Florida project, 230–236
Foege, William
on CDC HIV response, 107
on PHAs in Immunization Program, 104
post-retirement work, 209–210
on scientist-PHA pairing, 26, 31
smallpox eradication, 174, 180
Ford, Tracy, 129, 153–154
Foreign Quarantine Service, 104–105
Foster, Stan, 174
Fowler, James
Epidemiologic Consultation and Training Unit, *139*, 139–140
on hospital integration, 170, 171
on patient interviewing, 133–134
in polio immunization, *95*, 96
on professional attire/work environment issues, 70
and the Tuskegee experiments, 184
Francois, Rony, 232
Freckleton, Robert, 96
Friedberg, Penny, 69, 120, 258
FTE ceiling, 217–219

G

Galaska, Louise, 149, 158–159
Gallo, William, 21
Gerberding, Julie, 11, 23, 33, 117, 229
Getz, Henry, 46

Gill, Lamont, 58
Gimson, William
as CDC Deputy Director, 22, 229
on PHA hiring at CDC, 230, 233, 234
qualifications/training, 11
temporary duty assignments, 166
Giordano, Joseph
on co-op job confidence, 66
on Lida Usilton, 42
on PHAs in RTCs, 48–49
on the Physician Visitation Program, 87
Glenner, Sam, *76*
Global Programme on AIDS, 20. *See also* HIV/AIDS
gonorrhea
control, history of, 46, 81–83, 142
high-risk pregnancy, recognition of, 14
patient interviewing, 142–146
PPNG, 192–195
prevention efforts, 145
treatment issues, 145
Gonorrhea Control Program, 142–144
granuloma inguinale (GI), 72
Gray, Kent, 7–9, 196–197, 205
Great Midwestern Flood (1993), 196–197
Green, William, 184
Griggs, Billy, 84, 166, 174–176
Grubbs, Samuel, 50
Guinea worm, 28

H

Hagler, Robert, 75
Haitian refugees, 189
Hamlin, William "Luke"
assignment of, 61–63
on blood testing, 73
career, 64
described, *59*

hiring of, 58–60
on Lida Usilton, 41
Hammons, Delwin "Del," 64–65, 79
Hantavirus, 16, 28, 157, 167
Hassan, Margaret, 208, 209
Havlak, Russell
on the case management system, 140–141
on contact epidemiology, 193
Epidemiologic Consultation and Training Unit, *139*
on gonorrhea screening/interviewing, 145
HIV/AIDS work, 110–112
on Joe Moore, 160
on patient interviewing, 132–133, 137–138, 143, 145
post-retirement work, 225–228
on STD Division changes, 146
on syphilis' cultural value, 143–144
and the Tuskegee experiments, 184–185
Hayes, Woody, 75
Health Mobilization and Disaster Preparedness Program, 64, 105
Heath, John, 114–116
Henderson, D.A., 26, 166, 174, 177
Heningburg, Anne Renee
Buffalo landing, *31*
on problem-solving, 30
qualifications/training, 24–25
on racial/gender diversification, 123–124
temporary duty assignments, 165
Hicks, James, 174, 176
Hill, John, 193
Hilyer, Elvin, 104–105
Hinman, Alan, 25
HIV/AIDS, 20, 106–113, 153
Hobby, Oveta Culp, 80
Hogan, Robert, 176
hospital integration, 168–171
Hughes, Walter, 39, 64
Human papillomavirus virus vaccines, 26

Hurney, George, 184
Hurricane Andrew (1992), 16, 29
Hutchinson teeth, 72

I

Immunization Program
 challenges, 230
 development of, 96–98, 101–104
 Expanded Program on Immunization, 104
 measles, 102–103
 PHAs, demand for, 94
 PHAs in, statistic, 106
 polio, 94–96, 102, 104, 164
 in Puerto Rico, 10
 rubella, 103
 whooping cough, 102
incidence command, 23
influenza, 190–192, *191*
Irwin, Katy, 27

J

Jackson, Jack, 22, 184, 215–217, 223–224
Jarrar, Bassam, 148

K

Keegan, Robert, 156, 186
Kingon, Robert, 90, 109, *139*, 184
Kohmescher, Robert, 111–112, 159, 160
Koops, Glen, 230–237
Koski, Kathryn, 17–18

L

Lafayette-Bulwinkle Act of 1938, 37, 38
Lama, Jerry, 31–32
Lane, Michael, 175–178
Latimer, Kenneth
 on the case management system, 140–141

described, *136*
Epidemiologic Consultation and Training Unit, 138–140, *139*
on federal funding cuts, 80
on Lida Usilton, 41–42
on patient interviewing, 135–136, 138–139
Syphilis Follow-Up Program, 78
syphilis testing/treatment, 73–77, 76, 86
temporary duty assignments, 165
Lederer, Edith, 182
Lederman, Donald, 57, 58, 61, 64, 264
leprosy, 22
Little Red School House, 149, 150
Longenecker, Robert, 169, 170
Love, George, 69, 113

M

Madam. *See* Usilton, Lida J. "Madam"
Malone, Bernard "Bert," 12–14, 213
management
CDC philosophy, 26, 215–217
CDC requirements, 121–122, 214
incidence command style of, 23
Portfolio Management Project, 229–231, 238
senior, PHAs as, 10, 12, 16, 24–27, 92, 97, 124, 176, 212
Mancino, Peter, 226–227
Mann, Jonathan, 20
Mariel boatlift, 189
Martich, Fred, 112
Mason, Dean, 152, 212
Mason, James, 108
Masso, Anthony, *174*
Maternal Child Health (MCH) program, 101–102
Mauldin, Harold, 74–75, 101–102
McConnon, Patrick, 27–28, 178–179, 184, 212
McDowell, Dennis, 17, 165, 187–189
measles, 25, 102–103, 167, 174, 228, 230
medical case workers, 51

Medicare program, 168
Meyers, Frank, 199–200
microscopy, darkfield, 87–90, *88*
Miles, John, 150
Millar, J. Donald, 100, 174
Miller, Frank, 113–116, 160, 182–183
Montez, Ernest, 184
Moore, Joseph, 159–160
Mountin, Joseph, 56
Murphy, Kevin, 128

N

Narkunas, John, 114, 118–120
National Community Migrant Health Centers Program, 23
National Venereal Disease Control Act, 37, 38
Newberry, David, 207–209, *209*
Noble, Gary, 109
Nowicki-Lehnherr, Candice, 234

O

O'Conner, Kevin
  qualifications/training, 14–15
  syphilis epidemic, 194–195, *195*
  temporary duty assignments, 165
  100 Day Experiment, 52–54
Operation Pursuit, 138, 142, 181, 192

P

Parra, William
  administrative contributions of, 27, 33, 109, 146–147
  Epidemiologic Consultation and Training Unit, *139*
  on patient interviewing, 141–142, 145–146
  post-retirement work, 212
  on rapport building, 20–21
Parran, Thomas, *36*, 36–37, 56, 86
Patient confidentiality
  blood testing/screening, 78, 89

fieldwork, 152–155
patient interviewing, 137, 142
patient interviewing
behavior change model, 145–147
in case finding, 131–147
case management system, 140–141
challenges, 52–53, 135, 142, 151
changes in, 141, 145–147
confidentiality issues, 137, 142
in contact epidemiology, 131–147
gonorrhea, 142–146
Institute for Sex Research, *136*
as PHA role, 2, 67, 69, 71, 79, 124, 130
PHAs on, 132–139, 141–146
PHA training overview, 131–147
physician attitudes toward, 50, 133
in RTCs, 117
state methods of, 97
syphilis, 117, 131–138, 142–144
technique, alternative applications of, 171
training in, 65, 131–132, 138–141
two-way mirrors in, 136–137
Pendleton, John "Jack"
on co-ops, 56
on Lida Usilton, 40–41, 43, 264
in diabetes, *107*
penicillin, 46, 62, 66, 77–78, 80
Penicillinase-Producing Neisseria Gonorrhea (PPNG), 192–195
Peppy Epi, 82, 143
Phlebotomy, 61, *72*, 83, 130, 155-157. (*See also* Blood Testing/Screening)
physicians
patient interviewing, attitudes towards, 50, 133
syphilis control, attitudes/issues in, 62, 69, 80, 86–91
Physician Visitation Program, 87–92, *91*
Pietz, Harald, 21
polio
Babies and Breadwinners campaign, 94–96, *95*, 164

control, contact epidemiology in, 37, 48–50
immunization programs, 94–96, 102, 104, 164
National Immunization Days, 30
PHA assignees, 24, 30-31, *95*, 165,
retired PHA roles in, 221–223
treatment, history of, 24–25, 30
Portfolio Management Project (PMP), 229–231, 238
Posey, Lawrence, 91–92
Posid, Joseph, 21
Powers, Ed, 11–12, 14
PPNG (Penicillinase-Producing Neisseria Gonorrhea), 192–195
pregnancy, high-risk, 15, 20, 158–159
problem solvers/problem solving
fieldwork and, 152
PHAs as, 10, 29–33, 100
as qualification, 10, 29–33
Public Health Advisors (PHAs)
academic credentialing of, 215–218, 238, 285–286
classification of, 67, 256, 258
contributions of, 100–101, 124–125, 163–168, 176, 229
core skills, 155
creation of series, 67, 256–257
culture, 21, 23–24, 69–72, 85, 158–159, 167, 179, 238
diversification of
gender, 117–122, *118, 119*, 258
racial, 69, 113–116
statistical overview, 123
dress code, 70–71
early PHAs, 22, 38, 42, 48, 56, 58–67, 69
enculturation of, 238
field program dismantling, 231
human resource capacity of, 92
models of, 243
original list of, 253–254
post-retirement work, 207–213, 221–226
as problem solvers, 10, 29–33, 100
qualifications/training (See Training of PHAs)

racial equality issues, 93, 113–116
rapport building by, 17–20, 51, 89, 152–155
recruitment of (See Recruitment of PHAs)
reputation, 22, 25, 28, 215–216, 229–230
roles (See Roles of PHAs)
supervisors, 150–152
Public Health Apprenticeship Program, 230–238, *236*, 269–270
Public Health Prevention Specialist, 219, 220
Public Health Service,
move to Communicable Disease Center, 93-94
regional offices, 22, 38-39, 42, 45-46, 64, 94, 103-104, 116,163
Venereal Disease Division, chapter 2
Puckett, Dave, 118
Puerto Rico
immunization programs in, 10
syphilis control efforts in, 75–77, *76*

R

Rábia Balkhi Hospital Project, 202–205
Rapid Treatment Centers (RTCs)
closure of, 66, 79
establishment of, 38, 40, 47
female interviewers in, 117
funding for, 46, 47
PHA training in, 52, 70
roles of, 48–49, 77
transportation needs, meeting, 44
U.S.S. *Ernest Hinds*, 49
rapport building, 17–20, 51, 69, 89, 152–155
recruitment of PHAs
candidate qualities, 129–130
by CDC, 229–234
early history, 55–58, 64–66
issues in, 129, 213–214
Red Dog Program, 193
refugee resettlement, 165, 166, 185–190, *187*
reinventing government initiatives, 217

Rheubotham, Mary "Mother Mary," 46
Riley, Casey, 184
roles of PHAs. *See also specific disasters*; specific tasks
 anthrax scare (2001), 21–22, 29
 case finding as, 10, 14, 69, 92, 130, 167
 in CDC, 104–106, 163–168
 Chronic Disease Program, 105
 consultancies, 208, 223
 as Federal employee, 79
 hospital integration, 168–172
 overview, 2, 10, 20–22, 167
 patient interviewing as, 2, 67, 69, 71, 79, 124, 130
 PHA-scientist pairing, 26–29, 31, 166
 PHAs on, 25–26
 polio immunizations, 94–96, 102, 104, 164
 Public Health Apprenticeship Program, 234
 refugee management, 165, 166, 185–190, *187*
 retired PHAs, 221–225
 as senior management, 10, 12, 16, 24–27, 92, 97, 124, 176, 212
 syphilis prevention, 140–141, 160
 Tuberculosis Elimination Program, 99–102, 106, 130
 WHO, 20, 27, 104, 222
Roper, William, 26–27
Roy, Sally, 258
RTCs. See Rapid Treatment Centers (RTCs)
Rushing, Wilmon, 108–109, 112

S

Sabrero, Larry, 101
Sage, Michael, 228, 233, 234
Saigon, fall of, 165, 166, 185–190, *187*
Salinas, Louis, 134–135
SARS, 166, 198–201
Satcher, David, 116–117, 215
Scardaci, Anthony, 104–105, *106*, 221–223, 224
Scherzer, Norman, 120, 282
Schindler, Steve, 202–204, *204*

Schrader, Mark, 193–194
scientist-PHA pairing, 26–29, 31, 166
Seggerson, John, 99–100
Sencer, David
as CDC Deputy Director, 96, 105
described, *42*
hiring of, 264
on hospital integration, 168–169
on Johannes Stuart, 45
on patient interviewing, 133
on PHA acceptance, 98
on PHA usefulness, 97
on scientist-PHA pairing, 26
in smallpox eradication, 174
and the Tuskegee experiments, 182–183
September 11, 2001 attacks, 7–9, 166, 205, 227–228
Sexual contacts. *See* Contact epidemiology
sexually transmitted diseases (STDs). *See* Venereal Disease (VD) Program; specific diseases
Shannon, Robert, 46
Shelby, Laura, 148–149
Sheppard tubes, 87, 157. *See also* Blood testing/screening
Shimmens, John, 70–71, 98–99, 102–103, 190–191, 213
smallpox eradication, 84–85, 166–167, 173–180
Smallpox Program, 25–26, 105, 120, 222
Smith, Clarence "Larry," 96
Smith, Joseph, 118
Sorenson, Bonnie, 232
Speissegger, Lisa, 154–155
Spencer, Jack, 151, 218–220
St. Louis Encephalitis, 172
STD Division
changes, implementing, 146
HIV/AIDS work, 109–110
on PHA training, 216, 218
racial diversification in, 116
TEC group, 141–147 (*See also* Training of PHAs)

STDs. See Venereal Disease (VD)
Stenhouse, Don, *191*
Strategic National Stockpile (SNS)
  development of, 225–228
  history, 22, 240
  September 11, 2001 attacks, 7
Stuart, Johannes "Doctor"
  Bracero Program, 83
  on contact epidemiology benefits, 62–63
  described, *42*, 44–45
  in gender diversification, 117
  problem-solving abilities, 44, 49
  qualifications/training, 43
  retirement, 93
  syphilis control, history of, 33, 35
  VD Division role, 41, 43–44, 62
  worker recruitment by, 55–58, 64–66
Stubbs, Jack, 228
Supinski, John, 184, 193
surveillance containment, 175–176
Swank, Robert
  case management system, 140–141
  described, *60*
  patient interviewing development by, 60–61
  in patient interviewing training, 65, 131–132, 138–141
swine flu, 190–192, *191*
syphilis
  blitzing, 193–194
  blood testing/screening (*See* Blood testing/screening)
  Blue Start Research Program, 77-79
  case finding, 49–50, 85
  control
    Bracero Program, 83–85, 262–263
    case management system, 140–141
    contact epidemiology, 37, 48–54
    early history of, 33, 35–38, 46–54, *47*, 69
    eradication, 138–139, 146

federal funding cuts, 80–81
100 Day Experiment, 52–54
patient interviewing in, 117, 131–138, 142–144
Peppy Epis, 82
physician attitudes/issues in, 62, 69, 80, 86–91
cultural value of syphilis interviewing, 143–144
syphilis epidemic, 110, 194–195, *195*
epidemiology, 1935, 37
eradication, 138–139, 146
epidemics, 34-37, 110, 192–195, *195*
high-risk pregnancy, recognition of, 15, 20, 158–159
patient interviewing, 117, 131–138, 142–144
prevention efforts, 140–141, 160
Rapid Treatment Centers (*See* Rapid Treatment Centers)
recognition of, 14, 20, 86–88
risk identification, 60, 73
screening announcement, *74*, 99
tracking, by computer, 160
treatment
access, 19
arsenotherapy, 46
penicillin, 46, 62, 66, 77–78, 80
relapse issues, 77
Tuskegee Syphilis Study, 137, 181–185
Syphilis Follow-Up Program, 78–79

T

Talboy, Phillip
anthrax scare (2001), 21–22, 29
on blood testing, 157
hantavirus, work on, 167
qualifications/training, 16
SARS, 201
temporary duty assignments, 165–167
Terry, Luther, 138
tetanus immunizations, 102
thalidomide, 171–172

Thomas, Ron, 184
Thompson, Ed, 100–101
Three Mile Island, 163, *164*, 167
Tomlinson, Victor, 128
training of PHAs. *See also* Fieldwork
  academic credentialing, 215–218, 238, 285–286
  in blood testing/screening, 14, 60, 61, 72, 155–157
  case management system, 140–141
  chalk talks, 152
  competitions, 160–161
  in contact epidemiology, 14, 60 (*See also* Contact epidemiology)
  cross-training, 233
  dropout rates, 127, 161–162
  early co-ops, 69
  fieldwork (*See* Fieldwork)
  motivation issues, 150–152, 159–162
  overview, 10–18, 23–26, 52, 57, 85, 124–128
  patient interviewing (*See* Patient interviewing)
  in RTCs, 52, 70
  subject areas, general, 130–131
trust issues, 17–20, 51, 69, 89, 152–155
tuberculosis
  control, contact epidemiology in, 37, 48–50
  drug-resistant, 100
  fieldwork in, 14
  screening for, 48, 73, 83
  vs. syphilis, 37
Tuberculosis Elimination Program
  CDC, move to, 94, 97
  overview, 97
  PHA acceptance by, 97–99
  PHA roles in, 99–102, 106, 130
  screening announcement, *99*
Tuskegee Syphilis Study and Follow-up, 137, 181–185
typhoid, 37, 48–50

U

Urban Rat Control, 16, 105
U.S. Public Health Service (PHS)
culture, 69–70
physicians as emergency responders, 164
staffing issues, 269–270
STD career ladder systems, 282
Venereal Disease Division (*See* Venereal Disease Division)
worker retirement issues, 213–214, 231
Usilton, Lida J. "Madam"
described, *40*, 41–44, *42*
qualifications/training, 39
retirement, 93, 264
in RTC establishment, 40, 47
syphilis control, history of, 33, 35, 53–54
VD Division roles, 39–41, 62, 66–67, 74–75, 79
worker recruitment by, 55, 57, 58

V

Vaccine Assistance Act of 1962, 96, 102, 103
Vandermeer, Don, 184
Venereal Disease (VD) Investigators, 51–53, 56–57, 61, 78, 118. *See also* Public Health Advisors (PHAs)
Venereal Disease Division. *See also* Centers for Disease Control and Prevention; specific individuals; specific programs
Atlanta, move to, 92–98
culture, 45–46
establishment, 35
federal funding for, 80–81, 92, 142
interview process, 42, 60–61
penicillin evaluation by, 77–78
roles of, 35–38, 46, 62
structure, 39, 66
worker recruitment, 55–58
Venereal Disease Program. *See also* Gonorrhea; HIV/AIDS; Syphilis
changes, implementing, 141–142
diversification of
gender, 117–122, *118, 119*

racial, 69, 113–116
statistical overview, 123
fieldwork requirements, 19, 72
history
federal/state efforts, 35–38, 50–56, 138–139, 242
treatment, 14, 18, 35–38, 79–80
100 Day Experiment, 52–54
PHA acceptance by, 97–98
Rapid Treatment Centers (*See* Rapid Treatment Centers)
as training for CDC staff, 124

W

Wallace, George, 170
Ward, Donald, 193
Wasserheit, Judy, 215, 216, 218, 238
Watkins, Charles, 115–116, 173, *174*
Watkins, Wendy, 194–195, 195
Watson, William
assignment of, 61–63
on Babies and Breadwinners, 94–96
Bracero Program, 83–85, 262–263
career, 63–64
on CDC culture, 97
as CDC Deputy Director, 22, 26, *211*
on community screenings, 73
on contact epidemiology, 53
described, 59, *136*
on federal funding cuts, 80–81
on government job registers, 56
hiring of, 58
on Johannes Stuart, 43–44, 49, 57, 58, 117
on Lida Usilton, 264
on PHA roles, 25–26
post-retirement work, 209–210
smallpox eradication, 174
and the Tuskegee Syphilis Study, 181, 183
on the VD Division in Atlanta, 93

on VD Program, 39
on VD regional staff, 46, 55
Webb, Charles Joseph, 19–20
Weir, Stefan, 197–198
Weisner, Paul, 107
Wenger, Robert, 282
West, Gary, 212
Wheeler, Jerry, 178
Wolff, Wendy, 18–19, 122
World Health Organization (WHO)
culture, 20
PHA roles in, 20, 27, 104, 222
polio treatment by, 24
in smallpox eradication, 177
World Trade Center. See September 11, 2001 attacks
Wroten, Jack, 82, 88–89, 132, 192–194, 213

Z

Zyla, Larry, 109

About The Authors

BETH MEYERSON is founder and president of Policy Resource Group, LLC; a health policy consultancy with domestic and international emphases. Dr. Meyerson's work is informed by years in the public, private and non-profit sectors. For several years, she served as the state AIDS and STD Director for Missouri. It was in this capacity that she first became acquainted with Public Health Advisors and their contributions. Beth was born in Kalamazoo, Michigan and grew up in Shaker Heights, Ohio and Ann Arbor, Michigan. She received her baccalaureate degree from the University of Michigan (Go BLUE!), conducted master's study at Harvard Divinity School, and received her Master of Divinity degree from Christian Theological Seminary in Indianapolis. Beth earned her doctorate from Saint Louis University in Public Policy Analysis and Administration. Dr. Meyerson's most recent work has taken her to Kenya, Nigeria, Botswana, India, Russia and throughout the Caribbean with focus on HIV/AIDS and community development. She has authored several papers and books. Her most recent research appears in Sexually Transmitted Diseases, Public Health Reports, AIDS Care, and the American Journal of Public Health. Beth lives with her family in Indianapolis, Indiana.

FRED MARTICH was born in Johnstown, Pennsylvania and grew up in a nearby small coal mining community called "Charles." He graduated from Duquesne University in Pittsburgh. Fred married his college sweetheart, Joan, and together, they raised five children. He joined CDC's Syphilis Eradication Program in 1963 in Akron, Ohio, with subsequent field assignments in Columbus, Chicago, Milwaukee, and Montgomery, Alabama. In 1986, Fred joined the STD Program headquarters staff, serving as Program Consultant for numerous states. He became the Deputy Chief of HIV/AIDS prevention field operations services and finally the Deputy Chief of STD's Behavioral Interventions and Research Branch. Fred was a charter member of the Watsonian Society, an organization of CDC Public Health Advisors. He also served as the organization's Treasurer (2000-2001). In January 2002, Fred retired from CDC and now lives in Atlanta.

GERALD "JERRY" NAEHR was born in 1942 at Fort Benning, Georgia - the youngest of nine children. He graduated from Archbishop Curley High school (Miami, FL) and received a degree in Sociology from Spring Hill College in 1964. Jerry joined the U.S. Army and became a Preventive Medicine Specialist which included venereal disease investigation. He met his wife, In Ae (Debbie), while on military assignment to South Korea; they have four children. In 1967, Jerry completed military duty and joined CDC as a co-op in the Chicago VD program. He also had field assignments in Minneapolis and as the senior PHA in New York City. He had numerous roles including STD consultant, PHA recruiter, the Deputy and Director of the Field Services Office, Associate Director for Governmental Affairs with the National Center for Environmental Health (NCEH), Deputy to the Associate Director for Emergency Response and International Health (NCEH), Deputy Chief and Acting Deputy Division Director of the Environmental Health Services Branch (NCEH), and Assistant to the Director, National Center for HIV, STD, and TB Prevention. Jerry was a charter member of the Watsonian Society, an organization of CDC Public Health Advisors. He also served as the organization's President (1996-1997). After his retirement in 2002, Jerry has done contractual work on a part-time basis, mostly with CDC.